Qualitative Analysis
of Human Movement

Duane V. Knudson, PhD
Baylor University

Craig S. Morrison, EdD
Southern Utah University

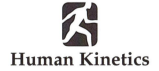

Human Kinetics

Library of Congress Cataloging-in-Publication Data

Knudson, Duane V., 1961-
    Qualitative analysis of human movement / Duane V. Knudson and
Craig S. Morrison.
        p.   cm.
    Includes bibliographical references and index.
    ISBN 0-88011-523-8
    1. Kinesiology.   I. Morrison, Craig S., 1946-   .   II. Title.
QP303.K59   1997
612.7′6--dc21   96-48347
                                                          CIP

ISBN: 0-88011-523-8

Chapter opener photographs for: chapters 1 and 6 are by Terry Wild Studio; chapters 3 and 4 are by Jack Vartoogian; chapters 7 and 8 are by Mary Langenfeld; chapter 9 is by CLEO Photography; and chapter 11 is provided by Neat Systems, Inc.

Acquisitions Editors: Rick Frey, PhD and Scott Wikgren; **Developmental Editor**: Judy Patterson Wright, PhD; **Assistant Editor**: Andrew Smith; **Editorial Assistant**: Jennifer Jeanne Hemphill; **Copyeditor**: Judith Gallagher; **Proofreader**: Pam Johnson; **Graphic Designer**: Robert Reuther; **Graphic Artist**: Sandra Meier; **Photo Editor**: Boyd LaFoon; **Cover Designer**: Jack Davis; **Photographer** (cover): Don Manning; **Cartoonist**: Dick Flood; **Line Illustrator**: Susan Carson; **Mac Artist**: Jennifer Delmotte; **Medical Illustrator**: M.R. Greenberg; **Printer**: Braun-Brumfield

Printed in the United States of America

10 9 8 7 6 5 4 3 2 1

Human Kinetics
Web site: http://www.humankinetics.com/

United States: Human Kinetics, P.O. Box 5076, Champaign, IL 61825-5076
1-800-747-4457
e-mail: humank@hkusa.com

Canada: Human Kinetics, Box 24040, Windsor, ON N8Y 4Y9
1-800-465-7301 (in Canada only)
e-mail: humank@hkcanada.com

Europe: Human Kinetics, P.O. Box IW14, Leeds LS16 6TR, United Kingdom
(44) 1132 781708
e-mail: humank@hkeurope.com

Australia: Human Kinetics, 57A Price Avenue, Lower Mitcham, South Australia 5062
(08) 277 1555
e-mail: humank@hkaustralia.com

New Zealand: Human Kinetics, P.O. Box 105-231, Auckland 1
(09) 523 3462
e-mail: humank@hknewz.com

CONTENTS

PREFACE

Several professions rely on qualitative analysis for improving the movement of their clients. The athletic coach, physical therapist, dance instructor, and physical education teacher are all examples of professionals who use qualitative analysis. How do these professionals make the diagnostic decisions that affect people's lives? This book was written to answer that question by assembling information from the many subdisciplines of kinesiology that contribute to the qualitative analysis of human movement.

The development of qualitative analysis as a subject area and professional skill has been hurt by the lack of a unified approach. The contributions of many subdisciplines of kinesiology to qualitative analysis have not been brought together. Formalizing these largely intuitive processes is very important in improving the professional's development of skill in qualitative analysis. Training future kinesiology professionals in an integrated approach to qualitative analysis is essential to maximizing the movement potential of people of all ages, from athletes to accident rehab patients.

This book presents a four-task model of qualitative analysis, integrating the many subdisciplines of kinesiology that contribute to the process. The model is comprehensive in scope but simple enough that it can easily be applied to all kinds of human movement. The major purposes of this text are to

- summarize the research and scholarly writing on the qualitative analysis of human movement from the various subdisciplines of kinesiology,
- illustrate the interdisciplinary nature of qualitative analysis,
- provide a four-task integrated model of qualitative analysis of human movement,
- provide tutorials that illustrate the integrated model of qualitative analysis, and
- increase interest in the development of qualitative analysis training in the kinesiology curriculum.

AUDIENCE AND SCOPE

Most scholarly work in qualitative analysis has been limited to the perspective of a single subdiscipline of kinesiology (biomechanics, motor development, motor learning, pedagogy, or sport psychology). This text, however, reviews major research and scholarly papers from all these subdisciplines, integrating the strengths of these separate views. The qualitative analysis of human movement is an interdisciplinary skill relevant to many professions. This book is designed for upper-level undergraduate or graduate courses on the qualitative analysis of human movement. Current and future professionals will find a wealth of information on qualitative analysis and many application examples throughout the book.

Few books are available that guide readers through the *process* of qualitative analysis of human movement. This book provides sequence illustrations of actual performances and written tutorials, guiding readers through the diagnostic process. It shows several fundamental human movements and sport skills and includes subjects of all ages and ability levels. The case studies and examples realistically illustrate what professionals encounter every day.

ORGANIZATION AND FEATURES

Organized into three parts, *Qualitative Analysis of Human Movement* reviews relevant literature demonstrating the need for an integrated approach to qualitative analysis, provides a detailed discussion of the four tasks of an integrated qualitative analysis, and then leads you through practical examples of how to perform an integrated qualitative analysis of several human movements. Throughout the text, we explain points by using real-world examples and show how the many subdisciplines of kinesiology contribute to each of the four tasks of qualitative analysis.

Each chapter begins with a *preview box* that showcases the topic of the chapter and its importance to qualitative analysis. The major topics of each chapter are highlighted in a list of *chapter objectives*. Examples are given throughout the text, and a longer discussion of a practical example is presented in the *practical applications* section of each chapter. Like the previews, practical applications use real-world examples and emphasize how all the subdisciplines of kinesiology contribute to qualitative analysis of human movement.

Three features that are especially important for helping readers master key concepts in qualitative analysis are the *key points*, the *chapter summaries*, and *discussion questions*. Key points are small sections that summarize an important concept that has emerged from the qualitative analysis literature. Each chapter concludes with a review that summarizes its major themes and a list of open-ended questions that are designed to stimulate discussion and interaction among various points of view.

The book also provides a *glossary* of key terms and an extensive *bibliography* of qualitative analysis literature. It is our hope that readers will find themselves thinking critically about their future or present professional practice. We also hope these kinesiology professionals will take steps to improve their skills in qualitative analysis and to help expand the knowledge base on the qualitative analysis of human movement.

ACKNOWLEDGMENTS

The authors are indebted to many people who helped in the development of this book. The comments of the reviewers, Jerry Wilkerson and Moria McPherson, are greatly appreciated. We are also indebted to all the professionals at Human Kinetics who improved the quality of this book immeasurably. Dr. Knudson would like to thank the most important people in his life, his family (especially Lois, Josh, and Mandy), scholars on whose work this book is built, and his Lord Jesus Christ. Dr. Morrison is indebted to the scholars who have come before him and to those who have been instrumental in his contribution to this book, in particular, Joyce Harrison, Jean Reeve, and Paul Dunham.

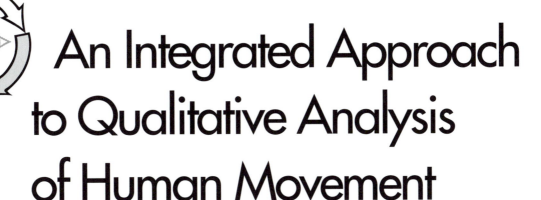

PART ONE

An Integrated Approach to Qualitative Analysis of Human Movement

Qualitative analysis is the primary method used to improve human movement of clients in many kinesiology professions. Good qualitative analysis requires an integrated and interdisciplinary approach. This view of qualitative analysis and a brief history of qualitative analysis in kinesiology are presented in chapter 1. Chapter 2 reviews important models of qualitative analysis in kinesiology and shows how the literature supports our integrated model of qualitative analysis. This integrated model of qualitative analysis includes four main tasks: preparation, observation, evaluation/diagnosis, and intervention. Chapters 3 and 4 show how the senses and the brain gather and interpret information about the status of performance within the process of qualitative analysis.

Introduction and History of Qualitative Analysis in Kinesiology

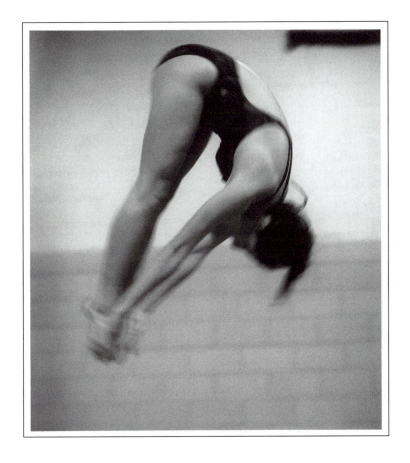

PREVIEW

A diver is having difficulty learning a new dive in the off season. You are the coach helping to improve execution of the dive. Essential to this improvement is your ability to analyze the dive qualitatively. You use your knowledge of diving to systematically observe the movement, evaluate and diagnose the diver's strengths and weaknesses, and then provide intervention that will help her improve. Observation and evaluation of several dives leads you to believe that the athlete does not create enough height and rotation at take-off. How can you help this athlete?

Chapter Objectives

1. Define qualitative analysis.
2. Explain the difference between qualitative and quantitative analysis in kinesiology.
3. Identify subdisciplines of kinesiology that provide information relevant to qualitative analysis of human movement.
4. Summarize major contributors from selected subdisciplines of kinesiology to the development of qualitative analysis.

The diving coach in the preview above faces a challenge that many kinesiology professionals must meet every day, the qualitative analysis of human movement. This chapter will introduce you to the many important aspects and subdisciplines of kinesiology that contribute to the qualitative analysis of human movement. Qualitative analysis may be the most important skill that kinesiology professionals need to improve the performance of their clients.

QUALITATIVE ANALYSIS IN KINESIOLOGY

Kinesiology is the term used to describe the academic discipline interested in the study of human movement, replacing what was often called physical education (Arnold, 1993; Newell, 1990). The premier scholarly society in this area (American Academy of Kinesiology and Physical Education) recommends the use of the term kinesiology to describe this academic discipline in higher education. Kinesiology professionals in a wide variety of careers (for example, teaching, coaching, dance, athletic training, sports medicine, physical therapy, fitness, ergonomics) all use qualitative analysis to improve human movement. Athletic coaches use qualitative analysis to make judgments on technique, strategy, and team selection. Physical education teachers often use qualitative analysis to evaluate student performance and to assign grades.

THE DEFINITION OF QUALITATIVE ANALYSIS

Qualitative analysis must be defined for the purposes of this text, since many terms have been used in the kinesiology literature that are not quite synonymous. Movement analysis, clinical diagnosis, skill analysis, error detection, observation, eyeballing, observational assessment, systematic observation, and other terms have all been used in the same context. We define *qualitative analysis* as the systematic observation and introspective judgment of the quality of human movement for the purpose of providing the most appropriate intervention to improve performance (Knudson and Morrison, 1996:17). Since the terms "observation," "intervention," and "performance" are used in this definition, it is necessary to define them also.

Observation is the process of gathering, organizing, and giving meaning to sensory information about human motor performances. This definition is very similar to Sage's (1984) definition of perception, and in qualitative analysis observation is closely related to perception. *Intervention* in qualitative analysis is defined as the administration of feedback, corrections, or other change in the environment to improve performance. Both observation and intervention are key tasks within the larger process of qualitative analysis of human movement. We will use the term *performance* in a broad sense to mean both the short-term and long-term effectiveness of a person's movement in achieving a goal.

> **KEY POINT**
>
> *Many words have been used to describe the process of the qualitative analysis of human movement. We define qualitative analysis as the systematic observation and introspective judgment of the quality of human movement for the purpose of providing the most appropriate intervention to improve performance.*

Observation in qualitative analysis is *not* limited to the use of vision only. All the senses that a teacher/coach can employ to gather information should be used. For example, a gymnastics teacher may rely on kinesthetic information from her arms in spotting early trials of a new skill. Since she is too close to the movement to make reliable visual checks of some phases of it, the information from hand placement and muscular effort to assist the learner complete the skill is critical to qualitative analysis. Auditory information about the rhythm of learners' impacts with the mat can also be an important point of observation in qualitative analysis for a gymnastics teacher, a dance teacher, or a therapist evaluating gait.

> **KEY POINT**
>
> *Good observation involves the use of all the senses to gather information about performance. Observation is not limited to visual inspection of human movement.*

QUALITATIVE VERSUS QUANTITATIVE ANALYSIS

Qualitative analysis is by nature a subjective judgment call. This does *not* mean that it is unorganized, vague, or arbitrary in nature. In fact, we will see that qualitative analysis requires extensive information from many disciplines, planning, and systematic steps to be most effective.

Figure 1.1 illustrates a continuum of human movement analysis. Any analysis of human movement can be located somewhere along the continuum from qualitative to quantitative. Analyses of baseball pitching can vary from broad statements by television color commentators to statistical breakdowns of pitches and their locations to radar measurements of ball speed. The qualitative end of the continuum involves the nonnumerical analysis of movement data or a judgment on the quality of an aspect of movement.

Quantitative analysis, however, is based on some *measurement* of performance. If performance can be expressed in numbers, then the analysis is based on quantified data. Quantification of data (in seconds, feet, meters, degrees per second) moves the analysis further to the right on the continuum. But even research measurements (quantification of a very controlled nature) cannot be purely objective. There is some subjectivity in deciding where to place the tape measure or where to take a skinfold measurement. Quantification does not automatically ensure validity and reliability, and the lack of quantification in a qualitative analysis does not automatically mean the assessment is less valid or reliable.

Information from traditional qualitative analysis in kinesiology falls near the left side of the analysis continuum. Most teachers or coaches use qualitative analysis in everyday practice situations to diagnose and correct errors. Other movement analyses are midway along the continuum. Evaluation of skill or developmental level using a rating scale or timing a 40-yard dash is at the beginning of quantified performance.

The highest levels of quantitative analyses in sport sciences, such as biomechanics and exercise physiology, are primarily being performed in university research settings or at the Olympic Training Centers for elite athletes. Biomechanists measure instantaneous values of velocity, acceleration, or force for various parts of the body. Physiologists measure oxygen consumption, body fat, or amounts of lactic acid in the blood. Generally, these measurements of human movement have been too expensive for widespread use in teaching and coaching settings.

A situation where a qualitative analysis would be helpful is illustrated in figure 1.2, where an athlete has missed a fly ball during outfield practice. A good qualitative analysis of this situation would include specific feedback to the performer to help improve subsequent performance. Many teachers might attempt to correct the hand position, which is clearly not the best hand position for fielding balls above the waist. The real question is whether a qualitative analysis integrating all sources of information would suggest

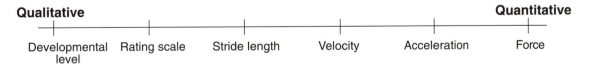

Qualitative   **Quantitative**

Developmental level   Rating scale   Stride length   Velocity   Acceleration   Force

Figure 1.1 Sample continuum of human movement analysis for analyzing running.

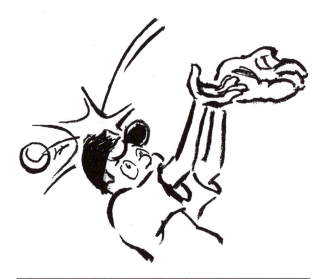

Figure 1.2 One attempt to catch a fly ball. A qualitative analysis of this situation would help the instructor provide appropriate intervention. What do you think is the most appropriate intervention?

correcting hand position as the most important feedback.

In the real world, several other factors might contribute to missing a fly ball. The athlete could have poor vision and require glasses. Environmental factors such as the sun or wind may have affected his performance. The psychological pressure of a critical time in the game may have impaired his concentration and perception. Maybe the player has an attention deficit disorder. If he was alert but did not attend to the right information (sound, ball trajectory, and spin), he could have misjudged the ball. If he missed several fly balls in a row, the analyst could begin to evaluate the size and direction of errors and decide whether lack of attention was the problem. This example illustrates the many factors that may have to be weighed in qualitative analysis and shows why qualitative analysis involves integration of the many subdisciplines of kinesiology.

THE INTERDISCIPLINARY NATURE OF QUALITATIVE ANALYSIS

Within kinesiology, there are many subdisciplines that study qualitative analysis with their own unique interests and outlook. Scholars interested in motor development have done extensive work in identifying and validating developmental sequences for fundamental movement patterns

(Roberton and Halverson, 1984; Wickstrom, 1983). Psychology and motor learning specialists have studied how skills are learned and the conditions of feedback that are related to performance and learning (Ammons, 1956; Magill, 1994; Newell, 1976; Newell, Morris, and Scully, 1985; Schmidt, 1991).

Experts in the field of biomechanics have formulated general principles of human movement for the purpose of qualitative analysis (Bunn, 1955; Groves and Camaione, 1983; Kreighbaum and Barthels, 1985; Luttgens and Wells, 1982; Norman, 1975; Piscopo and Bailey, 1981). Biomechanists have also proposed specific methods of qualitative analysis, since this subdiscipline was commonly assumed to provide the basis for qualitative analysis ability in students (Brown, 1982; Hay and Reid, 1982; Hudson, 1990a, b, and c; Norman, 1975). Scholars interested in sport pedagogy have recommended approaches to qualitative analysis (Barrett, 1979a, b; Hoffman, 1974, 1977a; Pinheiro, 1994; Pinheiro and Simon, 1992).

The problem is that qualitative analysis in the real world requires the simultaneous *integration* of all these and other bodies of knowledge, not many separate views of the same action. *Qualitative analysis is an interdisciplinary process* because all the subdisciplines of kinesiology contribute to all the tasks of qualitative analysis (see figure 1.3). Good qualitative analysis requires that

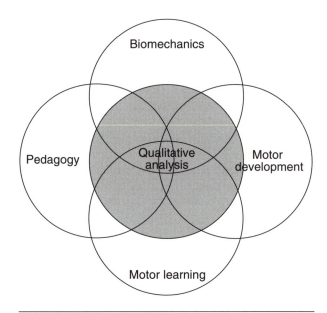

Figure 1.3 The interdisciplinary nature of qualitative analysis requires the integration of various subdisciplines within kinesiology. Only four subdisciplines are illustrated here to prevent confusion.

the professional be knowledgeable about—and able to integrate—information from all the subdisciplines of kinesiology.

A qualitative analysis that bases technique changes solely on principles of biomechanics (the science of technique) is not ideal because it overlooks the relevant information other disciplines provide for making these judgments. In the outfielder example, the athlete's hand position may not be typical performance or the most important correction. Knowledge of strength, maturation, and stages of motor development may apply to the situation being evaluated. The motor development literature would provide information about the typical stages that people go through in learning to catch. Motor learning and pedagogy research would also help in shaping the communication of corrections and the appropriate practice schedule. Knowledge of psychology could help in the motivation necessary to sustain the practice and short-term decrease in performance needed for long-term improvement.

> **KEY POINT**
>
> *Qualitative analysis requires the integrated use of information from many subdisciplines of kinesiology. The diving coach in the preview must combine information from many disciplines to help the diver learn the new skill. The coach's knowledge of the performer's strength and flexibility (exercise physiology) must be integrated with knowledge of the various aspects of the technique (biomechanics), the practice required (motor learning), and the nerve of the performer (sport psychology).*

The paradox of qualitative analysis in kinesiology is that it has emerged directly from the major subdisciplines, yet it has not been recognized as a distinct area of inquiry in its own right. Some kinesiology scholars believe that the profession has suffered due to lack of recognition of the importance of qualitative analysis (Huelster, 1939; Hoffman, 1974; Norman, 1975). It may seem odd that it has taken so long for qualitative analysis to emerge as an entity in kinesiology, but there are several plausible explanations as to why kinesiology has been so slow to formally address this important ability. Inadequate technology (high-speed film, video equipment, computers) has made

it difficult to create knowledge at a deep enough level to affect instructional practice. It has also been assumed that qualitative analysis ability arises from the undergraduate biomechanics course.

Another problem in the last few decades is that most of the research in kinesiology has become highly specialized by subdiscipline. A professional joining the American Alliance for Health, Physical Education, Recreation and Dance (AAHPERD) must select from six national associations and 87 different interest areas. Since qualitative analysis is based on the integrated use of many of these subdisciplines of kinesiology, it has been difficult to work across these boundaries. An excellent example of how the development of qualitative analysis has been fragmented by having a variety of different approaches rather than an integrated approach is the variety of terms used by the various subdisciplines to mean the qualitative analysis of human movement (Barrett, 1979a; Hoffman, 1977a; Radford, 1989).

It is likely that scholars from any three subdisciplines of kinesiology would use different terms for the qualitative analysis of human movement. We will see that early qualitative analysis scholars used terms like *observation* (Barrett, 1979c), or *error identification/detection* (Armstrong and Hoffman, 1979; Cloes, Premuzak, and Pieron, 1995; Vanderbeck, 1979) almost synonymously with qualitative analysis. Terms like *qualitative assessment* (James and Dufek, 1993) and *clinical diagnosis* (Hoffman, 1983) have also been used. This confusion is also apparent in the variety of "analysis" terms: *skill analysis* (Gangstead and Beveridge, 1984; Hoffman, 1974; Wilkinson, 1992b), *movement analysis* (Biscan and Hoffman, 1976), *visual analysis* (Wilkinson, 1992a), and *subjective analysis* (Arend and Higgins, 1976).

Another recent problem is that the term *systematic observation* has come to be used in sport pedagogy to mean the observation and classification of teacher and student behaviors for the evaluation of teaching (Siedentop, 1991), not the qualitative analysis of performance as would seem appropriate.

The consistent use of qualitative analysis terminology across the subdisciplines of physical education would be very useful in the development of qualitative analysis. This fragmented development of qualitative analysis makes the understanding of its origins in kinesiology more important. The next section will summarize some key contributions to the development of qualitative analysis in kinesiology.

THE HISTORY OF QUALITATIVE ANALYSIS IN KINESIOLOGY

This section will review some of the important contributions and developments in the art and science of qualitative analysis in the kinesiology literature. The literature is divided into contributions from the subdisciplines of biomechanics, motor development, motor learning, and pedagogy (in alphabetical order) to illustrate their unique contributions and to show the fragmented nature of qualitative analysis research. This is a brief summary of selected subdisciplines of kinesiology. Other subdisciplines, for example sport sociology and sport psychology, also contribute to the process of qualitative analysis. Readers should study these and other subdisciplines when they are relevant to a particular qualitative analysis. Readers should also take note of the timing of these contributions and think about how changes in the sciences of kinesiology have influenced the development of qualitative analysis in each subdiscipline.

Biomechanical Contributions

Early leaders in the subdiscipline of kinesiology/biomechanics were interested in the qualitative analysis of human movement and wrote textbooks for their courses emphasizing qualitative analysis (Broer, 1960; Cooper and Glassow, 1963; Scott, 1942). Remember that the term kinesiology is used to refer to the course in the physical education curriculum on applied anatomy and mechanical analysis of human movement. Early quantitative biomechanical analysis was labor intensive, involving a great deal of hand tracing and calculation from 16-millimeter film, so qualitative analyses of movement were more common and accepted.

Quantitative analyses of movement became more common than qualitative analyses in undergraduate preparation for two main reasons. Quantitative analyses grew in power and automation with improvements in computers and measurement systems, and physical education in higher education focused on research and academic credibility for survival. However, interest in qualitative analysis in professional preparation has been continued by biomechanists who have called for more emphasis on principles and application of course content to qualitative analysis (Berg, 1975; Brown, 1982, 1984; Davis, 1984;

Hay, 1983, 1984, Norman, 1975, 1977). Qualitative analysis has been a recurring topic of presentations and discussions at the national conferences on teaching kinesiology and biomechanics in sports held in 1977, 1984, and 1991. There is a consistent history of biomechanical scholars applying research to qualitative analysis and contributing to the knowledge about qualitative analysis in kinesiology.

At the first National Conference on Teaching Undergraduate Kinesiology in 1977, the Kinesiology Academy appointed a task force to survey kinesiology/biomechanics instructors and to draft guidelines for the teaching of undergraduate kinesiology. The "Guidelines and Standards for Undergraduate Kinesiology" were approved by the Kinesiology Academy in 1980.

This proposal of a standard approach to undergraduate kinesiology/biomechanics coursework in physical education had two main objectives: first, to provide a knowledge base for systematic analysis of human movement, and second, to provide "experience in applying that knowledge to the execution and evaluation of both the performer and the performance in the clinical and educational milieu," (Kinesiology Academy, 1980:19). This essentially qualitative emphasis in undergraduate preparation supports the implementation of qualitative analysis of movement in undergraduate kinesiology/biomechanics courses.

At the second national symposium on Teaching Kinesiology and Biomechanics in Sports, Marett and colleagues (1984) reported on another national survey of kinesiology/biomechanics courses. Undergraduate kinesiology/biomechanics courses were now placing a greater emphasis on teaching mechanical principles and applying qualitative analysis at the expense of anatomical kinesiology. Several papers were presented on strategies for teaching qualitative analysis in the undergraduate kinesiology/biomechanics courses (Brown, 1984; Daniels, 1984; Hay, 1984; Hoffman, 1984; Hoshizaki, 1984; Kindig and Windell, 1984; Phillips and Clark, 1984; Stoner, 1984). The latest technological advance in interactive instruction, the interactive videodisk, was also demonstrated at this meeting (Zollman and Fuller, 1984).

At the third national symposium on Teaching Kinesiology and Biomechanics in Sports, more papers were presented on qualitative analysis in undergraduate kinesiology/biomechanics. Research on the effect of biomechanics instruction and qualitative analysis (Dedeyn, 1991; Knudson, Morrison, and Reeve, 1991) and introductory experiences in qualitative analysis (Bird and Hudson, 1990) were presented. Several other presentations described experiences teaching biomechanical principles in a qualitative way (Wilkerson, Kreighbaum, and Tant, 1991). After a discussion session, a committee was formed to revise the guidelines and standards. In 1993, standards adopted by the renamed Biomechanics Academy of the National Association for Sport and Physical Education (NASPE) also advocated that undergraduate kinesiology/biomechanics emphasize qualitative analysis.

There has been no recent survey like Marett and colleagues (1984) on the content of undergraduate kinesiology. It is not clear how many undergraduate biomechanics lab or course hours are devoted to applying biomechanics in qualitative analysis situations. Many undergraduate biomechanics labs and lab workbooks still focus on quantitative biomechanical analyses.

Recent biomechanical contributions to qualitative analysis have been mostly in the realm of scholarly papers (Hay, 1984; McPherson, 1990; Schleihauf, 1983) and textbooks designed for implementing the qualitative nature of the guidelines and standards (Adrian and Cooper, 1995; Hay and Reid, 1988; Kreighbaum and Barthels, 1985). It is clear that biomechanics has contributed to the development of qualitative analysis, and these contributions must be integrated with contributions from other subdisciplines of kinesiology.

Motor Development Contributions

Scholars interested in motor development have documented the typical changes in movement patterns as children mature and become more skilled in many movements. The nature and description of these developmental changes in movements have been studied in several ways (Seefeldt and Haubenstricker, 1982). The developmental changes in movement have been called developmental sequences and tend to be described using either the *whole body* (Haubenstricker et al., 1983; Seefeldt and Haubenstricker, 1982) or various *components* of the movement (Halverson, 1983; Roberton, 1983; Williams, 1980).

Motor development research on typical changes of children learning motor skills is invaluable for the kinesiology professional qualitatively analyzing the movement of children. For example, a youth sport coach would benefit from knowing when growth spurts may influence changes in strength and coordination, or when most children attain mature levels of many fundamental movements.

Qualitative analysis based on decades of motor development research are summarized well in many motor development books (Roberton and Halverson, 1984; Wickstrom, 1983). Motor development within kinesiology traces its roots to psychology and educational research on human development. Motor development textbooks often review this early research on the cognitive, perceptual, social, and motor skill changes that occur with development. Several qualitative analysis systems incorporating developmental sequences of fundamental movement patterns have been proposed (Roberton and Halverson, 1984; Michigan Education Assessment Program, 1984; Ulrich, 1985; Wickstrom, 1983).

These systems are very effective in elementary physical education settings. Like youth sport coaches, physical educators need to know developmental milestones of many movements and the typical variability in children reaching these milestones. Maturation rates are typically plus or minus two years of chronological age. Physical educators must individualize teaching and feedback, because children of the same chronological age differ in developmental level and physiological age.

Recent research in motor development has been expanding the scope of the field. Studies are now focusing on the application of developmental sequences to more specific tasks, like sport skills (Haywood, Williams, and Van Sant, 1991; Messick, 1991; Rose and Heath, 1990; Rose, Heath, and Megale, 1990). Motor development theory and research are also focusing on changes in development across the life span by documenting movement changes in older adults (Haywood and Williams, 1995; Williams, Haywood, and Van Sant, 1996).

Motor Learning Contributions

Research in motor learning has focused on issues related to the speed and permanence of learning new motor skills. This research has often used simple motor tasks with goals that could be precisely quantified. The major contribution of motor learning research to qualitative analysis in kinesiology is the wealth of information on the effect of many kinds of feedback on learning motor skills.

Feedback is the primary mode of intervention in qualitative analysis. Teachers of discrete movements (for example, a golf swing) may provide immediate feedback as part of qualitative analysis. An understanding of motor learning research on summary feedback might help a track coach provide good feedback in continuous events like sprinting or distance running. There are several good review articles dealing with movement feedback (Annett, 1993; Bilodeau, 1969; Lee, Keh, and Magill, 1993; Magill, 1993; Magill, 1994; Newell, 1976; Newell, Morris, and Scully, 1985).

Pedagogy Contributions

One of the earliest authors to comment on the need for qualitative analysis of movement was Huelster (1939). She suggested that courses like anatomy, body mechanics, and kinesiology were not enough to give physical education graduates the ability to do real-time qualitative analysis of human movement. Many of Huelster's suggestions were well ahead of her time and could be incorporated into the current physical education curriculum. Some of her ideas will be reviewed in chapter 2.

The next major call for the development of qualitative analysis came from research suggesting that good performers do not necessarily make good analyzers of movement (Kretchmar, Sherman, and Mooney, 1949). This view that the kinesthetic sense of skilled athletes may not transfer into qualitative analysis ability has been validated in recent studies (Girardin and Hanson, 1967; Osborne and Gordon, 1972; Armstrong and Hoffman, 1979).

More research on qualitative analysis in physical education began to appear in the late 1960s and 1970s (Armstrong, 1977a and b; Biscan and Hoffman, 1976; Girardin and Hanson, 1967; Hoffman and Armstrong, 1975; Hoffman and Sembiante, 1975; Landers, 1969; Moody, 1967; Osborne and Gordon, 1972). In 1974, Shirl Hoffman wrote a watershed article about the inability of people who had taken the undergraduate kinesiology/biomechanics class to analyze movement qualitatively. Other scholars have agreed with Hoffman's position that traditional biomechanics courses alone do not adequately prepare students for qualitative analysis and that specific instruction is necessary (Barrett, 1979a, b, and c; Hoffman, 1974, 1977a, b, and c, 1984; Locke, 1972). This position has been supported by some research (Knudson, Morrison, and Reeve, 1991; Morrison and Reeve, 1988), although there is evidence that

applied and conceptual instruction in kinesiology/biomechanics can affect the physical education teacher's selection of feedback to students (Dedeyn, 1991; Knudson, Morrison, and Reeve, 1991; Nielsen and Beauchamp, 1992). Neilsen and Beauchamp (1992), for example, found that conceptual instruction improved the amount of corrective, accurate, and specific feedback provided by students qualitatively analyzing videotaped performances of volleyball and team handball skills.

Other important developments in the 1970s were the scholarly reviews of observation literature by Barrett (1977, 1979a, b, c), and a thorough model of human movement analysis by Arend and Higgins (1976). The model presented a comprehensive picture of movement analysis, both qualitative and quantitative. It tried to integrate the many subdisciplines of kinesiology, from planning analysis to providing intervention to the performer. Siedentop (1991) also identifies this as the time period when the pedagogical literature changed from methods of teaching research to research documenting teaching and learning behaviors. Remember that the term systematic observation refers to the observation and classification of teacher behaviors in the process of evaluating teaching, not the qualitative analysis of performance. Pedagogy within kinesiology also contributed to the development of qualitative analysis by identifying feedback patterns and behaviors of effective teachers and coaches.

Pedagogical interest was shifting from an emphasis on observation to a broader picture of qualitative analysis. By the end of 1979, demand for the implementation of qualitative analysis in the undergraduate physical education curriculum had slowly grown. The initial call to address this need had been made, research had begun, a theoretical basis had been framed, and specific changes in undergraduate preparation had been proposed.

Pedagogical research on qualitative analysis continued to grow in the 1980s. Bayless (1980, 1981) reported studies indicating that several styles of instruction could improve the error detection of undergraduate students. In 1983, two important scholars summarized their research in key papers. Barrett (1983) proposed her model of observation as a teaching skill, and Hoffman (1983) proposed two models for the analysis of movement. Hoffman, Imwold, and Koller (1983) applied the taxonomy developed by Fitts (1965) to analyze children's movement. Research began to use eye-tracking recorders to document visual search patterns (Bard, Fleury, Carriere, and Halle, 1980; Petrakis, 1986, 1987) and the influence of perceptual style on qualitative analysis was investigated (Beveridge and Gangstead, 1984; Gangstead, Cashel, and Beveridge, 1987; Morrison and Reeve, 1989, 1992; Swinnen, 1984a).

Other issues investigated were experience (Allison, 1987; Barrett, Allison, and Bell, 1987; Imwold and Hoffman, 1983; Pinheiro, 1990), transfer to other skills (Morrison and Reeve, 1986), transfer to teaching (Nielsen and Beauchamp, 1992), teaching qualitative analysis to classroom teachers (Allison, 1985a and b; Morrison and Harrison, 1985), instruction in qualitative analysis (Gangstead, 1987; McPherson, 1988; Morrison, Gangstead, and Reeve, 1990; Morrison and Reeve, 1988; Morrison, Reeve, and Harrison, 1992; Pinheiro, 1994; Wilkinson, 1990, 1991, 1992b), and retention of qualitative analysis ability (Wilkinson, 1992a; Morrison, 1994; Morrison and Harrison, 1985).

Petrakis and Romjue (1990) examined the process of mental strategies of experienced observers to see if there were any similarities common to all observers. Procedural knowledge of qualitative analysis appeared to be the same for experienced observers, but their observation strategies appeared to be different. Some observers looked for specific parts of a skill to evaluate proficiency; others scrutinized the overall performance. The former approach indicates an analytic perceptual preference, while the latter points to a gestalt approach. Perceptual style (how a person takes in and organizes sensory information for interpretation) does appear to make a difference in qualitative analysis. The effect of perceptual style is a focus of recent research on qualitative analysis.

In a major theoretical leap, Kniffin (1985) took qualitative analysis to the next logical step. He showed that videotape instruction in the qualitative analysis of movement could produce positive results in the gymnasium. Although these results had been hypothesized by researchers in the field, this was the first real evidence that specific film and videotape training in qualitative analysis would lead to improvement in movement diagnosis in the classroom. Other research has shown insignificant differences in live qualitative analysis proficiency of kinesiology students after videotape training (Eckrich, Widule, Schrader, and Maver, 1994). Interactive videodisks have recently been used for instruction in qualitative analysis (Chung, 1993; Harper, 1995; Kelly, Walkley, and Tarrant, 1988; Klesius and

Bowers, 1990). The transfer of video training in qualitative analysis to live settings is a topic that needs more research so that instruction in qualitative analysis can be designed.

A manuscript by Morrison and Harrison (in press) described how the qualitative analysis of movement could be integrated into the total undergraduate physical education curriculum. The model for this integration was taken from DePauw and GocKarp (1989) and was based on her successful attempt to integrate adapted physical education into as many courses as possible at the undergraduate level. Radford (1988, 1989, 1991) added to the review literature on qualitative analysis by attempting to define movement observation and propose ways of linking observation, feedback, and assessment. Pinheiro and Simon (1992) proposed a model of information processing that is a useful first step in understanding how perception works in qualitative analysis.

Pedagogical contributions to the understanding of qualitative analysis are significant. Scholars have focused attention on qualitative analysis instruction in the curriculum and enlarged the scope of qualitative analysis inquiry beyond the observation of movement.

Recent Developments

A growing body of literature and interest in qualitative analysis has originated from a disciplinary perspective within kinesiology. Many subdisciplines of kinesiology have contributed to the development of qualitative analysis, but no consistent terminology or curricular implementation of qualitative analysis training has been agreed upon. Some recent developments in kinesiology show promise for the further development of qualitative analysis preparation of undergraduates.

Several recent trends have begun to focus more attention on how kinesiology curricula address professional preparation. One is the philosophical debate over name changes for departments of physical education (Newell, 1990). Another is the restructuring of academic schools and departments in higher education. The 1992 National Association for Sport and Physical Education/ National Council for the Accreditation of Teacher Education (NASPE/NCATE) guidelines require (number 22) that qualitative analysis be part of the undergraduate curriculum for physical education teacher preparation (NASPE, 1992). Finally, there is a distinct trend toward interdisciplinary and cooperative approaches to teaching, learning, and research. Funding agencies and journals are encouraging interdisciplinary research, and there is even a new journal with this focus (*The Journal of Interdisciplinary Research in Physical Education*).

In the last few years, several doctoral dissertations have focused on qualitative analysis (Chung, 1993; Eckrich, 1991; Harper, 1995; Leis, 1994; Matanin, 1993; Pinheiro, 1990; Rush, 1991; Taylor, 1995; Williams et al., 1996). Professional

journals like *Strategies* and the *Journal of Physical Education, Recreation and Dance* (*JOPERD*) have been publishing papers on how to analyze specific sports skills (Jones-Morton, 1990a, b, c, d, 1991a, b; Hudson, 1990b; Knudson, 1991, 1993; Knudson, Luedtke, and Faribault, 1994; Knudson and Morrison, 1996; Tant, 1990). Further interdisciplinary research and dedicated instruction related to qualitative analysis can only improve the preparation of kinesiology students for a variety of human movement professions.

PRACTICAL APPLICATION: A Tale of Three Coaches

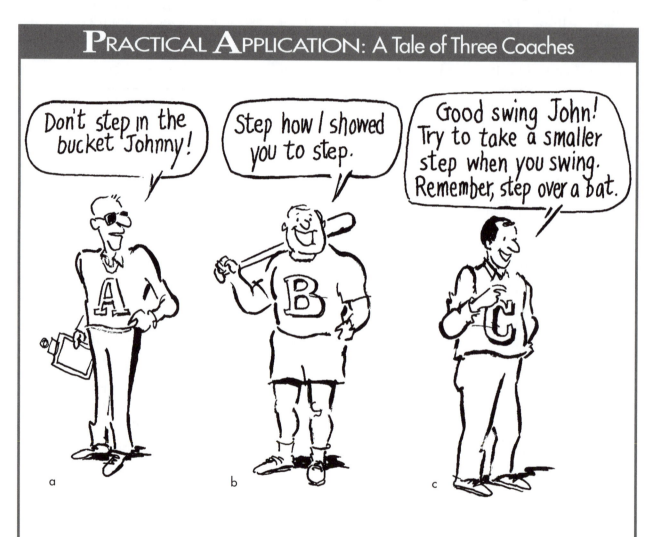

Three Little League teams started practice for the summer season on the same day. The teams had the same number of players, the same level of skill and talent, the same number of practices, and games against the same opponents. The volunteer coaches appeared to be similar, but they had slightly different approaches to qualitative analysis.

Coach A had a treasury of time-honored baseball cues and a keen eye for finding problems in his player's performances. As soon as an error was observed, the related correction was provided. During batting practice, fielding practice, and competition the children were bombarded by a barrage of corrections and helpful pointers. Classic "paralysis by analysis" was occurring. The children on the team had difficulty improving despite all of Coach A's advice. But even though they didn't win the championship or break any league records, the team had an enjoyable season. Parents were not sure why their children were not picking up all the gems of advice from Coach A. Why did it seem their children played below potential, and the other teams had most of the good luck?

Coach B had been a good ballplayer in his day. The game came easily to him because he was a natural athlete. Coach B presented the fundamentals of the game as he remembered them from his playing days, but he didn't have Coach A's keen eye. He couldn't seem to find the problem in a child's throw or swing. Often Coach B focused on errors he was familiar with and did not notice that these errors were symptomatic of other problems in technique or strength limitations. The parents were impressed with Coach B's demonstrations and believed the children were lucky to have such a skilled coach. But the team didn't make the playoffs, and they never seemed to look as good as the demonstrations Coach B gave.

Coach C knew there was a lot the children needed to work on to become skilled players, and he knew they needed to work together to make a good team. He often wanted to help each child with personal coaching, but he knew this wasn't possible. Coach C thought he had better choose his words carefully to communicate effectively and to protect his players' self-esteem and confidence. Almost unconsciously, Coach C praised effort and often found only one thing each child should work on. Parents were concerned that Coach C didn't look as active, involved, or technical as Coach A. He sure didn't look as good in action as Coach B. But the children learned quickly and trusted Coach C because he always seemed to find the one thing that helped them hit the ball or get the throw to the right spot. The players had a great season. They hit, ran, and fielded with confidence. Skill and luck came together, and the team won the post-season tournament. Somehow Coach C must have known that analytical skill was needed to evaluate technique and decide how best to help improve performance.

The astute reader may have noticed that Coach A was a skilled observer and diagnostician of movement errors, but he did not use knowledge from the disciplines of psychology and motor learning to provide the most appropriate feedback. Coach B was knowledgeable about baseball skills but lacked the knowledge and experience to develop his own observational and diagnostic skills. Coach C was a good example of an *integrated approach* to qualitative analysis. The story suggests that Coach C was skilled in all of the four tasks of an integrated approach to qualitative analysis: preparation, observation, evaluation/diagnosis, and intervention. Neglect of any one of the four tasks limits a teacher's or coach's effectiveness in improving players' performance. The next chapter will outline several models of qualitative analysis and show how these four tasks form the basis for an integrated model of qualitative analysis of human movement.

SUMMARY

Many professions use qualitative analysis to improve human movement. Qualitative analysis of human movement is interdisciplinary, requiring the integration of information from many subdisciplines of kinesiology. Important subdisciplines include (among others) biomechanics, motor development, motor learning, and pedagogy. Unfortunately, most research and professional literature on qualitative analysis has not been interdisciplinary; it has been written from the perspective of only one subdiscipline.

DISCUSSION QUESTIONS

1. What kinesiology professions rely most heavily on qualitative analysis to improve human movement?

2. How has terminology been a barrier to the development of qualitative analysis in kinesiology?

3. Why is qualitative analysis an interdisciplinary process? Give examples.

4. In what situations are qualitative analyses more appropriate than quantitative analyses? Why?

5. Why have particular subdisciplines of kinesiology contributed more to the development of qualitative analysis than others?

6. If two teachers disagree on the correction to give a child, could you give a logical explanation of why they might differ?

The Role of Models in Qualitative Analysis

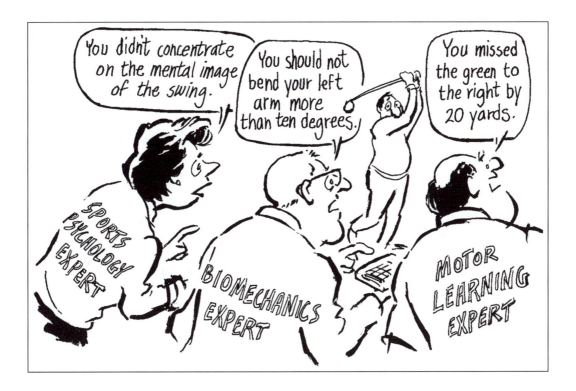

PREVIEW

There is a humorous fable about three golf coaches who tried in vain to agree on what would improve a golfer's swing. The conflict arose because each person had a different perspective on how to analyze performance qualitatively. This story is analogous to the search for the best approach to qualitative analysis of human movement.

Chapter Objectives

1. Distinguish between comprehensive and observational models of qualitative analysis.
2. Identify major observational models and major comprehensive models within various subdisciplines contributing to the qualitative analysis of human movement.
3. Identify tasks that are common to approaches and models for the qualitative analysis of human movement.
4. Describe the tasks and characteristics of a comprehensive, integrated model for the process of qualitative analysis of human movement.
5. Discuss the validity and reliability of qualitative analyses of human movement.

There are a number of approaches or models for the qualitative analysis of human movement in kinesiology. This variety stems from the many subdisciplines of kinesiology that contribute to qualitative analysis. Scholars from several subdisciplines have developed models to explain the important components of the qualitative analysis process. Researchers interested in motor development have documented approaches to qualitative analysis based on phases or levels of motor development. Biomechanics researchers have proposed models to apply the principles of mechanics to the qualitative analysis of human movement. Scholars in sport pedagogy and motor learning have also contributed models for the qualitative analysis of human movement.

A COMMON STRUCTURE FOR QUALITATIVE ANALYSIS

Are there similarities between models for qualitative analysis that originate in different subdisciplines of kinesiology? Can a football coach, dance instructor, and physical therapist be doing similar tasks in qualitatively analyzing movement? The purpose of this chapter is to synthesize the various models of qualitative analysis in the kinesiology literature into a comprehensive, integrated, and yet simplified model for the qualitative analysis of human movement. We will see that there are four similarities among different models of qualitative analysis. These four tasks are the basis for the interdisciplinary and integrated model of qualitative analysis in this book.

It is not possible to review all the books or articles that deal with this subject. Many authors have contributed to this area, but this book can review only selected models. Readers are encouraged to read these original sources and others that can be found in the bibliography. Dance educators may be interested in the application of Laban movement analysis to qualitative analysis (Allison, 1986; Hamburg, 1995). Health professionals in physical medicine, physical therapy, or athletic training would profit from studies of the qualitative analysis of gait (Bampton, 1979; Craik and Oatis, 1995; Lehmann, 1982). An example of qualitative analysis of gait is presented in chapter 9.

Before specific models are reviewed, we remind you that the terminology, scope, and complexity of the qualitative analysis models varies. Scholars from a particular subdiscipline often emphasize the aspects of qualitative analysis to which their subdiscipline is strongly related. Table 2.1 categorizes selected qualitative analysis models in kinesiology into two kinds of models, comprehensive and observational.

Comprehensive models deal with the big picture of qualitative analysis, laying the groundwork for the whole process. These models usually provide information on movement goals, preparation for observation, stages of motor development, observation, evaluation, diagnosis of errors, and appropriate feedback. Comprehensive models attempt to summarize all the important tasks relevant to qualitative analysis of human movement.

Observational models of qualitative analysis are focused on the task of observation within

Table 2.1
Scope of Selected Models for Qualitative Analysis

Comprehensive	Observational
Abendroth-Smith, Kras, and Strand, 1996	Barrett, 1979c, 1983
Allison, 1985b	Brown, 1982
Arend and Higgins, 1976	Cooper and Glassow, 1963
Balan and Davis, 1993	Dunham, 1986, 1994
Hay and Reid, 1982, 1988	Gangstead and Beveridge, 1984
Knudson and Morrison, 1996	Hoffman, 1983
McPherson, 1990	Hudson, 1985, 1995
Norman, 1975, 1977	Pinheiro, 1994
Pinheiro and Simon, 1992	Radford, 1989
	Roberton and Halverson, 1984
	Seefeldt and Haubenstricker, 1982

qualitative analysis. They therefore fit into comprehensive models. Observational qualitative analysis models tend to fit into what we call the observation task of a comprehensive model of qualitative analysis. We will see that some observational models include parts of other tasks within a comprehensive model of qualitative analysis; a continuum probably exists moving from a strictly observational model of movement to a comprehensive model of qualitative analysis.

OBSERVATIONAL MODELS FOR QUALITATIVE ANALYSIS

Observational models of qualitative analysis in kinesiology are important because they focus on a professional skill that has been ignored in the past—the immediate, live observation of people trying to learn various movements. They typically emphasize how to observe, critical features of the skill, the sequence or phases of movement to be observed, and possible errors and cues. These models have traditionally focused the observer's attention to particular parts of a skill or body actions. Some models attempt to analyze or break down a motor skill for a systematic observation. Others use a more gestalt approach, in which the analyst builds a total picture or feeling about the movement from all sources of information, producing a general assessment of that movement. Many of these models will be ex-

panded on in other relevant sections of this text. Observational models are dealt with first because they have been the focus of research in recent years.

Pedagogical Observational Models

Pedagogy is the subdiscipline of kinesiology that has focused attention on the development of observational models to improve the qualitative analysis of teachers (Barrett, 1979c; Dunham, 1986, 1994; Gangstead and Beveridge, 1984; Hoffman, 1983; Pinheiro, 1994). Chapter 1 mentioned how the work of Huelster (1939) and Barrett (1979c) increased interest in the development of observation training in the kinesiology curriculum. A recent paper by Pinheiro (1994) proposes an observational model as part of his larger comprehensive model of qualitative analysis (Pinheiro and Simon, 1992). The models of Gangstead and Beveridge (1984), Dunham (1986, 1994), and Hoffman (1983) will be summarized to illustrate how observational models contribute to qualitative analysis.

Gangstead and Beveridge's Model

A model proposed by Gangstead and Beveridge (1984) emerged from the traditional qualitative analysis models in kinesiology/biomechanics courses (Cooper and Glassow, 1963). This model is a true observational model focusing on the observer's attention on the temporal and spatial aspects of the movement. The temporal foci are the preparation, action, and follow-through phases of the movement. The spatial foci are the performer's body weight, path of the hub (slowest moving part), arms, legs, trunk action, head action, and impact/release parameters. Figure 2.1 presents this model as modified from Cooper and Glassow (1963). The Gangstead and Beveridge model is designed to concentrate the analyst's attention on the sequence of the movement and the critical features. This observational framework is useful for observers who have difficulty diverting their attention to different parts of a movement.

Hoffman's Model

Hoffman (1983) proposed a diagnostic prescriptive model of qualitative analysis. The fundamental requirements are a good mental picture of what a performance should look like and a clear goal/purpose for the movement. The teacher focuses on the difference between the observed response and the mental image of the correct response. If a discrepancy exists between what is seen and what should be, the observer is charged with diagnosing (the extent of discrepancy and possible cause) and prescribing a remedy.

This model was further developed into a hypothetical-deductive model of qualitative analysis. Differences between observed and desired performance could be related to a lack of a critical ability, a deficiency in skill, or a psychosocial problem. The Hoffman model significantly extends many observational models, hypothesizing on the evaluation and diagnosis of movement errors. The important task of evaluation and diagnosis of performance will be fully discussed in chapter 7.

Dunham's Model

Dunham (1986, 1994) proposed the use of task sheets for qualitative analysis and emphasized the importance of getting an overall feeling about the quality of the movement before observing specific components. This gestalt impression in the observational process is different from traditional observational models, which focus on temporal or spatial information first. Dunham instructed the observer to get an overall feel for the way the skill is performed. The basic ideas of a gestalt are that the whole is greater than the sum of its parts and that the best way to analyze movement is to observe the whole and decide on its quality. If quality is lacking, then analyze the skill by temporal or spatial means or use one of the other models proposed in this chapter to find the specific problem. An example of Dunham's task sheets, which form the basis of the gestalt, is presented in our discussion of the preparation task of qualitative analysis on pp. 77-80 in chapter 5.

Body components	Temporal phasing		
	Preparation	Action	Follow through
Path of hub			
Body weight			
Trunk action			
Head action			
Leg action			
Arm action			
Impact/release			

Figure 2.1 The Gangstead and Beveridge (1984) observational model of qualitative analysis.
Reprinted, by permission, from S.K. Gangstead & S. Beveridge, 1984, "The implementation and evaluation of a methodological approach to qualitative sport skill analysis instruction." *Journal of Teaching in Physical Education*, 3 (62).

Biomechanical Observational Models

Biomechanics scholars have also proposed observational models that translate abstract biomechanical principles into observable actions in human movement. Two excellent examples of these approaches are the work of Brown (1982) and Hudson (1985).

Brown's Model

Brown (1982) proposed 19 visual evaluation techniques that were developed with the Youth Sports Institute in preparing volunteer youth sport coaches. These qualitative analysis techniques are organized into five areas: vantage point, movement simplification, balance and stability, movement relationships, and range of movement. The observation and evaluation of movement are based on application of the 19 techniques in a general to a specific way. One observes multiple trials by first considering the vantage point, observing slower parts of the movement to simplify observation, and then focusing on faster, more complex parts of the movement.

Hudson's Model

Another biomechanist (Hudson, 1985) proposed an approach to qualitative analysis called POSSUM (purpose/observation system of studying and understanding movement). In the POSSUM approach, the movement is classified according to its purpose (maintenance of balance or maximum effort). A strength of the Hudson observational model is that the purpose *must* be associated with some observable dimensions of the movement. These dimensions are the variables that the observer must evaluate visually. The Hudson model is based on selecting visual variables that are important. They must distinguish between skill levels, be observable qualitatively by the naked eye, and be subject to change by the performer.

Figure 2.2 illustrates how a purpose is linked with visually observable variables. Each visual variable has a continuum that assists in evaluating performance. The visual or spatial analysis of these dimensions is achieved with two kinds of visual foci. The observer may focus at the whole-body, or *somatic*, level or on the *sectional* (segmental) level.

Hudson has continued to develop these analyst-friendly descriptions of biomechanical variables. In 1990 she proposed six generic dimensions of *value*, or visual variables. Her research has also focused on examining how experienced and novice observers visualize variables in unfamiliar motor skills and on studying how long and in what phase of the movement visual variables are observed (Hudson, 1990c).

Recently Hudson (1995:55) expanded this idea and identified 10 *core concepts* of kinesiology (table 2.2). These concepts are the variables that an analyst can evaluate and give feedback about in order to improve performance. The core

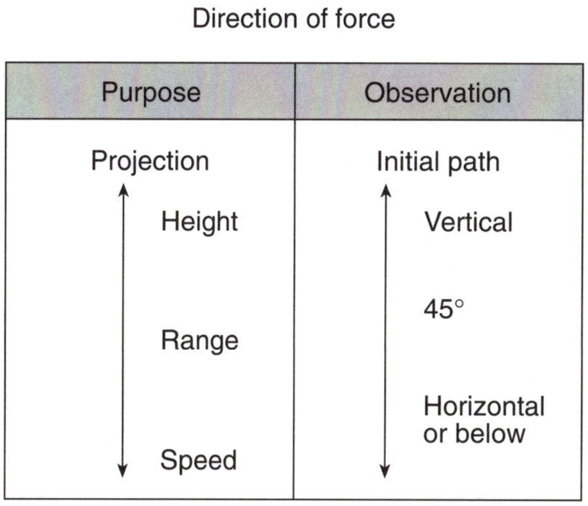

Direction of force

Purpose	Observation
Projection	Initial path
↑ Height	↑ Vertical
	45°
Range	
	Horizontal or below
↓ Speed	↓

Figure 2.2 Examples of the principle of direction of force from the POSSUM model of qualitative analysis. The purposes of motor skills are linked with observable variables for the evaluation of performance.
Adapted, with permission, from Jackie Hudson (1987), *What goes up . . . .* Paper presented to the Kinesiology Academy, AAHPERD National Convention, Las Vegas, NV.

Table 2.2
Core Concepts of Kinesiology

Range of motion
Speed of motion
Number of segments
Nature of segments
Balance
Coordination
Compactness
Extension at release
Path of projection
Spin

From "Core concepts of kinesiology" by J. Hudson. Reprinted with permission from the *Journal of Physical Education, Recreation & Dance*, June, 1995, 54-60. JOPERD is a publication of the American Alliance for Health, Physical Education, Recreation and Dance, 1900 Association Drive, Reston, VA 22091.

concepts are, in essence, the technique knobs that an analyst can turn in helping performers improve their movement. Hudson's work is important because it has stimulated discussion of visualizable biomechanical variables and focused attention on the issue of coordination.

> **KEY POINT**
>
> *Models that have been proposed for qualitative analysis within kinesiology have either focused on the process of observation or had a more comprehensive view of the tasks within qualitative analysis.*

COMPREHENSIVE MODELS FOR QUALITATIVE ANALYSIS

This section reviews the contributions from kinesiology scholars proposing comprehensive models of qualitative analysis, which develop an overall picture of all the tasks that are involved in the qualitative analysis of movement. This broad, interdisciplinary view is important to understanding how a comprehensive and integrated model of qualitative analysis was developed for this book. The comprehensive models presented here are also organized by the subdiscipline with which they are associated.

Pedagogical Comprehensive Models

Sport pedagogy scholars have proposed several comprehensive models for the qualitative analysis of human movement. Remember that these models are different from the large body of pedagogy research on systematic observation. In sport pedagogy, *systematic observation* refers to the method of preference for *evaluating teaching*. Systematic observation is a way to categorize student and teacher behaviors in the classroom in order to gather valid data on the teacher and teaching techniques. But qualitative analysis is a professional skill focused on the learner, not the process of teaching or coaching. Qualitative analysis is the systematic observation and introspective judgment of the quality of human movement for the purpose of providing the most appropriate intervention to improve the learner's performance.

Arend and Higgins' Model

One significant model for the qualitative analysis of human movement was proposed by Arend and Higgins (1976). They advocated an *integrated approach* and presented a comprehensive model for analyzing human movement with several strategies, depending on whether the purpose of the analysis was skill or performance. They saw skill analysis as an evaluation of learning, or how human movement changed over time. Performance analysis was the evaluation of the execution of a task or subphase of a task. The Arend and Higgins model is so comprehensive that it was designed to accommodate *any* kind of analysis of human movement. Their model, for example, can be used for subjective, anatomical, or quantitative analyses of human movement. The model is also described in a book (Higgins, 1977).

The Arend and Higgins (1976) model of analysis breaks qualitative analysis down into three phases: preobservation, observation, and postobservation. Preobservation has three levels of decomposition, or levels of the factors important in the movement. Each level provides more specific background information on the movement being analyzed. The third level of decomposition identifies the precise biomechanical, tactical, and morphological factors related to the movement. This model and paper were very important because previous articles on qualitative analysis had focused on the observation task, with little discussion of the preparatory activities or analytical activities after observation.

The Arend and Higgins (1976) paper was also important because it provided a comprehensive summary of an *integrated* analysis of human movement. Issues from biomechanics, pedagogy, motor development, and other kinesiology subdisciplines are included in the plan for analysis. This discussion cannot do justice to the quality or depth of the issues discussed in the paper. Arend and Higgins proposed that the concept of *critical features* be understood as parts of a movement that can be least modified to be successful. The model was general enough to allow a flexible approach, so the strategy used should be based on the purposes of the analysis.

Pinheiro's Model

Recently, several comprehensive models of qualitative analysis models have emerged with a pedagogical heritage (Balan and Davis, 1993; Pinheiro 1990, 1994; Pinheiro and Simon, 1992). Pinheiro has proposed models that describe the overall processes of qualitative analysis (Pinheiro and Simon, 1992), as well as the observational model previously described (Pinheiro, 1994). Their comprehensive model is based on an information processing approach.

The three levels in this model are cue acquisition, cue interpretation, and diagnostic decision. Cue acquisition is like the observation task in our integrated, comprehensive model of qualitative analysis. Cue interpretation is analogous to our evaluation step. And the diagnostic decision is analogous to the diagnosis step within the evaluation/diagnosis task of qualitative analysis. All of these processes can also be viewed as part of information processing in qualitative analysis.

Balan and Davis' Model

Balan and Davis (1993) presented an ecological task analysis approach to teaching physical education derived from the work of Davis and Burton (1991). Their approach includes qualitative analysis as an essential component of the teaching, learning, and evaluation process. Their model also differs from others in emphasizing performer responsibility and control of the observational environment. Responsibility for finding movement solutions is shifted to performers/students, which is appropriate for individualized styles of instruction. The analyst is charged with controlling the physical (practice, equipment, etc.) and social environment to facilitate analysis of the movement. This model is almost like a style of teaching (the pedagogy connection again).

Biomechanical Comprehensive Models

Since undergraduate kinesiology/biomechanics has been the course traditionally associated with developing qualitative analysis skills, many comprehensive models of qualitative analysis have been developed by biomechanics scholars. Some recent proposals that represent the field and show the variety of contemporary biomechanical analysis approaches will be reviewed here.

Hay and Reid's Model

One of the most complete discussions of qualitative analysis in a biomechanics textbook may be by Hay and Reid (1982, 1988). They differentiate qualitative analysis from quantitative analysis based on the subjectivity of the evaluation of the movement. Their model for qualitative analysis involves four steps: development of a deterministic/biomechanical model of the skill, observa-

tion of performance and identification of faults, ranking of the priority of the faults, and instructions to the performer.

Develop a Model of the Skill. The first step in the Hay and Reid (1982) model for qualitative analysis is the development of a *deterministic model* of the skill. First the mechanical purpose or result is identified—for example, time in a 100-meter dash, horizontal distance for a javelin throw, or height in a vertical jump.

Then the factors that directly influence or determine the result are identified. Figure 2.3 illustrates a deterministic model of a long jump. For this step, knowledge of qualitative analysis and the careful reading of research literature are important. Hay and Reid illustrate the point of background knowledge with examples of incorrect opinions concerning correct form held by coaches and by champion performers who are successful despite inefficient form.

Another recent comprehensive model of qualitative analysis called biomechanically based observation and analysis for teachers (BBOAT) expands the use of these deterministic models by applying them to traditional phases of the movement and skill level of the learner (Abendroth-Smith, Kras, and Strand, 1996).

Observe Performance and Identify Faults. The second step in Hay and Reid's qualitative analysis model is observation of performance and identification of faults. It is important to use all sensory information: visual, aural, tactile, and kinesthetic. The model proposes several suggestions for the observation. The setting for the performance should be controlled to minimize distractions and should be as realistic as possible.

They also suggest that the position of the observer be at right angles to the direction of body motion. This position can vary depending on the skill or part of the skill that is of interest to the observer. The distance they recommend from which to observe slow and fast movements is 10 to 15 meters and 20 to 40 meters, respectively. The authors argue that the focus of observations generally follows a pattern. Two or three trials will yield a general impression (a gestalt, which will be discussed at length in chapter 4). Then the separate parts of the movement can be observed systematically in later trials.

Hay and Reid (1988) suggest that there are two ways observers identify faults in human movement. The traditional approach is to break the movement down into phases and compare the performer's movement to a mental image of the

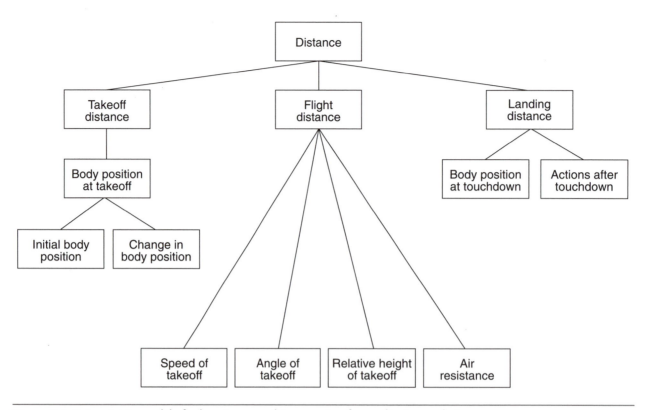

Figure 2.3 Deterministic model of a long jump used in preparing for qualitative analysis.
Reprinted, by permission, from J.G. Hay, 1983, "A system for the qualitative analysis of motor skill." In *Collected Papers on Sports Biomechanics*, edited by G.A. Wood (Nedlands, Western Australia: University of Western Australia Press), 106.

appropriate movement. They call this the *sequential method*. They suggest that flaws in this method are the assumption of an ideal form, the lack of any valid rationale for determining ideal form, and the typical assumption that champion athletes use ideal form.

Instead, Hay and Reid suggest that the *mechanical method* be used to identify performance faults. The mechanical method is based on using the deterministic, biomechanical models to systematically evaluate the model factors to see if performance can be improved. This evaluation begins by identifying the lowest factors on each path. These are the underlying determinants of the effectiveness of the performance. The factors that cannot be changed by the performer are eliminated from consideration, and the observer evaluates what factors can be improved.

The authors claim that the mechanical method does not rely on any visual model of ideal form. They do suggest that the method uses the form of skilled performers as a guide for what is effective and what correction may be appropriate. It appears that the mechanical method proposed is another structure or paradigm on which to base qualitative analysis. In the end, it may still rely

on the same mental image comparisons as traditional qualitative analyses. Chapter 4 deals with some of these perceptual issues from an information processing perspective.

Rank the Priority of Faults. The third step in the model is the evaluation of faults. Priorities should be set so that one or two corrections can be selected to work on. Hay and Reid advocate that faults be prioritized using two rules. Faults are excluded if they are related to or result from other faults, and faults should be corrected in the order that generates the most improvement in the time available. If an observer cannot prioritize some faults based on these rules, they should be ranked in the order in which they occur in the skill.

Instruct the Performer. The final step in Hay and Reid's model for qualitative analysis is providing instruction to the performer. This is a critical step; the results of the analysis can be wasted if feedback is poorly delivered. It is important to check the performer's understanding of the information. Hay and Reid strongly suggest that instructions to the performer be limited to one fault at a time. They also advocate direct corrections or literal descriptions of what the performer should do (drill approach) first. If this is unsuccessful, more figurative feedback that leads indirectly to the correction (problem-solving approach) should be used.

The Hay and Reid (1982, 1988) text provides their conception of a comprehensive method of qualitative analysis of motor skills. Their approach relies on a strong knowledge of biomechanics to break down motor skills and analyze the movements of performers. Their book provides several insightful examples of qualitative analysis of sport skills using their model.

Norman's Model

A biomechanics researcher who called for a qualitative analysis emphasis for the undergraduate kinesiology course (Norman, 1975, 1977) also proposed that 10 biomechanical principles of motion be used to analyze movement qualitatively (table 2.3). These principles were generated from a decade of experience and from the many kinesiology textbooks that identified principles of biomechanics that could be applied to human movement. Some of the principles are similar and are based on the same mechanical variables. This approach has become part of the extensive Canadian coaching effectiveness programs.

Table 2.3
**Biomechanical Principles
for Qualitative Analysis**

Summation of joint torques

Continuity of joint torques

Impulse

Reaction

Equilibrium

Summation and continuity of body-segment velocities

Generation of angular momentum

Conservation of angular momentum

Manipulation of moment of inertia

Manipulation of body-segment angular momentum

From "Biomechanics for the community coach" by R. Norman. Adapted with permission from the *Journal of Physical Education, Recreation & Dance*, March, 1975, page 52. *JOPERD* is a publication of the American Alliance for Health, Physical Education, Recreation and Dance, 1900 Association Drive, Reston, VA 22091.

In effect, Norman's model for qualitative analysis is based on these underlying mechanical factors that create human movement. Again, the first step in the analysis is identifying the mechanical purpose or objective in the movement. The mechanical purpose should focus not just on the desired outcome (for example, the distance of a punt) but on the mechanical *cause* of the outcome as well. In the javelin throw, the athlete wants to maximize release velocity and optimize release conditions (height and angle). The qualitative analysis is then based on identifying errors or violations of the biomechanical principles. A diving instructor who observes an overrotated entry position in a dive must decide whether the diver's error was the generation of too much angular momentum or the poorly timed manipulation of the *moment of inertia* of the body segments.

Many other biomechanics textbooks base qualitative analysis on the evaluation of mechanical principles related to the particular skill (Groves and Camaione, 1983; Kreighbaum and Bartels, 1985; Luttgens and Wells, 1982). A series of articles by Sanders and Wilson (1989, 1990a, b) proposed 12 biomechanical concepts and their application in teaching and coaching motor skills. Remember that Hudson (1995) has recently provided a user-friendly list of observable biomechanical variables related to movement.

McPherson's Model

An excellent comprehensive model of qualitative analysis based on previous biomechanical models was proposed by McPherson (1990). Her model of a systematic approach to skill analysis has four steps: preobservation, observation, diagnosis, and remediation, as shown in figure 2.4. Her article provides excellent discussions of the importance of mechanical principles and their relationship to critical features. Her discussions on observational plans and diagnosis of errors are also very thorough. A biomechanical qualitative analysis model similar to McPherson's was also developed by Philipp and Wilkerson (1990).

Motor Development Comprehensive Models

The field of motor development is concerned with documenting the changes in motor skill over the human life span. Several researchers have extended their work to include models for observing and classifying the developmental level of various motor skills. These models are

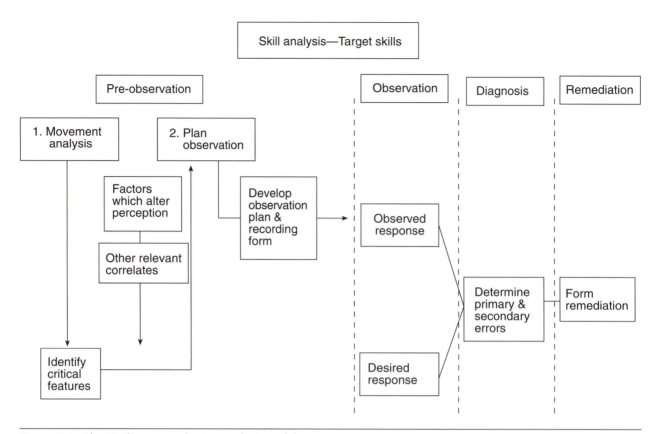

Figure 2.4   The McPherson qualitative analysis model.
Reprinted, by permission, from M. McPherson, 1990, "A systematic approach to skill analysis," *Sports*, 11(1), 2.

PRACTICAL APPLICATION

To see the difference between comprehensive and observational models of qualitative analysis, consider the qualitative analysis abilities of a student and an instructor. The dance student is busy learning to be a skilled dancer and has limited observational abilities. The novice dancer observing a demonstration may not realize all the complexities that go into creating the safest and most aesthetic movement. The dancer's observation of another dancer is limited to what someone else has told him/her is important. Does the dancer have much basis on which to interpret or decide what is correct or incorrect about a fellow dancer's performance? Would the dancer observe movement in a systematic way?

Contrast the dancer with an experienced dance instructor. Would a veteran dance instructor be skilled in both an observational and a comprehensive model of qualitative analysis? Would the instructor be knowledgeable in all aspects of dance and qualitative analysis?

based on either classification stages of whole-body action (the Michigan State University approach) or classifications of stages of various movement components (legs, trunk, arms, etc.) developed at the University of Wisconsin. The following sections will illustrate these different approaches to evaluating the development of the overarm throw.

Movement Component Developmental Models

The motor development literature has many movement component models for the observation and classification of fundamental movement patterns and skills (Halverson, 1983; Roberton, 1983; Williams, 1980). The text by Roberton and Halverson (1984) summarizes many of the component developmental models of fundamental movement patterns studied at the University of Wisconsin.

These authors have studied the development of overarm throwing longitudinally and cross-sectionally and have validated developmental levels in six components of the overarm throw. A child's developmental level for various body parts of overarm throwing can be observed from the point of view of the trunk, backswing, humerus, forearm, stepping, and stride actions. Roberton and Halverson (1984) propose that the trunk action be evaluated first in throwing and striking qualitative analysis. They suggest that the key developmental changes in the other components of throwing and striking are timed to changes in the use of the trunk.

Since the overarm throw is important to many sports, the component model of motor development has also been applied to other sport skills. Rose et al. (1990) developed a component model for observation of the tennis serve, a skill related to the overarm throw. The tennis serve was broken down into developmental levels within six components of the movement. Messick (1991) also reported a prelongitudinal screening study of the motor development of the tennis serve based on six components.

Whole Body Developmental Models

There are also several examples of the whole-body developmental sequence analyses of fundamental movement patterns (Haubenstricker et al., 1983; Seefeldt and Haubenstricker, 1982). The classic text by Wickstrom (1983) provides several examples of whole-body motor development sequences that can be used for observational assessment. Several editions of this text have outlined the stages of motor development of most fundamental movement patterns.

The classic whole-body developmental sequence for overarm throwing, documented by Wild (1938), is reviewed by Wickstrom (1983). The development of overarm throwing in children from two to seven years old generally shows four stages. Stage I throwing involves a flexion and extension of the elbow, essentially in a sagittal plane and without a change in foot position. Stage II throwing generally occurs from age three to five and has several characteristics. There still is no foot movement, but some transverse plane trunk rotation is added to an elbow flexion and extension that may be in a more oblique or horizontal plane. Stage III throwing is usually seen

in five- and six-year-olds. The movement begins with a step with the same-side leg (which limits the potential trunk rotation) and arm preparatory movements that are usually straight back. Stage IV throwing is commonly found in boys and girls around six and a half years of age. This mature throwing movement involves a forward step with the opposite side foot, a downward arm back-swing, trunk rotation, horizontal adduction of the upper arm, and elbow extension.

Figure 2.5 illustrates stage II and stage IV in the whole-body development of the overarm throw. An analyst can use this approach to know what actions to look for and the typical changes to expect in young throwers.

Motor development models for the visual analysis of motor skills provide important information on the sequences and changes people go through in learning motor skills. Analysts should be aware of the developmental levels for the skills they study. Motor development research could be of even greater value to qualitative analysis if we could learn what corrections and practice are most effective in accelerating motor development. Should corrections be focused at the next developmental level, or should cues related to mature form be used as intervention?

Four Commonalities

All of the observational and comprehensive models of qualitative analysis in kinesiology have commonalities and could be used by almost any profession in the qualitative analysis of human movement. Good qualitative analysts are very knowledgeable about the movements and the performers. They use this knowledge to plan the observation of performance. They evaluate the strengths and weaknesses of performance and diagnose the steps needed for improvement. Then they provide intervention to improve performance. These four tasks and their inter-relationships are shown in figure 2.6. This model illustrates an integrated approach to qualitative analysis of human movement that will be expanded on in the next section.

A COMPREHENSIVE, INTEGRATED MODEL OF QUALITATIVE ANALYSIS

Figure 2.6 illustrates our comprehensive, integrated model of qualitative analysis, and some

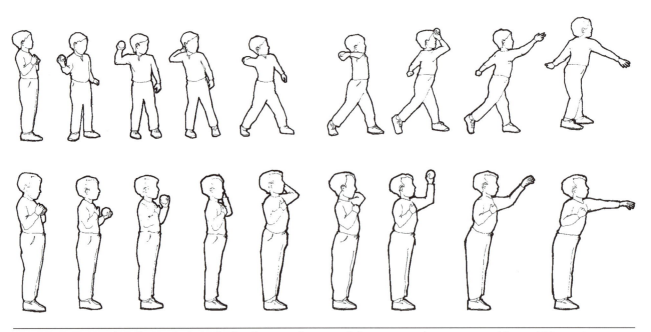

Figure 2.5 Examples of two whole-body developmental stages of the overarm throw proposed by Wild (1938). Courtesy of Steven Barnes, Multimedia Laboratories, Florida State University, Tallahassee.

of the important issues within each task. This model synthesizes many of the important aspects of models just summarized (Arend and Higgins, 1976; Hoffman, 1974, 1983; McPherson, 1988, 1990; Hay and Reid, 1982) and gives a simple, logical sequence and flow to the qualitative analysis process. The four tasks of an integrated qualitative analysis should be viewed as equally important. A weakness in any one task diminishes the effectiveness of the whole qualitative analysis.

Some important features of the integrated model of qualitative analysis should be apparent. First, the model is circular, emphasizing the continuous learning and improvement that are part of professional growth. Second, there is a way to move from intervention directly to observation. For example, an analyst may provide feedback to a performer and immediately begin another observation to continue the qualitative analysis. Third, intervention may be postponed until more information is obtained through observing the performance again. A skilled analyst may adjust the observational strategy based on an evaluation of information in early observation of a performer.

We believe that an integrated model of qualitative analysis should be viewed as part of the teaching process in kinesiology. Qualitative analysis is a key teaching skill that should be systematically addressed by the curriculum in

teacher preparation and other kinesiology programs. Practicing professionals should continuously read and think critically about how they apply qualitative analysis in the classroom, field, or lab. They should also serve as mentors or teachers of qualitative analysis to students in field experiences.

The following chapters will outline significant issues in each of the four tasks in an integrated qualitative analysis. Analysts will need to research and think critically about the key features of the movement, cues, the typical steps in motor development, developing observational strategies, and the common errors that clients exhibit in order to complete the preparation task of qualitative analysis. The second task involves systematically observing human movement to gather appropriate information about the performance. The third task, evaluation and diagnosis, involves identifying and ranking possible corrections or feedback. The fourth task, intervention, often involves providing feedback or changes in practice conditions that will lead to improved performance.

There are four important tasks in a comprehensive view of qualitative analysis: preparation, observation, evaluation/diagnosis, and intervention.

KEY POINT

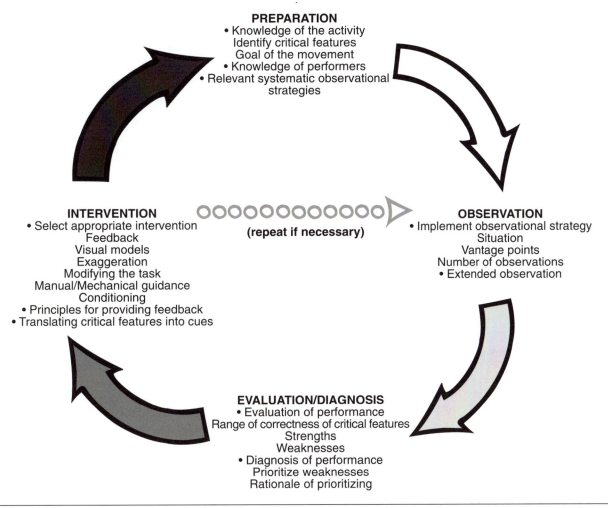

Figure 2.6　The comprehensive, integrated model of qualitative analysis. Some of the important issues for each task are listed.

The integrated model is broad enough to include all the major tasks of qualitative analysis yet simple enough not to be overwhelming. Like performers, analysts can also be overcome by paralysis by analysis (see figure 2.7). Analysts may try to apply a very complicated qualitative analysis approach or attend to unimportant information. A simple model based on critical features of the movement reduces the observational and analytic demand on the analyst (though it may increase the demands of preparing for qualitative analysis). The next section, on validity and reliability of qualitative analysis, also supports the need for a focused, simple model of qualitative analysis. Our integrated model combines expertise and knowledge from many relevant disciplines to form a new approach to qualitative analysis. At any step, knowledge from all relevant subdisciplines of kinesiology may be applied to improve performance.

Whichever approach or model of qualitative analysis is used, the question often arises as to the accuracy of an analyst's assessment and intervention. A few studies have examined the validity and reliability of such analyses. The results will be discussed in the next section of this chapter. It is important to note that these studies typically focus on the observational task of qualitative analysis.

VALIDITY AND RELIABILITY OF QUALITATIVE ANALYSIS

Important questions in any assessment relate to the issues of validity and reliability. In qualitative analysis, *validity* typically refers to the analyst's ability to correctly identify strengths and weakness of a performance. *Reliability* refers to

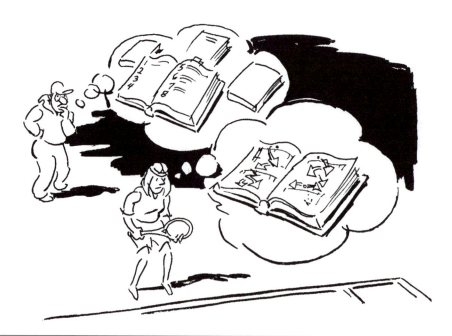

Figure 2.7　Like a performer, an analyst may be susceptible to paralysis by analysis. Both parties in qualitative analysis should focus their attention on only a few specifics at a time and should continue to communicate with one another.

the consistency of these subjective ratings. These issues can be even more complex within the context of a comprehensive model. The validity of a qualitative analysis may be affected by the diagnosis of which weaknesses are most important or by which intervention the analyst selects. The research has typically not dealt with this larger view of the validity of qualitative analysis.

Validity

Validity in qualitative analysis has two important levels. The first level is *logical validity*, which is established by the consensus of the literature and expert opinion on the movement being analyzed. An example of logical or face validity would be if the qualitative analysis accurately identified the critical features of the movement being analyzed. This first level of validity is very important, although there have been no interdisciplinary conferences that have been organized to establish the important aspects of human movements or their analysis.

The next important level is *criterion-referenced* validity, or checking the qualitative evaluation and diagnosis of some critical feature of performance with a criterion measurement of that feature. For example, you could check the criterion-referenced validity for visual estimation of knee angle in landing by comparing ratings of coaches to high-speed video or goniometric measure-

ments of athletes' knee angles. A qualitative analysis of a movement must be valid to be of any value to the performer.

Qualitative analysis models have typically used panels of experts to provide logical validity for the components used in the analysis, but few studies have documented the criterion-referenced validity of qualitative analysis in kinesiology. Studies are clearly needed to document whether observers trained in a qualitative analysis system agree with quantification of the same variables. Studies of the criterion-referenced validity of qualitative analysis in ergonomics and physical therapy literature provide a clue to the probable validity of qualitative analysis in kinesiology, where few studies have been done.

Validity Studies Within Ergonomic/Human Factors

Engineers in the field of ergonomics/human factors routinely develop observational models for evaluation of the physical demands of various work tasks. The field of ergonomics/human factors studies the optimum design of facilities, tools, and tasks for humans. Ergonomic studies have demonstrated that visual estimation of static body-segment angles in posture assessments are accurate to within 3 to 5 degrees (Douwes and Dul, 1991; Ericson et al., 1991). In a recent study, untrained observers who visually estimated static shoulder angle from videotapes had slightly greater errors (mean absolute errors of 9 degrees) (Genaidy, Simmons, Guo, and Hidalga, 1993). The subjects tended to overestimate the true angle in low shoulder angles and underestimate the true angle in medium and high shoulder angles.

A study by de Looze et al. (1994) examined the agreement between two observers' visual estimation of body actions in a materials handling task and measurements of the same variables. Coefficients of agreement were not acceptable for torso flexion or for the position of the arms and legs. Only subjective ratings of gross body posture had acceptable agreement ($k = 0.79$) with the criterion measurements. In summary, the ergonomics literature suggests there is criterion-referenced validity of qualitative analysis for some variables but not for others. However, few validity studies have included large numbers of subjects who have been systematically trained in qualitative analysis.

Validity Studies Within Physical Therapy

In the field of physical therapy, several studies have attempted to develop valid qualitative analysis models for evaluating movement quality (Boyce et al., 1995). One study found that observers could estimate step length in walking at slow to normal speeds to within 1.2 to 2.4 inches of accuracy (Stuberg et al., 1990). The best accuracy in visual assessment of step length occurred from close observational distances (0 to 3 meters); errors were two to three times larger if faster walking speeds were evaluated. Clearly, the validity of qualitative analysis depends in part on the speed and complexity of the movement.

One possible reason that visual assessments do not have consistently strong criterion-referenced validity is the perceptual limitations of observers. Saleh and Murdoch (1985) found that biomechanical measurement systems identified more gait abnormalities than skilled visual gait analysts. The perceptual limitations of observing fast and complex human movements are discussed in chapter 4. Another validity problem documented in the physical therapy literature is the tendency of assessments to be influenced by previous assessments (Eastlack et al., 1991; Miyazaki and Kubota, 1984). More research is needed that presents important performance variables (joint angles, muscle stretch, step lengths, trunk lean) on videotape to be analyzed qualitatively and quantitatively. Studies using a variety of human movements, conditions, and speeds of execution could begin to provide evi-

dence for the criterion-referenced validity of qualitative analysis.

Reliability

There have been more studies of the reliability of the qualitative analysis of human movement than studies of its validity. Intra-rater reliability is the consistency of the qualitative analyses performed by a single analyst. *Inter-rater reliability* is the consistency or agreement of the qualitative analyses of several analysts assessing the same performer. There is much reliability research on qualitative analysis in the physical therapy and physical education/kinesiology literature. Reliability issues are important to consider when planning qualitative analysis or interpreting the qualitative analyses of others.

Reliability Studies Within Physical Therapy

Physical therapy studies have examined the reliability of qualitative analysis of human gait and other clinical measurements. Observational gait assessment has had low to moderate interobserver reliability, with intraclass correlations between 0.6 and 0.7 (Goodkin and Diller, 1973; Krebs et al., 1985; Eastlack et al., 1991). The reliability of qualitative assessments of gross motor function in people with cerebral palsy, however, has been good (Gowland et al., 1995). A summary of these studies will shed some light on the issue of the reliability of qualitative analysis of human movement.

Attinger et al. (1987) studied the inter-rater reliability of visual assessment of gait asymmetry with a jury of eight medical professionals. Reliable identification of the foot on the ground the longest was 80% probable and rose to 87% probable when the asymmetry was greater than normal. The experts were unable to rate the amount of asymmetry, or to reliably identify a limb that was loaded more than the other.

Krebs and colleagues (1985) evaluated the inter- and intra-observer reliability of three expert observers with videotapes of 15 disabled children. Intra-rater reliability was moderately reliable. Mean agreement of repeated ratings was 69% (31% of assessments disagreeing with assessments made a month earlier by the same therapist). For a clinician to be 95% sure he/she had observed a change, there had to be a 10% difference in leg kinematics. Mean inter-rater agreement was 67.5%, with a mean intraclass correlation of 0.73. A 33% difference in walking kinematics would be required to detect differences in walking with different analysts. These results were supported by Keenan and Bach (1996) who found poor ($k = .59$) intra-observer agreement of five clinicians' ratings of rearfoot motion in gait.

In a study of the inter-rater reliability of the qualitative analysis of gait reported by Eastlack et al. (1991), 53 physical therapists rated 10 gait variables (knee kinematics and temporospatial variables of the gait cycle) during the 4 phases of stance from videotapes of patients. Notably, this study was the first to allow the use of slow-motion replay by the observers. The inter-rater reliability of the gait variables was slight to moderate ($< .69$). Joint kinematics had less agreement than temporal or spatial variables. These poor results may be related to the fact that 32 of the 53 physical therapists involved in the study were unfamiliar with any of the 4 major models for the qualitative analysis of gait in physical therapy.

Other sources of information on the reliability of qualitative analysis in physical therapy include studies of visual estimation of joint range of motion and gross motor performance. Studies of the reliability of visual estimation of joint range of motion have had mixed results. Studies of the qualitative analysis of foot and ankle motion in gait have shown poor (Keenan and Bach, 1996) to moderate (Youndas et al., 1991, 1993) inter-observer agreement, while other studies have documented inter-observer reliability of visual assessment with intraclass correlations above .82 (Watkins et al., 1991). Gowland and colleagues (1995) reported good reliability ($r > .92$) for overall ratings and attribute ratings ($r > .84$) of the movement of cerebral palsy patients by 19 physical therapists.

Reliability Studies Within Kinesiology

Kinesiology research has supported the moderate reliability of qualitative analysis observed in the physical therapy literature. Motor development and adapted physical education studies have used the generalizability study (G study) approach. This is important because a G study is designed to examine all variables that affect reliability of any measurement or assessment (observers, occasions, different performers).

Ulrich (1984) reported acceptable reliability (*K*s between .62 and .84) of a standardized assessment of 12 fundamental motor skills. Ulrich, Ulrich, and Branta (1988) reported a G study of the qualitative analysis using the Michigan State developmental stages of the hop, horizontal jump, and running. Subjects received minimal instruction (1 hour) in qualitative analysis of the whole-body developmental level of the three skills. One observer watching three trials could reliably analyze the hop ($G = .88$). Reliably assessing the developmental level of the horizontal jump and running required multiple observers and trials. These two skills showed potential observer bias with 20% to 30% of the variance in the ratings being related to interaction between the subject and the observer. The observers had been warned against this error, but there may have been a tendency to relate the age of the subject to the developmental level assigned. For example, some observers may have been inclined to rate a younger-looking subject lower or an older-looking subject higher.

> *Although qualitative analysis has been shown to have content validity, studies show only moderate validity and poor to moderate reliability.*
>
> KEY POINT

Bias was also observed by Painter (1990) even after training in qualitative analysis. This G study examined the effect of training, academic major, and kind of motor development model (whole-body or component) used to identify 20 female college students' developmental level of hopping. A key finding was that focusing on hopping components resulted in greater reliability than a whole-body approach to qualitative analysis. By focusing on components (arm or leg action) of hopping, one observer looking at one performance could reliably identify the developmental level.

Mosher and Schutz (1983) also found that slow components of the overarm throw (foot placement and body rotation) could be reliably observed in one trial by one observer. Fast and complex movements are difficult to observe reliably. These studies found that the action of the arms during hopping (Painter, 1990) and throwing (Mosher and Schutz, 1983) was difficult to observe reliably. Painter concluded that one kinesiology student would need at least five trials to observe and rate the arm action in hopping. A single kinesiology student analyst would have to observe 10 trials to reliably rate the whole-body developmental level of hopping.

The physical therapy and kinesiology literature suggests that the reliability of qualitative analysis in actual practice (different analysts, students, number of observations, variable conditions) is likely to be poor to moderate. There are, however, ways to increase the potential reliability of qualitative analysis. Increasing the number of observers or the number of trials observed tends to increase reliability. Another approach is to increase the specificity of the system/model by analyzing discrete events and providing a simple rating for them (Kerner and Alexander, 1981). Identifying specific critical features and defining rules on how they will be evaluated can help build in the potential for agreement in multiple observations of human movement.

SUMMARY

The problem with the three golf coaches at the beginning of the chapter is that they do not have a comprehensive approach to qualitative analysis and they do not have a specific process of observation (as illustrated by the observational models in this chapter) to analyze movement in real time. The result is that they all come up with different information on which to base decisions. Good qualitative analysis must be based on an interdisciplinary approach that integrates all the subdisciplines of kinesiology.

This chapter reviewed key models of qualitative analysis in the kinesiology literature. These models either had a *comprehensive* view of qualitative analysis or focused on the *observation* task. Four tasks that are common to a comprehensive view of qualitative analysis are preparation, observation, evaluation/diagnosis, and intervention. These four tasks are the basis for the comprehensive, integrated model of qualitative analysis that this book is based on.

A review of the research showed only moderate criterion-referenced validity for qualitative analysis of human movement. Studies in real-world conditions showed only poor to moderate reliability. This literature suggests that qualitative analyses must be carefully planned and implemented to maximize their validity and reliability. The greater the complexity of the qualitative analysis model and critical features of the movement analyzed, the greater the potential for disagreement among analysts. A compromise must be reached between the depth and complexity of the most accurate model and the simplicity that will reduce the analyst's perceptual overload and improve reliability.

DISCUSSION QUESTIONS

1. What features of qualitative analysis are similar in models from different disciplines or specializations within the fields interested in human movement?

2. How complex a model of qualitative analysis is necessary for good professional practice? Can there be too much complexity in preparing for qualitative analysis?

3. What tasks of qualitative analysis are emphasized by models from sport pedagogy? biomechanics? motor development? gait analysis?

4. How does a qualitative analysis model relate to different approaches to teaching motor skills?

The Role of the Senses in Qualitative Analysis

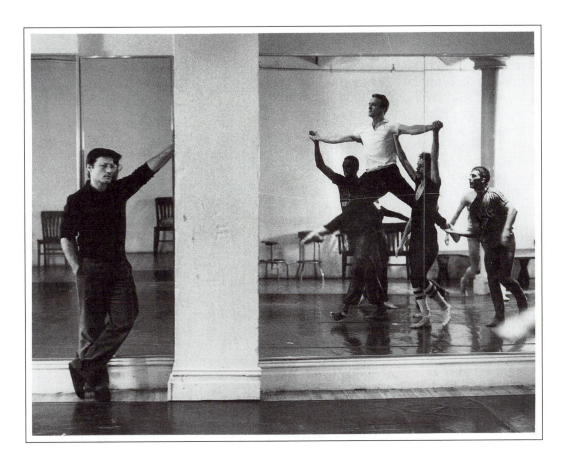

PREVIEW

A modern dance instructor is working hard with his company to finish a piece he created. Movements in this piece must be precise to prevent collisions and to make sure everyone is in time with the music. To make the piece come together, the instructor relies on many of his senses. He watches to look at dancers' placement as well as their body alignment and limb position. He listens carefully to make sure everyone is in time. Occasionally he participates in the class so that he can gather tactile and kinesthetic information about the progress of the piece. Without information from all of his senses, he would not have a complete picture of what happens in the new dance piece.

Chapter Objectives

1. Describe the structure of the sense organs used in qualitative analysis.
2. Describe the function of the sense organs associated with qualitative analysis.
3. Discuss some of the limitations of the senses in gathering information for qualitative analysis.
4. Describe the integration process of the senses used in qualitative analysis.

The complexities of each sense and their contribution to qualitative analysis are staggering even before we consider the simultaneous interaction of several senses. The senses provide the information from which qualitative analysis decisions about human movement are made. They are to the qualitative analysis of movement what instruments are to the quantitative analysis of movement; they gather information about performance. *Perception* is the organization and interpretation of stimuli from our environment, mediated by our senses. Perception involves making "sense" of our sensory information (Sage, 1984). This chapter will provide an overview of the senses and their role in perception. It will review each sense's contribution to qualitative analysis and the integration of sensory information.

Although this chapter will examine the four major senses—vision, audition, touch (haptic), and kinesthetic proprioception—individually, they work closely with each other. The senses work together in the observation task of qualitative analysis to provide a basis for the evaluation and diagnosis of human movement (Hay and Reid, 1988; Hoffman, 1983; Radford, 1989).

Different senses provide unique information that the observer puts together to improve the observation of performance. The kinesthetic proprioceptive sense an analyst uses while spotting a gymnastic tumbling run may tell more about the forces being exerted by a performer than vision or audition. Audition may be the best sense for gathering temporal information on the timing of the tumbling, while vision is most sensitive to spatial changes in the position of the body in flight. All this sensory input must be interpreted and evaluated to gather relevant information for the evaluation and diagnosis task within qualitative analysis. The most dominant sense is typically vision.

VISION

The primary sense used in the qualitative analysis of human movement is vision, so most of the information in this chapter focuses on vision. Until the late 19th century, visual observation was the primary method for studying the biomechanics of movement. This section will review important information about the capabilities and limitations of human visual perception of motion.

There are major limitations to our ability to see fast movements. In fact, the improvements in observational power created by photography and cinematography have dominated the science of biomechanics for the century since their development (Cappozzo, Marchetti, and Tosi, 1992). The initial furor created by the cinematographic photographs of moving people and animals made by Muybridge and Marey in the late 19th century are a testament to the limited perceptual power of the naked eye.

The sensory receptor involved in vision is the eye. This receptor takes energy from the visual spectrum of electromagnetic radiation and converts it into nerve transmissions directed to the appropriate parts of the brain. It is important to understand the structure and function of the eye.

> *Understanding the structure and variety of sense organs used in qualitative analysis will make an analyst aware of the limitations and strengths of sensory information.*
>
> KEY POINT

Structure of the Eye

In general terms, each eye has a lens, which focuses the light onto the retina at the back of the eye. Here, the light energy causes chemical changes, which in turn stimulate the optic nerve leading to the vision centers of the brain. The important structures of the eye are illustrated in figure 3.1.

There are several important structures related to eye function. The sclera is a tough membrane that composes the majority of the outer eye. It helps maintain the eye's shape and structure. The cornea is a transparent continuation of the sclera over the area where the light is allowed to enter. Irregularities in the shape of the eye (near- and farsightedness) and the cornea (astigmatism) contribute to problems with visual acuity.

The structures immediately below the cornea are the iris and the pupil. The iris is a colored membrane with circular muscles that allow it to contract or dilate, which makes the pupil shrink or enlarge. In bright light, the pupil contracts, screening out some light energy; in limited light, the pupil dilates, allowing more light in.

The lens is the structure immediately behind the iris and pupil. The lens is suspended by ligaments attached to ciliary muscles, which contract and relax to allow the lens to change shape. This change in shape allows clear images to be focused on the back of the eye. The lens is a clear, transparent structure with a convex shape.

The next important structure is the retina, which forms the inner surface of the eye. This is where light is converted into chemical energy. This structure is extremely complex. The conversion of light energy takes place in two different types of cells: rods and cones. These cells have different purposes and function differently. Rods are about a thousand times more sensitive than cones. Rods are primarily used in black-and-white (achromatic) vision and are very useful for seeing at night. Cones are less sensitive to light and allow us to see colors (chromatic). This color vision is the result of chemical interactions of rhodopsin, retinene scotopin, and vitamin A.

The fovea centralis is a pinhead-sized indentation in the back of the retina, where there is a dense gathering of rods. This portion of the eye allows for the best visual acuity because of the concentration of rods and their one-to-one innervation. Axons from the rods and cones exit to the optic nerve at the optic disc. This area of the eye is called the blind spot because it has no rods or cones. The areas in front of and behind the lens are filled with clear fluid designed to help maintain the shape of the eye while allowing light to pass through. The fluid in front of the lens is called the aqueous humor, while the fluid behind the lens is called the vitreous humor.

From the optic nerve of each eye, information is transmitted via the lateral geniculate body to the visual cortex of the occipital lobe in the brain. From here, information is transmitted to various

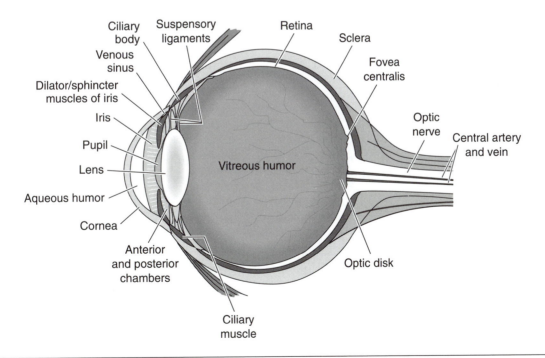

Figure 3.1 Diagram of the eye and its functional components.

association areas of the brain so that visual information can be integrated with other sensory information as well as stored in memory.

Functional Components of the Eye

The eye has many functions that allow it to gather information from our surroundings. The major functions are accommodation, static visual acuity, dynamic visual acuity, convergence/divergence, depth perception, eye dominance, tracking, peripheral vision, and fusion. The rest of this section will review how vision functions, beginning with visibility.

Visibility

The *visibility* of any object or event is its detectability by the human eye. This is a complex phenomenon because there are many levels of detectability that are important in qualitative analysis. The lowest level could be just noting or recognizing an event. Chapter 4 examines the processes of perception, including detection, in greater depth. At higher levels, the ability to discern information about an event puts greater demands on the visual system. At the lowest level, the two most important factors in visibility are lighting conditions and contrast (McCormick and Sanders, 1982). These two factors will be discussed in the following section on visual accuracy.

Accuracy of Visual Perception

The ability to see details in an object is called *visual acuity*. This ability is strongly related to the adjustment of the eye's lens (*accommodation*) and the shape of the eye. There are many measures of visual acuity; the most common is minimum separable acuity. A good example of this is the common Snellen eye chart, in which the smallest features discernible (usually letters) are evaluated. This is the most common measure of *static visual acuity* (SVA). Besides an individual's innate SVA, many factors affect visual discrimination, among them contrast, lighting, motion, time, color, and age.

Contrast is the percentage difference in illumination of the features of an object being viewed. The contrast between the black letters and the white paper of the Snellen eye test (or this book) is very high. The contrast between a dark uniform and a poorly lit athletic field is considerably worse. If the contrast between an object and the background is low, the object must be larger to be as detectable as a smaller object with greater

contrast. Professionals selecting colors for uniforms or clothing should think about the potential contrast among the colors selected, the environment, and the equipment.

> *Good vision for qualitative analysis is a very complex phenomenon, involving more than just static visual acuity. Other factors affecting vision in human movement are dynamic visual acuity, perception of color, contrast, accurate eye movements, eye dominance, and peripheral vision.*
>
> **KEY POINT**

The amount of light, or *illuminance*, is an important factor that interacts with contrast to determine the visibility of an object or event. There is extensive research on the effects of lighting on human performance in many tasks. In general, the more illumination, the better the performance (McCormick and Sanders, 1982). There can be too much illumination, however; glare or brightness reflected from the object and background make it difficult to see the object. It is also important to remember that the eye's sensitivity to light changes with illuminance. The transition of sensitivity from darkness to light is relatively quick (less than a minute), while adjustment from light to dark can take 30 minutes or more (McCormick and Sanders, 1982). Current research in visual discrimination in varying lighting conditions is based on contrast sensitivity function (Kluka, 1991).

Another factor influencing visual discrimination is the perception of color. Recall that the retina has two types of light sensitive receptors: rods and cones. A human eye has about 130 million rods that are primarily sensitive to light intensity and about 7 million cones that are primarily sensitive to the wavelength of light and are responsible for our perception of color (McCormick and Sanders, 1982). Some people have difficulty discriminating between red and green or between blue and yellow. True color blindness is very rare, but color deficiency is usually found in about 8% to 10% of males and less than 1% of females (Gavriyski, 1969). Although these are not large percentages of the population, it would be wise to plan sporting events with contrasting colors that are not combinations of red/green or blue/yellow.

The time available to focus on an object strongly affects SVA. The greater the viewing time, the better the chance of making visual discriminations. If either the object or the observer is in motion, that reduces the time the eyes will be able to focus on the object. This brings us to *dynamic visual acuity* (DVA), or the visual discrimination of an object when there is relative movement between the object and the observer. A person's DVA deteriorates rapidly as the eye's angular velocity exceeds 60 or 70 degrees per second (Bahill and LaRitz, 1984; Burg, 1966). The less time an object is in our visual field, the less able we will be to see and judge the motion of that object.

Our DVA increases from ages 6 to 20 and then tends to decrease (Burg, 1966; Ishigaki and Miyao, 1994; Morris, 1977). This is why it is developmentally appropriate for baseball/softball leagues for small children to use a batting tee rather than machine-pitched balls. As children's visual and hitting skills improve, coaches can incorporate pitched balls and more realistic batting tee drills. For example, older players practicing with a batting tee can focus their eyes forward, quickly saccade their eyes to the ball, and then hit the ball.

Unfortunately, good SVA does not guarantee that a person will have good DVA. Studies have found weak correlations ($r<.6$) between SVA and DVA at slow speeds (Burg, 1966; Kluka, 1994) and no correlation at faster speeds (Morris, 1977). The weak association between SVA and DVA is not surprising, since SVA is the ability to observe detail in ideal conditions (static, two dimensions, good lighting and contrast), while DVA is observational ability in less than ideal conditions (motion, three dimensions, and poor contrast).

Research suggests that DVA can improve with training (Long and Rourke, 1989) and finds large differences between individuals (Morris, 1977). Some people are velocity resistant and are not strongly affected by the relative motion of an object. Others are velocity susceptible; their visual perception is easily disturbed by relative motion of the object (Morris, 1977). Clearly, relative motion and DVA influence the qualitative analysis ability of a teacher or coach. Research on ball catching has also shown that the temporal constraints of the environment affect how the eyes track the object's motion (Montagne, Laurent, and Ripoll, 1993).

There are many examples in sport where the relative motion of people or objects past the observer is so great it cannot be observed reliably. Officiating in sports like basketball and American football has been controversial for many years. The National Football League experimented with instant replays to make final judgments on difficult calls in the late 1980s. In tennis, the controversy over calling balls in or out (Vincent, 1984) led to the development of photoelectric sensors to help call the service line in professional matches.

Another problem related to time and DVA is sporting events of very short duration. Examples are collisions or release events in high-speed sports. In most striking sports (for example, baseball and tennis), coaches use cues to have the players watch the ball until it hits the bat or racquet. Since ball/bat collisions in baseball and softball last only 1 or 2 milliseconds, it is highly unlikely that any athlete can see the ball hit the bat. Watts and Bahill (1990) reviewed their studies of vision in baseball and concluded that batters cannot track the ball to the point of impact even in slow-pitch softball! Ball speeds in most sports exceed the eyes' ability to track the trajectory smoothly (Ripoll and Fleurance, 1988). Braden (1983) studied the accuracy of judging where tennis balls landed from various court positions and found that the players were less reliable (11 percent error rate with a mean error of 5 inches) than the line persons or umpire.

Events occurring faster than about 1/4 of a second usually cannot be seen (Eastman Kodak, 1979). If humans had very fast vision, there would be no illusion of motion when we watch movies, which are really the flashing of 24 distinct pictures each second. There is a clear time limitation in our eyes' ability to perceive motion of objects in our field of view. Knowledge of this limitation is critical to planning for qualitative analysis and what aspects of performance we can observe reliably. A complete description of eye motions to track moving objects is presented in the following section on important eye movements. After reading that section, you will know many good reasons why an official could appear to be looking right at a key play and still miss the call.

Important Eye Movements

There are many kinds of movements the eyes use to view moving objects. These movements are coordinated to keep the two eyes working together. Kluka (1991) classifies eye movement into four types: saccadic, vestibulo-ocular, vergence, and smooth pursuit. Saccadic eye movements are for scanning rapidly and jumping to various points in the visual field. Vestibulo-ocular movements are coordinated with head motion to keep the eyes on some object. *Vergence* eye movements allow the eyes to focus on objects at different distances, while *smooth pursuit* eye movements are used to follow slow-moving objects.

Eye movements that make it possible to view objects up close and at a distance are called *convergence* and *divergence*, respectively. Accommodation and convergence relate to the eye's ability to focus quickly, smoothly, and accurately as objects approach or recede from it. This ability is especially important in sports because objects and individuals are always changing their relationships to us. It is equally important in qualitative analysis. These functions are achieved by changes in the tension of the muscles of the lens and the muscles that move the eyes.

To observe this aspect of vision, hold a pencil at arm's length and slowly move it toward your nose. As the pencil gets closer, your eyes move from an almost straight-ahead position in the sockets to a position where they seem to be touching the nose. You are now cross-eyed. Your eyes have converged. At the same time, the lens has changed shape to keep the pencil in focus. The same process takes place as we analyze skills that involve movement that is close to us.

Depth perception is the ability to judge how far away objects are from you or the relative distances objects are away from you and each other. At a distance, we generally judge depth by comparing object size. As objects get closer, this perception is mainly a function of eye position as sensed by kinesthetic proprioceptors in the eye muscles as the eyes look toward the nose or farther outward to the side of the head.

When something has our visual attention, we carefully focus both eyes on the object; this is called *fixation*. One reason fixation is so important is that the focus of visual field is limited to 3 degrees (Kluka, 1991). As you read this text, you smooth-pursue eye movements to keep the focus of your vision on the words you are reading. If you were to focus closely on a word in the middle of the page and not move your eyes, the words in your peripheral vision would be blurry and less recognizable. To get a feel for how small this area of visual focus is, extend your arm forward. Hold it straight out with your thumb extended vertically. The width of your thumb in this position (the thumb rule) is a good approximation of the focus of your visual field (Groot, Ortega, and Beltran, 1994).

Because information from one eye reaches the brain faster and is processed more quickly, that eye becomes dominant (Kluka, 1991). The *dominant eye* guides the other eye in direction of movement and fixations. The use of the dominant eye in sports requiring accuracy has been studied for many years. The combination of eye and hand dominance has been a topic of recent studies of hockey, batting, and golf putting (Morrison, 1976; Steinberg, Frehlich, and Tennant, 1995; Tieg, 1983). It is easy to establish which eye is the dominant eye. A typical test is to extend your arms forward, making a small (1 square inch) hole between your hands (figure 3.2). Pick a distant object (such as your partner's right eye) and center it in the hole formed by your hands. Without moving, close one eye at a time. The eye that still has the object lined up in the hole is your dominant eye.

The use of the eyes to *track* moving objects is a very complex phenomenon. Let's look at the eye movements of smooth pursuit and the saccade to illustrate how visual limitations affect qualitative analysis.

Smooth Pursuit. When there is slow relative movement between an observer and an object,

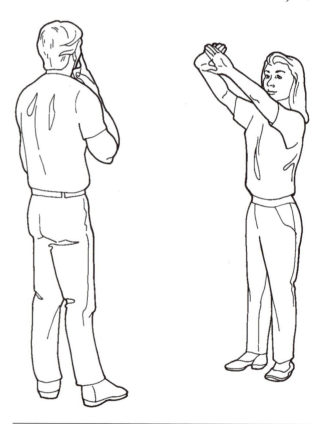

Figure 3.2 Simple test to establish eye dominance. (See description in text.)
Reprinted, by permission, from K.M. Haywood and C.F. Lewis, 1989, *Teaching Archery: Steps to Success* (Champaign, IL: Leisure Press), 14.

the eyes can smoothly move together following the object until eye angular velocity reaches between 40 and 70 degrees per second (Bahill and Laritz, 1984; Ripoll and Fleurance, 1988; Robinson, 1981). People can become skilled at visually tracking objects and predicting their landing or bounce location.

A good way to illustrate the accuracy of visual tracking in estimating ball impact or intercept is to toss a person a tennis ball softly from 2 or 3 feet away. Have her catch the ball with one hand. After a couple of trials, ask her to close her eyes when you say "close" early or in the middle of the ball trajectory. Most people will be able to catch the ball with their eyes closed.

Unfortunately, many sports or other movements require eye movements beyond our ability for smooth pursuit. In volleyball, eye angular velocities of more than 500 degrees per second are needed to track the trajectory of a spiked ball (Kluka, 1991).

Saccade. Sports like tennis, badminton, basketball, and baseball generate ball speeds that require another kind of eye movement to be able to track the ball. The quick motion of both eyes from one fixation to another is called a saccade. While the eyes are rotating to the next fixation, they are essentially turned off to prevent a blur of light and images as they move. This down time has been called saccadic suppression or omission (Campbell and Wurtz, 1978).

Recent research on saccadic eye movements in normal subjects has shown that there is no significant difference between men and women, but saccadic eye movement parameters decrease significantly with age (Wilson, Glue, Ball, and Nutt, 1993). Sports studies have shown anticipatory patterns of saccades relative to the kind of motion of the object that is being tracked (Bahill and Laritz, 1984; Haywood, 1984; Hubbard and Seng, 1954; Ripoll and Fleurance, 1988). Saccades can reposition eyes at angular velocities exceeding 700 degrees per second (Carpenter, 1988).

Limitations of Eye Movements. The limitations of eye motions in tracking of moving objects, visual suppression, and fixations all have implications for sports and qualitative analysis. The analyst must realize that some high-speed events simply cannot be observed. If a key event occurs when the analyst's eyes are in a saccade, it will not be seen. If an observational strategy is not followed, the analyst's eyes may be drawn (fixate) to an extraneous action, causing the analyst to

miss an important error in performance. The selection of a viewing distance for observation in qualitative analysis has a major impact on the eye angular velocities required to track a performer.

If vision is part of remediation, it is important not to ask the performer to do things that his eyes cannot do. The actions relating to the cues, "keep your eyes on the ball" and "watch the ball hit your bat/racquet," clearly do not occur (Watts and Bahill, 1990) and may be miscues (Kluka, 1991). *Sports Illustrated* is filled with photos of baseball hitters or tennis players who usually have their eyes focused forward of ball impact. Coaches making qualitative analyses of officiating should now understand how such terrible/fortunate (depending on which bench you are on) calls are made in sporting events.

Peripheral Vision

Peripheral vision is our ability to gather information from the environment other than the point of visual focus. This is a function primarily of the rods in the eyes, as they are situated in areas not central to where light is focused. This ability is particularly sensitive to slight movement and is processed faster than vision requiring color.

Peripheral vision directs our attention to movement in the environment around us so we can process this information. It also sets the stage and orientation of events so they can be mapped or matched to general backgrounds (Alfano and Michel, 1990). Restriction of peripheral vision, especially in qualitative analysis, can lead to fewer meaningful reference points and poorer analysis.

Fusion

Although the eye has often been compared to a camera, research on visual perception led Johnsson (1975) to conclude that the eyes act more like motion detection systems than still cameras. The eyes do not in a sense capture photos; rather, they constantly evaluate a changing flux of light focused on the retina to generate a three-dimensional (3-D) image of the visual field. In normal vision, both eyes send information to the brain, where it is blended and interpreted as a three-dimensional phenomenon. This blending of each eye's essentially 2-D visual information into a 3-D whole is called *fusion*.

Kluka (1987) presents a way to demonstrate this phenomenon. Tape two 8 1/2- × 11-inch pieces of paper, one white and one red, in a corner at eye level. The white piece is placed in front of you while the red piece is on the wall next to your left shoulder. Place a pocket mirror in front of your left eye touching your nose, so that you can see the red piece of paper in the mirror. Look at the white piece of paper with your right eye. If you are the same distance away from both pieces of paper, you should see a single piece of pink paper instead of one white and one red piece. Another way to illustrate fusion is to hold your thumb vertically at arm's length and aligned with another object in the distance. By focusing your eyes on the thumb (seeing two distant objects) or the object in the distance (seeing two thumbs) you can "see" how information from two eyes are blended to create a three dimensional representation.

Selective Nature of Visual Attention

Our senses have variable levels of sensitivity, and vision may be the most variable and selective of all the senses. Without a conscious effort to attend to one object, the eyes will dart about the visual field, moving to unusual or quickly moving objects. In short, normal vision will pay attention to any number of things in a person's view. Chapter 4 gives some examples of how the eyes search the visual field in order to make sense of visual stimuli.

The implications of this fact for qualitative analysis are interesting and varied. One perspective is to consider this selectivity a barrier to systematic observation and therefore plan a specific observational strategy to compensate. The other perspective is to use this sensitivity to locate and focus on unusual features of a movement. A problem with this approach is that we are not always conscious of what our eyes are focused on. We may waste observational time looking at un-

important aspects of performance and not noticing important ones.

Biases in Visual Perception

There are several biases in visual perception that may be hardwired into the 3-D perceptual set of vision. Many of these phenomena are related to the geometry of the situation. The farther an object is from the viewer, the smaller it appears and the smaller the displacement past the observer, compared to a similar object moving at the same speed close to the observer. For example, on a late-night walk, nearby objects move past at the speed of your gait while distant objects appear to move past slowly. This is why people tend to overestimate the speed of objects close to them and underestimate the speed of objects at a great distance (Johnsson, 1975).

The large horizontal perspective of our visual field also leads to a tendency to overestimate the lengths of vertical lines compared to horizontal lines (Prinzmetal and Gettleman, 1993). A novice coach, for example, might more readily perceive that the up-and-down motion of a runner is exaggerated before perceiving overstriding. Other biases are a tendency to underestimate object size with an inward shift of accommodation (Meehan and Day, 1995) and a tendency for dimmer objects to appear farther away (Kluka, 1991).

Many readers are familiar with some of the many images that can be interpreted as two different things (for example, two faces or a vase). You can see only one interpretation of the image at a time. An example of the 3-D bias of vision is illustrated in figure 3.3. What two things does it show? The image is literally two lines that touch

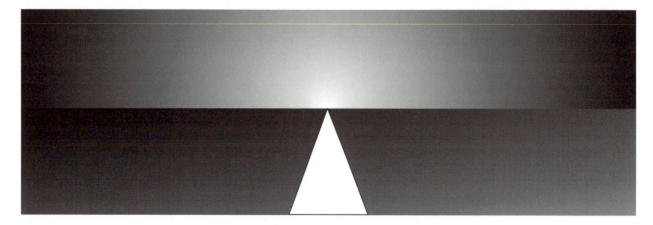

Figure 3.3 What objects do you see in this image? Do the lines intersect or are they parallel? Even simple drawings tend to be interpreted as three-dimensional objects.

at a point. The objects are typically interpreted as parallel lines (a road stretching to the horizon).

Sports Vision

As the interest in vision in sports has grown, several articles have been written on visual skills in sports (Blundell, 1985; Fisk, 1993; McNaughton, 1986; Sherman, 1980). Research has also been conducted on commercial programs for training DVA, like Eyerobics (Cohn and Chaplik, 1991; Long, 1994; MacLeod, 1991) and Dynavison (Klavora, Gaskovski, and Forsyth, 1994, 1995). The International Academy of Sports Vision, established in 1984, is an organization that encompasses many professions interested in vision in sport. It sponsors professional meetings, *Sportsvision* magazine, and the *International Journal of Sports Vision*. Kluka (1991) summarized the research, noting that there are 14 important visual skills relevant to learning motor skills and other factors affecting visual perception. Another organization interested in vision in sport is the Sports Vision Section of the American Optometric Association.

Coaches need to observe how performers use their eyes in many sport skills. Knowledge of how the eyes work and their limitations is important for analysts so they know what is observable and what feedback on the use of the eyes is helpful. For example, the miscue of "keep your eye on the ball" may not interfere with performance in some sports, even though it can't be done. But the cue "watch the ball hit your bat" could adversely affect performance by encouraging head motion and less visual attention earlier in the trajectory of the ball. Cues on ball tracking should emphasize focused attention, minimal or smooth head motion, and characteristics of the ball (seams, spin, etc.). The adage to coach "from the eyes down" may be very important in some skills. It is also important that any intervention regarding vision be accurate and effective, not just a cliché.

THE AUDITORY SYSTEM

The gross anatomy of the auditory system is less complex than that of the visual system. The auditory system converts the energy of sound waves into the sensation of sound and can be an important source of information for qualitative analysis. The rhythmic sounds of a movement or the discrete sound of a collision all provide relevant information to qualitative analysis.

Structure of the Ear

There are three main sections to the auditory system: the external ear, the middle ear, and the inner ear. The *external ear* is essentially made up of the external skin and cartilage. This is what we normally refer to as the ear and is technically called the auricle. From this structure emanates the external acoustic meatus (figure 3.4). This section of the ear ends in the tympanic membrane, or the eardrum.

The *middle ear* is a cavity that transfers the mechanical energy of sound waves. The lateral side is made up of the eardrum, while the medial side consists of the oval window. Three small bones called the ossicles—the malleus (hammer), the incus (anvil), and the stapes (stirrup)—are suspended in the middle ear and reach from the

---

PRACTICAL APPLICATION

You are a cross-country skate-skiing instructor qualitatively analyzing skate skiing in an activity class. Your students want to have fun, but you also have them focused on improving. What sensory information should you attend to the most? Are there specific senses that are most appropriate for the critical features of skiing?

Assume you are skiing behind a skier who needs a push-off correction. As you begin observing again, what senses are most relevant? A good approach would be to give feedback on the important sounds from the skis and then give verbal cues/prompts on when to signal the next weight shift or pole plant. Your auditory senses monitor the force and duration of the push-off, while your sense of vision provides information on balance during the next glide. You need to pay attention to these senses and integrate the sensory information to provide good qualitative analysis in this situation.

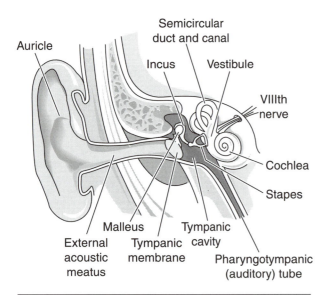

Figure 3.4 Diagram of the ear and its functional components.

eardrum to the oval window. As sound waves press on the eardrum, these three small bones transfer this energy mechanically to the oval window. Contraction of the small muscles suspending these bones helps to lessen the effects of sound overload on this organ.

The pressure of the stapes on the oval window moves the perilymph (fluid in the semicircular canals of the *inner ear*), which causes movement picked up by hair cells in the cochlea. These hair movements are converted into nerve impulses that, taken to the brain via the eighth cranial nerve, give us the sensation of sound.

Functional Components of the Ear

The interaction of the ears and the brain allow us to perceive sound. From what we hear, we can make sense of the frequency of sound waves (interpreted as pitch) and the amplitude of sound waves (interpreted as loudness). The small muscles in the ear attached to the ossicles can contract or relax to modify the sound. This is analogous to the way the muscles of the eye work with the lens to focus light in vision. This ability is demonstrated in the case of loud noises such as departing jet aircraft. The ossicle muscles tighten to reduce vibration and sound transmission.

We can also best determine the tempo of activity from the input gathered by our ears. This information comes from alterations in frequency and pitch. Dance provides many examples of combining these elements of sound as factors for qualitative analysis. The desirable timing of actions in a dance can be counted aloud (1, 2, 3 . . .). The loudness of each number can vary to show the emphasis placed on the action occurring at that time.

> *The information gathered by our ears (frequency and amplitude of sound) is vitally important to the qualitative analysis of rhythmic movements (dance, hurdles, etc.). Auditory information from discrete events is also very important. The sound of impact in baseball and the sound of a gymnast landing are important sources of information about performance.*
>
> **KEY POINT**

THE HAPTIC SYSTEM AND KINESTHETIC PROPRIOCEPTION

The last source of information about movement can be gathered by our kinesthetic proprioceptors and our haptic systems. Both performers and analysts can use these senses to gather information about the quality of performance. A wrestling coach teaching a new move can feel the strength of a wrestler in resisting the move, while the wrestler can feel the body position and action of the move as the coach executes it. When the wrestler tries the move on the coach, the coach can use proprioceptive and haptic information to observe the timing and positioning of the new move for qualitative analysis.

Structure of the Haptic System and Kinesthetic Proprioception

The touch receptors of our *haptic system* involve encapsulated and unencapsulated receptors in the dermis just below the epithelial layer of the skin. They also involve nerves wrapped around the shafts of hair follicles. The two receptors of most interest to us, the tactile corpuscles (touch) and the pacinian corpuscles (pressure), are illustrated in figure 3.5. These two receptors can give an analyst valuable information about a performance when in direct contact with a performer, as when spotting a gymnast in a back handspring. An analyst might ask a performer to use her sense of touch; for example, having a golfer increase grip pressure in one hand over another.

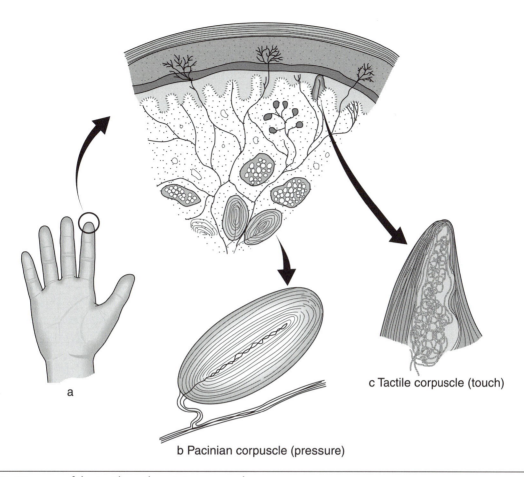

a

b Pacinian corpuscle (pressure)

c Tactile corpuscle (touch)

Figure 3.5 Diagram of the tactile and pacinian corpuscles.

Kinesthetic proprioceptors such as muscle spindles (stretch receptors) and golgi tendon organs (GTOs) can also provide important information about performance to the analyst and the performer. Muscle spindles sense velocity and length changes of muscle, while the GTOs gather information about the tension in a muscle. A muscle spindle is a fluid-filled capsule tapered at each end. The spindle is bulbous in the middle and has intrafusal muscle fibers at each end. These muscle fibers are called intrafusal because they are within the encapsulating membrane of the spindle. They regulate the length of the spindle.

Wrapped around the middle of the fibers are the primary nerve endings. The secondary, or flower spray, nerve endings are spread out in the muscle fibers next to the spindle and have different functions. The primary, or Ia, fibers are sensitive to dynamic movement at low thresholds and are extremely fast in conducting information to the brain. The flower spray endings have a higher threshold and conduct information more slowly.

They are less sensitive to movements than the Ia fibers.

The golgi tendon organs are located at the musculotendinous junction and form a series of branching nerve endings much like the flower sprays of the muscle spindles. When a muscle contracts or relaxes, it changes the tension on the tendons connecting it to a bone. This change in tension is detected by the GTO and transmitted to the brain. The GTO has a low transmission threshold, so it provides a constant flow of information about the current tension in a muscle and the change in tension in that muscle. GTOs usually send inhibitory stimuli to the brain to protect the body from making too much muscle force. An arm-wrestling match usually ends quickly, because one competitor fatigues and loses his ability to override GTO inhibition.

The last kinesthetic receptors are the joint receptors. There are three kinds: spray-type receptors, pressure-type receptors, and a GTO-type receptor. These receptors send information directly to the brain about movement occurring in joints. Rather than providing a great deal of specific information about movements as the GTOs and muscle spindles do, these receptors give general information about the limits of joint movement and joint angular position.

Functional Components of Touch

The haptic senses of touch (tactile corpuscles) and pressure (pacinian corpuscles) send information to the brain when they are stimulated. These receptors are found in the skin and attached to hair follicles. Either the gentle pressure (touch) on the skin or the movement of the hair in the follicles triggers these receptors. When these stimuli breach the threshold of the nerve, signals are transmitted to the brain indicating direct contact with an object or close proximity to an object.

The pressure receptors (pacinian corpuscles) have a higher threshold than touch receptors. They react when touch becomes pressure. Then information about the stimulus is sent directly to the brain. Pressure receptors, especially in the feet, tend to stimulate the extensor reflex.

> **KEY POINT**
>
> *The tactile system (sense of touch) can provide a great deal of information about performance to the analyst and the athlete. This information is gathered primarily by pressure and touch receptors.*

Functional Components of the Kinesthetic Proprioceptive System

The kinesthetic proprioceptors work to tell us about movement in our limbs and body. They do this by sending information to the brain from the stretch receptors in the muscles, the golgi tendon organs in the tendons, and the senses in the joints. The stretch receptors tell the brain about speed of contraction and muscle length. The muscle spindle works by stimulating the nerve wrapped around it. It is very sensitive to the slightest change in length. The flower spray endings associated with the spindle are less sensitive and harder to trigger. The contrast between the signals of these two sensory receptors gives us information about the speed of movement.

The GTO tells us primarily about the load on a muscle. It does this via the tendon's stimulation of the nerve endings. Joint receptors give

general information to the brain that movement has taken place. The combination of all of this information allows us to understand the relationships between body parts and muscle tensions.

> **KEY POINT**
>
> *Kinesthetic feedback is another source of information about performance. It is gathered by golgi tendon organs, muscle spindles, and other joint receptors. An analyst might ask an athlete to tell her how much knee flexion he used in the last trial and to focus on that sense in practice.*

FUNCTIONS OF THE SENSES UNDERLYING QUALITATIVE ANALYSIS

We all know that eyes allow us to see and ears permit us to hear, and that we can sense movement and recognize touch. However, our senses provide more than general information via vision, audition, kinesthesia, and touch. Each of them can elicit qualities from the energy forms it interprets to provide very specific information about what is occurring in our environment. The integration and interpretation of this information allow us to make decisions about how to proceed in qualitative analysis.

As you recall, we defined perception as the organization and interpretation of stimuli from the environment, mediated by our senses. Each of our senses provides us with a great deal of specific information from our environment, and this information becomes the basis for decisions. The following section gives examples of how the sensory system works.

Part of the work of these four major sensory receptor groups is done by either electrical, chemical, or mechanical energy. The other part of their work involves perception. For example, think of tracking the flight of a kicked ball. Electrical energy is used in nerve transmission, chemical energy for color vision, and mechanical energy for transmitting sound waves through the eardrum to the bones in the middle ear. The perceptual component is easily demonstrated by the adjustments of the eye and head movement to the direction of the energy received by the senses.

For an example of how all the senses might be used to understand movement and provide feedback to an athlete, consider a coach spotting an athlete vaulting in gymnastics. The athlete has a run-up approach, a hurdle onto a board, placement of hands on the horse, and flight to a landing. In this skill, the coach can use all of his senses to gain information about the performance so as to provide feedback.

Sound contributes to feedback decisions. The tempo, loudness, and pitch of the run-up, hurdle, placement of hands on the horse, and landing of feet on the mat all provide useful data. The tempo of the run-up, the different pitch from hitting the vaulting board, horse, or mats correctly or incorrectly, and the loudness of any of these parts tell the coach something about the quality of the skill.

The coach's visual system can track the athlete's movement and provide information about body position, body placement in relation to the apparatus, and the relationship of body parts to each other. Interestingly, the linear and angular velocities may be so great when the athlete is on the board and horse that the coach cannot get any usable visual information. This situation forces the coach to make decisions about performance based on data from the other sensory systems.

The coach will then have to rely on the systems of sound, touch, and kinesthesis to judge performance quality. During flight or landing, he will likely touch the athlete and may even push to help in rotation or flight. At this point, touch and pressure information will be added to the input being processed by the coach. Proprioceptive kinesthetic information will flow to the central nervous system as the coach moves his body parts to support the gymnast. Clearly, there is an incredible flow of data bombarding the brain. All of this information must be organized, given meaning, and then combined into a total picture to describe what has occurred.

To say the least, the perceptual process is an incredibly large and efficient system. It is even more amazing to think that we use all of these systems to gain information about a particular movement. Even if we use only two or three of these systems, we can imagine what the other systems would feel, look, or sound like. For example, if the coach in our gymnastic example moved away from the horse, he could still imagine what a good vault would feel like, kinesthetically and haptically, as opposed to a bad vault.

INTEGRATION OF THE SENSES

As you can see, the perceptual system is continually bombarded by sensory input. How do we pay attention to what is important? How do we use all the information available from the senses to make decisions? Welch and Warren (1980) define the complex process of *intersensory integration* as the perception of an event, as measured in terms of one sensory modality, being changed in some way by the concurrent stimulation of one or more other sensory modalities. Our perception of an event through one sense is affected by our perception of the same event through other senses.

It is even likely, as when spotting in gymnastics, that we will use our haptic and kinesthetic proprioceptive senses as well as vision and audition. The sound of the block on the horse could be compared to the visual or proprioceptive information the coach has just observed. The approach and block sounded vigorous, but there still was not enough rotation. What sense might a gymnastics coach put the most confidence in when sensory information conflicts?

> *With a great deal of practice, the brain can automatically integrate sensory information and prioritize it based on its importance to the qualitative analysis being performed. A skilled coach might hear an unusual rhythm in an athlete's performance and then visually observe the movement in qualitative analysis. A diving coach concentrating on observing the dive might use the sound of the diver hitting the water to aid her visual observation of the athlete's entry.*

KEY POINT

How does the brain deal with the input from competing senses, and how does this flow of information from the different senses interact? The types of information the brain deals with fall into three general categories: detection of an event, spatial stimuli, and temporal stimuli. The cognitive handling of inputs from these three sources can be explained by the information processing issues that will be discussed in the next chapter.

Detection of an Event

Relatively strong auditory and tactile stimuli take about 110 to 120 milliseconds to detect. Visual stimuli take slightly longer, about 150 milliseconds (Riggs, 1971). However, it appears that with intense training, analysts can speed up their visual detection and integration of stimuli to 33 milliseconds (Secrist and Hartman, 1993). Note that reaction time is inversely related to stimulus intensity. That is, the more prominent the stimulus, the faster the response. It might take concentrated effort for a coach to use auditory observation in a competitive environment with crowd noise.

Stimuli in the analyst's environment rarely act in isolation. The effect of accessory stimuli (stimuli to which we are not attending selectively) on a primary stimulus (the sense we are using selectively) is one of either inhibition or facilitation. If the accessory stimulus is low to moderate in intensity, it generally facilitates perception of the primary stimulus. If the accessory stimulus has a high intensity, it may have an inhibiting effect (Shigehia and Symons, 1973; Shigehia, Shigehia and Symons, 1973). For this effect to be optimized, these stimuli must occur close together.

These effects may be due to physiological reasons or selective attention (Welch and Warren, 1980). The physiological effects that seem to enhance detection relate to muscle tonus of sensory organs (the muscles of the ossicles in the ear or muscles of the pupil in the eye). Selective attention may cause someone to pay more attention to a particular movement because of a secondary stimulus.

Spatial Stimuli

For spatial stimuli, the order of dominance changes. The visual sense predominates, followed by audition, proprioception, and then touch (Welch and Warren, 1980). Another major difference is that audition is accurate only in the horizontal plane, while vision is accurate in all planes. It is interesting to note how closely auditory and visual perception interact in processing spatial information. Visual perception appears to provide a framework for auditory information (Warren, 1970, Platt and Warren, 1972). It seems that our visual memory provides a basic map to which auditory information can be applied. As mentioned, the left-right discrimination is most accurate for sound spatial information, even though it is mapped to the visual framework.

Kinesthetic proprioception of hand movements can detect spatial differences of about ± 1.25 centimeters (Magill and Parks, 1983), which suggests that we can gain quite accurate information concerning movement from our kinesthetic receptors. We can sense the slightest movement of a body part of someone we are spotting. That is, we can sense an arm or leg movement of less than an inch.

Temporal Information

When short-duration stimuli are processed, it seems that audition is most accurate, followed by touch and then vision (Welch and Warren, 1980). Auditory stimuli also appear to last longer than other stimuli (Behar and Bevan, 1961), so we can analyze auditory information for a longer time than other information. The temporal accuracy of kinesthetic proprioception relative to other senses is not clear. Thus, a qualitative analyst might want to have a visual focus for the take-off of the long jump, using the sound of the approach and take-off as supplementary information.

SUMMARY

All of the senses are extremely important in the qualitative analysis of movement. Too often, analysts disregard the importance of the various senses and how these senses work together to provide information. Vision is generally the sense that predominates in the qualitative analysis process, but the best observation incorporates auditory, haptic, and kinesthetic information as well. In some cases, analysts cannot use their sense of vision to gather information, so the other senses become the primary senses for observation.

Processing of information from the senses is primarily driven by the function of attention. Different senses process information at different speeds, and different senses may have primacy when dealing with certain types of information. The processing of input would be difficult if we did not know what stimuli to focus on in different situations. The cognitive information processing of sensory information (chapter 4) is very important for interpreting sensory information in qualitative analysis.

DISCUSSION QUESTIONS

1. What visual limitations are most strongly related to a blown call by a sports official? For a given sporting event, who is more likely to make a visual mistake: an athlete, an official, or a spectator? Why?

2. For the movements you analyze qualitatively, which sense provides the most relevant information? What are the limitations of this sense?

3. Go to a golf driving range and compare the distance the ball travels to kinesthetic (feel of swing and impact), auditory (impact sound), and visual (initial flight) information. What sense seems most accurate?

4. Experiment with a metronome or weights to determine the accuracy of your sense of audition or kinesthesis. Which sense is more sensitive?

CHAPTER

4

The Role of Information Processing in Qualitative Analysis

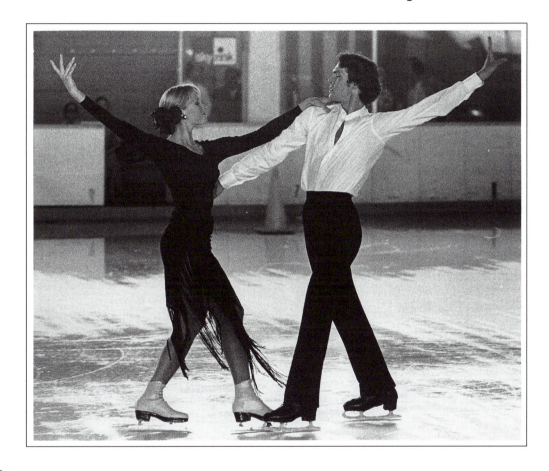

PREVIEW

The skaters in this photograph have a great deal on their minds. Above all, they want to perform their best. They need to precisely coordinate their moves with each other, the music, and the rink. They must cognitively process information about their performance coming from their eyes and ears. To most people this appears to be the only information important to the skaters' success. However, this is not true. Information coming from joint, touch, and pressure receptors as well as other sensory receptors must be integrated with vision and auditory information. The amount of information that the performers, coaches, and judges must process to evaluate the performance is enormous.

Chapter Objectives

1. Define information processing.
2. Explain major facets of information processing models.
3. Diagram a generalized flow chart for information processing.
4. List perceptual components and how they relate to qualitative analysis.
5. List tasks associated with perception.

Information processing is to qualitative analysis as precise measurement is to the sciences. Information processing is where information is gathered, organized, categorized, and sent on to decision-making centers in the brain. It is truly staggering to think that the human brain can handle all of these complex tasks as well as it does. It is also important to realize that the brain can adapt and improve its information-handling ability with instruction and practice. This chapter will examine tasks of perception, models of information processing, and research on information processing as it relates to qualitative analysis. In chapter 3 we found that all the senses work together to contribute to the task of observation in qualitative analysis. These themes can be taken a step further to information processing for a full understanding of the complex process of qualitative analysis of movement.

THEORETICAL BASIS FOR INFORMATION PROCESSING IN QUALITATIVE ANALYSIS

To understand how this complex task of information processing in qualitative analysis is achieved, let's review what is known about information processing in similar activities— like flying jet fighters. Hartman and Secrist (1991) wrote a seminal article explaining that situational awareness in flying involves more than exceptional vision and, in fact, more than the senses. The sense of vision is only a starting point for this complex perceptual activity. Pilots must take sensory information, organize it, interpret it, decide on the correct response, and then initiate the response.

For us, gathering information by the senses is only the beginning of qualitative analysis. We must go through processes like those the fighter pilots go through. The model we proposed in chapter 2, whose parts are explained in detail in chapters 5 through 8, underpins our approach to the processes analysts use to take in information and respond correctly to the observed performance. A review of information processing will help put the role of the senses in qualitative analysis into perspective. This review will look at perceptual tasks, models of information processing, and how these tasks and models relate to qualitative analysis.

KNOWLEDGE AND INFORMATION PROCESSING

Along with skill knowledge, information processing forms the basis of qualitative analysis. Knowledge of the components of a movement and their sequence is useless unless the analyst can resolve meaning from the performance being analyzed. Essentially, information processing organizes and gives meaning to information from the sensory receptors. Remember that this is essentially the definition of perception (Sage, 1984). The terms *information processing* and *perception* are used interchangeably in this chapter. Another way to explain information processing is the interpretation of sensations transmitted to the brain by sensory receptors.

The process of perception appears to have two major parts. The first is the organization of sensory information, which involves sending the information from the sensory receptors to the appropriate areas of the brain. The second part deals with the interpretation of this information and the assignment of meaning to it. Once this meaning has been established, the qualitative analysis tasks of evaluation and diagnosis can follow.

Information processing has two major components: organizing sensory information and assigning meaning to that information.

PERCEPTUAL TASKS

Perception has been studied primarily from the point of view of the types of tasks used in perception. These tasks or experimental conditions allow us to understand what is required of the cognitive processes that attempt to decode and organize environmental stimuli. According to Proctor and Dutta (1995), these tasks are detection, discrimination, recognition, and identification. People involved with qualitative analysis will readily associate with the different tasks described here.

In *detection tasks*, a person need only indicate when a stimulus has occurred. A typical subject might be asked to indicate if a light flashed on or not or whether there was a sound. Usually studies dealing with detection attempt to ascertain the lowest threshold at which a stimulus can be detected. These studies often go on to see if the person's detection ability can be adapted to stimuli that are below the initial thresholds. With training, this effect is often achieved.

An example of this type of task in sport might be this question: Did the offensive lineman move his hand? To a game official, detection of this event would lead to a penalty if it occurred before the snap of the ball. Similarly, a teacher's or coach's perception might work at the level of detection in skill analysis. For example, a teacher might decide whether or not a child's elbow preceded the forearm in an overhand throw. Either it did or it did not. Could the elbow/forearm relationship be detected?

Perceptual tasks have four levels: detection, discrimination, recognition, and identification. All four levels of perception are used in qualitative analysis.

Discrimination tasks generally require a subject to attend to various stimuli and to distinguish among them. Are the stimuli the same or different? Or do they have more or less of some qual-ity? A batter in baseball has to attend to the flight of the pitch and the spin on the ball and discriminate among possible types of pitches in order to adjust his swing. Generally speaking, good batters have this perceptual ability developed to a higher level than poor batters. They can discriminate among pitches and adapt. This ability is important for teachers analyzing movement. For example, did the hands land on the front, middle, or back part of the horse in a vault? The analyst knows the hands made contact with the horse but in order to provide correct feedback must discriminate where contact occurred.

Recognition tasks require more perceptual processing than either detection or discrimination tasks. This type of task usually involves stimuli that have been presented previously versus those that have not. A person can distinguish stimuli learned previously from stimuli with which he is not conversant. In a gymnastics floor routine, a spectator would be able to name some of the tumbling moves with which he was familiar. He would recognize these tricks. He would not be able recognize any moves he had not seen before.

Recognition implies that a good deal of knowledge is needed to help with the analysis. A spectator or coach who did not know the whole routine of a gymnast would not know if a part was missing or changed. In qualitative analysis, recognition is important because it is the level of perception that allows the analyst to start providing expanded feedback which helps in perfecting skill performance. It is the level where we look for complete matching of a performance and its critical features with a prototypic skill.

Identification tasks drive the perceptual processes even more than recognition. These types of tasks require that a person respond to a stimulus in a specific way, to make a judgment in response to a stimulus. These responses can be the same for different or similar stimuli. A guard in basketball might encounter the stimulus of a certain defense setup by an opponent. She might respond by running this play or that play in order to beat the specific defense. Once the player has identified the stimulus (defense), she can decide on the appropriate answer(s).

Similarly, a teacher or coach might identify a certain error in movement, such as a step on the wrong foot in a throw. The response correcting the error might differ based on the knowledge he has about the skill or performer. Skill-related feedback might be appropriate in one situation, while motivational feedback might be more effective in another situation.

As you can see, information processing and perceptual processes are complex and require a great deal of effort on the part of analysts. The complexities of analysis are far more intricate than most of us imagine. In truth, we have just begun to describe the cognitive-perceptual picture. This process is elaborated on throughout this chapter.

MODELS OF INFORMATION PROCESSING

Several models have been postulated to describe the way information is processed from the initiation of a stimulus to the completion of a response. These models are useful for both the description of motor responses and the principally cognitive solutions required by qualitative analysis. All these models attempt to explain *how* information is processed regardless of the level: detection, discrimination, recognition, or identification. Historically, two major categories of processing have been postulated: single channel and multiple resources (O'Donnell, Moise, Warner, and Secrist, 1994).

Single-Channel Models

Single-channel models have generally fallen out of favor because they do not explain the huge amount of information people are capable of handling. In 1958, Broadbent proposed the limited-capacity model of information processing, which described the processing activity of the stimulus as only one channel, similar to a one-lane, one-way street. Only so much information could pass through the brain in one direction at a time. The capacity model described by Kahneman (1973) supported this point of view.

In 1960 Treisman (in Anderson, 1990) said that a certain amount of processing must take place before information is filtered into a single channel. A screening process allows pertinent information to be attended to and passed on to higher levels of processing. Building on this line of thought, Deutsch and Deutsch (1963) proposed the pertinence model, which attempted to explain the filtering (screening) process as a matching of all stimuli with long-term memory.

> **KEY POINT**
>
> *Information processing models have evolved over the years from single-channel, limited-capacity models to multiple-channel, parallel-processing models. Practice and education allow us to develop information processing to its optimum. This development needs to be purposeful and focused.*

Multiple-Resource Models

Because the human brain can handle so much information, the limited-capacity models fell out of favor. But they did lead to two ideas carried forward to later models: filters and channels of information. *Filters* are explained as processes the brain uses to help organize information. They are believed to deal with information such as color, lines, language, spatial information, intensity of stimuli, and duration of stimuli, to name a few. Channels are seen as pathways for information and communication in the brain. These channels can be parallel or serial and can move information forward, sideways, and backward.

Multiple-resource models succeeded the limited-capacity models. Wickens' model (1984a, b) proposed that sensory input is processed by multiple parts of the brain. He also suggested that processing resources are separate from response processes. Pribram and McGuinness (1975) postulated the cognitive-energetic stage model, which depicts information processing as dependent on internal and external sources of energy.

Following this came the model of automaticity formulated by Schneider and Shiffrin (1977) and Anderson (1990). This model explains information processing as automatic for well-learned and highly practiced sensory input. Little or no concentration is required for familiar information.

Pattern recognition models were espoused as extensions of the multiple-resource explanation of information processing. The two types of pattern recognition models are template matching and feature interaction. Template-matching models (Anderson, 1990) indicate a continual matching process of stimuli to stored templates. The themes of template matching and feature integration will be discussed further later in this chapter. The feature integration theory (Treisman and Gelade, 1980) proposed preattentive and focused attention parts to information screening. The first level does not demand much attention, but the second is far more intensive if features are deemed important at the lower energy levels.

In 1992, Pinheiro and Simon presented a general information processing approach of how qualitative analysis proceeds. This theoretical explanation was the first attempt to apply an information processing model to qualitative analysis of movement. They based much of their model on schemas (ways of encoding and storing information in memory). They explain qualitative analysis as information processing at two levels: short-term and long-term memory. They add that information is stored as either semantic (information about things) or recognition (dealing principally with visual stimuli). They explain qualitative analysis as chunks of information being recognized as relevant in short-term memory and therefore being passed on to long-term memory for further processing. This involves a matching process with previously stored relevant data about the incoming information. They suggest various levels of processing in qualitative analysis, such as information acquisition (the senses), processing (short- and long-term memory), and decision making.

Schmidt's Information Processing Model

Perhaps the most familiar information processing model to many readers is the motor learning model proposed by Schmidt (1991) and shown in figure 4.1. This model explains motor control information processes concerned with human movement problems. It is presented here because it can illustrate points important to terms and ideas already expressed in this chapter. The lines from one section to another represent channels, mentioned in previous models (there are also channels within each box representing major functions or brain activities). For example, the filter system (or screening process) can be seen in the comparator part of Schmidt's model.

Schmidt's model has closed and open loops for intrinsic movement feedback. The closed loop represents feedback from skills that take longer to complete, such as the tennis serve, and indicates how the skill can be modified while in progress. For example, when serving into a strong wind, the server can adjust the ball toss movement due to wind pressure. The open loop in Schmidt's 1991 model indicates that the skill proceeds so quickly (such as a bat swing in baseball) that it cannot be modified while in progress.

O'Donnell et al.'s Information Processing Model

O'Donnell et al. (1994) proposed an information processing model that draws on much of the work already cited and provides an excellent structure on which to base a description of the complex activity of sensory organization and interpretation. This advanced theoretical approach posits a framework upon which the many components of qualitative analysis can be hung because it is so comprehensive. There are three major steps in the progression of this model: the energetics system, the attention allocation system, and the response system. Again, note the similarity of processing to the Pinheiro and Simon (1992) model. Figure 4.2 shows this model.

The Energetics System. The energetics system drives the information processing potential by the metabolic and psychological state of the individual. Metabolically, the body must provide energy to allow for the physiological processes to occur. Psychologically, emotions, neurological status, and motivation increase or limit the release of energy from the metabolic pathways, which allow sensory information to flow. The qualitative analyst must use energy to pay attention and focus that attention in observing human movement.

The Attention Allocation System. The filters in the model's attention allocation system are of great interest to qualitative analysis. This is where sensory information is organized so that it can be matched with the knowledge base. This organization process is extremely complex and not fully understood. It is hypothesized that this is where activity relating to spatial (verbal and nonverbal) perceptions, imagery, motion, topology, mental rotation, critical features, and more takes place to sort through sensory information. This is analogous to template matching (Anderson, 1990), short-term memory (Pinheiro and Simon, 1992), the comparator (Schmidt, 1991), and feature integration (Treisman and Gelade, 1980). It is here that information is organized and channeled for further processing so that the final filters deal with recognition of stimuli.

Again, it is difficult to say how much information is attended to and how much is stored. This model proposes multiple channels and parallel processing, so a great deal of information can be handled. However, at some point a single channel is used and the relevant information in this channel is what is attended to. Although we may

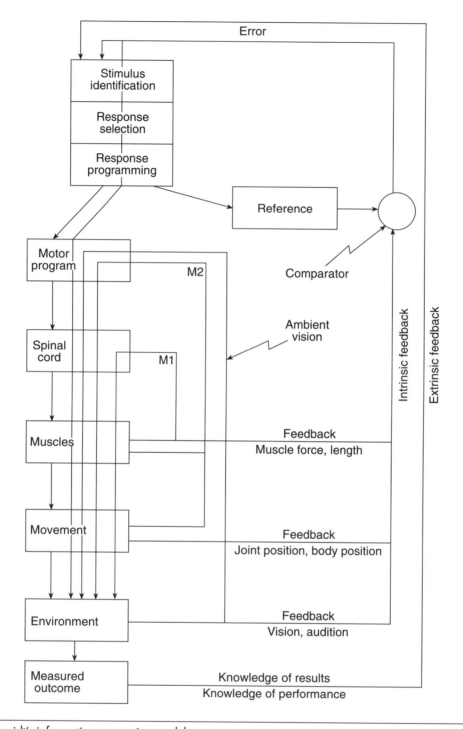

Figure 4.1 Schmidt's information processing model.
Reprinted, by permission, from R.A. Schmidt, 1991, *Motor Learning and Performance*. (Champaign, IL: Human Kinetics), 265.

retain multiple channels of information in our central nervous system, it appears we can attend *to only one thing at a time* in a controlled fashion. This is especially true when information is new and continually changing. When we deal with familiar, predictable information, we can attend to several stimuli simultaneously. These processes

are explained as controlled or automatic processing of information and will be discussed later in this chapter.

An Example of Information Processing in Qualitative Analysis. A teacher analyzing a skill using a gestalt (the sum is greater than its parts) approach to qualitative analysis exemplifies the

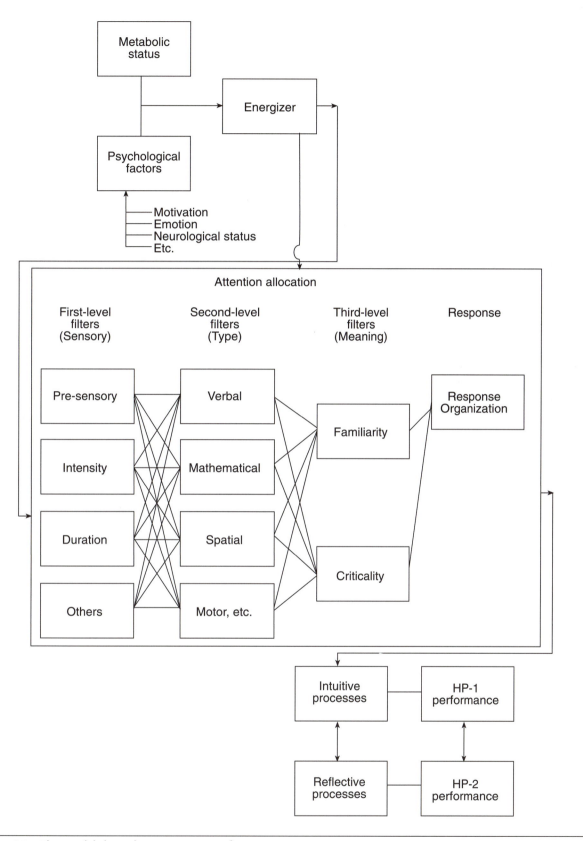

Figure 4.2 This model shows how we process information.

Reprinted, by permission, from R. O'Donnell, S. Moise, D. Warner, and G. Secrist, 1994, "Enhancing soldier performance: A non-linear model of performance to improve selection, testing and training," U.S. Army Research Laboratory, Report ARL-CR-174, 17.

parallel processing and incredible amount of information the brain can handle. The whole performance is examined and a feel for the quality of the performance is developed. We pick up many visual, auditory, kinesthetic, and tactile stimuli. We pass these stimuli through the filters in an attempt to organize and integrate them. At the next level, we try to match these stimuli with previous information from our knowledge base. In hurdling, sound information would be matched with expected visual information. If the match is not good, we need to gather more information or delay intervention until the differences can be resolved. This process moves forward, backward, and sideways in the filters until the stimuli have been organized to present a coherent, understandable picture.

If the stimuli cannot be resolved into a coherent picture, then the process is started again. In this case, the analyst may try to resolve the problem by focusing on a particular part of the skill (the arms or the legs). The observational model proposed by Gangstead and Beveridge (1984) was designed to help with this process. This back-and-forth sensory integration and interpretation process is neverending and is fundamental to qualitative analysis.

If one attentional focus is not useful, then we can switch to another and access the acquired information about that focus remaining in our memory. When processing stimuli, we must try to get the best information. This information is then sent on to the response area so the stimulus can be interpreted appropriately.

The Response System. The third stage of this model, the response domain, explains responses as either intuitive or reflective. Because the O'Donnell et al. (1994) system is designed to explain both slow and fast processing of information, both the intuitive and the reflective modes are presented. Most qualitative analysis responses pass through the reflective (slower) processing track. This would be true even if we quickly intuited the correct intervention from the analysis of a movement. Although we might want to respond to a movement quickly, it is crucial to consider types of feedback from different disciplines to optimize the intervention.

To illustrate how the O'Donnell et al. (1994) theoretical model might explain qualitative analysis, figure 4.3 presents a skill to be analyzed. The analyst observes the performance using as many senses as possible. The sensory input is then organized in the filters and passed along to the decision centers in the brain. A response is formulated and the specific type of intervention is given. Then the analyst begins the process again, perhaps by watching another performance or by pulling back from short-term memory information to develop appropriate feedback. This is why it is important to be aware that many senses gather information for qualitative analysis

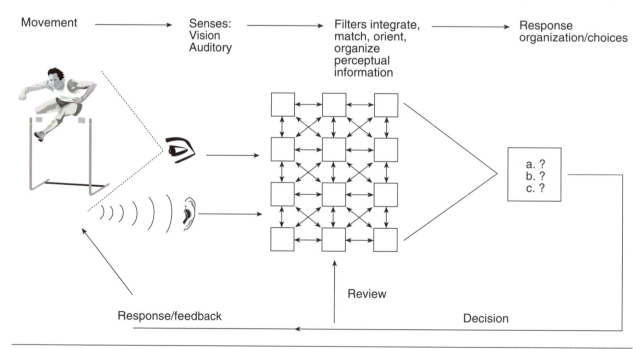

Figure 4.3 Information processing model with skill illustration.

and that memory can hold traces of performance information from the senses for short periods of time.

Comparisons Between Models.   In comparison, the closed loop in Schmidt's (1991) model is similar to the reflective (Type II) processing path of the O'Donnell et al. (1994) model. In the Type II O'Donnell et al. model, feedback would be given only after the observer had time to reflect on the movement and all possible types of feedback. The open loop in Schmidt's (1991) model would be like the fast processing in the O'Donnell et al. intuitive response (Type I), in which, in many cases, feedback is given before the skill performance has been completed. This type of feedback from the analyst may be correct, but it has limited value since the response has not been completely considered. This type of situation is seen in the case of a basketball player throwing up a desperation shot and having the coach respond by yelling out "oh, no, DON'T SHOOT" before the completion of the shot. We have all seen this situation and know that sometimes the shot goes in the basket. When it does, the coach, with egg on his face, then yells out "great shot." The fast response does not consider all of the relevant information. Whereas, the slow, reflective response considers many possible alternatives.

We suggest a *reflective* approach in qualitative analysis, that is, let the skill performer finish several performances and allow the analyst to reflect on the performances once they have concluded. Often, we appear to rerun the images of the movements in our mind before we respond. This is explained by Anderson (1990) as part of the short-term sensory memory and by Pinheiro and Simon (1992) as part of short-term memory. Therefore, we should really take time to consider responses when dealing with qualitative analysis information. Most experts recommend watching several skill performances before making feedback decisions.

RESEARCH ON INFORMATION PROCESSING IN QUALITATIVE ANALYSIS

Evidence for the importance of information processing in the qualitative analysis of movement has slowly accumulated over the years. The two major sources are investigations that use perception or facets of perception directly in various qualitative analyses of movement and those that examine perception in general. The information from these latter sources can be applied indirectly to qualitative analysis. They are undoubtedly the basis for investigations of perception in qualitative analysis. Analysts should realize that they deal with information based on many of the following processes. Understanding these diverse processing factors can expand and improve an analyst's abilities.

Again, we hypothesize that considerable complex cognitive activity takes place in the filter system. The research in qualitative analysis that examines filter function has dealt primarily with spatial ability, imagery, types of examples (correct only versus correct and incorrect), and observational models.

Research on information processing and qualitative analysis has been limited but should be an area of major concern in the future. Factors examined by research so far include perceptual styles, eye tracking, and imagery.

KEY POINT

Imagery and Qualitative Analysis

As part of the O'Donnell et al. (1994) information processing model, imagery is part of the filters. It appears that vivid mental images of performances can be used to match information in the filters. This process is like template matching (Anderson, 1990), feature integration (Triesman and Gelade, 1980), and Pinheiro and Simon's recognition (1992). This matching process is part of the analysis that decides the merits of a performance. Because verbal and visual information is stored differently, it is communication between the verbal and the visual abstract representations in the mind that allows for performance evaluation. As mentioned previously, the whole brain is used for qualitative analysis. This information is then fed to the response system, and feedback or other responses are formulated depending on the purpose of analysis.

We are not completely sure how images are stored. Farah, Hammond, Levine, and Calvanio (1988) believe there are two kinds of imagery: spatial and visual. These concepts are extremely complex and beyond the scope of this text. They are mentioned here to alert the reader that mental images are complex and can be different for different analysts.

The results of the studies of imagery and qualitative analysis are less than conclusive, but they do illustrate the importance of vivid mental imagery in the analysis of movement. In 1975, Hoffman and Sembiante studied whether a person analyzing movement does it by holding a mental image in memory. They concluded that the ability to formulate and hold a vivid mental image was related to qualitative analysis ability. In the second Hoffman study (Hoffman and Armstrong, 1975), visual imagery did not appear to be a discriminating factor in qualitative analysis ability. The factors under examination here relate directly to the question of how a person analyzes a skill. Although the jury is still out, intuitively imagery would seem to be a very important factor in matching a systematized skill performance with a prototypic skill performance. This topic deserves further research.

Spatial Ability and Qualitative Analysis

People's ability to deal with spatial information in qualitative analysis has been only superficially investigated. It seems obvious that the more easily a person can process visual-spatial information, the more easily she can analyze movement, since movement is nothing more than changes of position in space.

Researchers have assessed *spatial ability* solely by examining perceptual style (*field dependence/ independence*), whether or not subjects can use background cues to extract information from the environment. A tennis player who is very field independent does not need reference points such as court lines and the net or other environmental information. This type of player can gather sufficient information from the opponent to decide on appropriate responses. An analyst who can separate performers from background factors will be less susceptible to a disorganized sensory background and may not need to spend much time manipulating the observational situation. By contrast, an analyst who has difficulty analyzing movement without reference to floor lines or background markers is field dependent. This person must make sure the analysis environment is well organized.

Three studies (Gangstead, Cashel, and Beveridge, 1987; Morrison and Reeve, 1989, 1992) have looked at spatial ability from a verbal and nonverbal (nonanalog and analog) point of view. Gangstead, Cashel, and Beveridge found a rela-

tionship between qualitative analysis and field independence. They used the rod and frame test (Witkin, 1954) to determine analog spatial ability. Morrison and Reeve used the verbal-spatial group embedded figures test (Witkin, Oltman, Raskin, and Karp, 1971) to see if spatial ability was important to qualitative analysis. All of these studies concluded that spatial ability does have an effect on qualitative analysis. People appear to use a combination of analog spatial ability and verbal spatial ability to help organize movement information as part of the filter system. This suggests a need for explicit verbal skill descriptions (this concept will be discussed in chapter 5) as well as practice with movement examples to develop qualitative analysis.

Correct and Incorrect Examples as Types of Information

A number of authors have used correct and incorrect examples of skill performances to teach qualitative analysis (Beveridge and Gangstead, 1984; Gangstead, 1984; Kelley, Walkley, and Tarrant, 1988; Morrison and Reeve, 1989; Morrison, 1994). Only Gangstead (1984), Morrison and Reeve (1989), and Morrison (1994) attempted to differentiate between the two types of information and qualitative analysis ability. Gangstead found that for qualitative analysis instruction, examples of correct and incorrect performances were superior to correct examples only. The studies by Morrison and Reeve (1989) and Morrison (1994) found no significant difference for type of information.

These research projects were initiated to establish the value of more and contrasting instructional information to the development of analysis ability. The authors felt this information would be valuable in the filter stage of the O'Donnell et al. (1994) model or the comparator stage of the Schmidt (1991) model. Despite the conflicting results for types of examples, this book will present both correct and incorrect technique for examples and tutorials in qualitative analysis.

Observational Models

As part of the idea of the attention allocation system (O'Donnell, 1994) or the stimulus recognition stage (Schmidt, 1991), Gangstead and Beveridge (1984) developed an observational model for qualitative analysis. This model was designed to help focus an analyst's attention on specific parts of a performance and to reduce extraneous information. Those who recommend a gestalt approach to the initial analysis, such as Dunham (1986, 1994), tell analysts to first allocate their attention to the whole performance and then look for general stimuli upon which to judge the performance. A systematic observational strategy using a structured approach such as a gestalt or an observational model is crucial to the perceptual process in observation of movement.

Development of Spatial Perceptual Ability

These studies appear to be just the beginning of research that could lead to enhancement of qualitative analysis ability. Damos (1988) has demonstrated that visual spatial ability can be enhanced by training. Since spatial ability appears to be a correlate of analysis ability, development of spatial ability could underlie enhancement of analysis ability.

So far, there appears to be only one training system to train perceptual spatial abilities (Secrist and Hartman, 1993). This system is available only to F-15 and F-16 fighter pilots. Essentially, it is a rapid-fire presentation of visual situations normally encountered by pilots on combat missions. Short bursts of combat sequences (5 to 6 seconds) are presented, and subjects are required to make instantaneous decisions (in 0.33 to 0.67 seconds). All challenges are graded to the subjects' current level of performance. A similar system could be used with skill analysis instruction to sharpen information processing abilities. To some degree, systems like this already exist in videotape and videodisk presentations, but they are much slower and are not purposefully matched to the live environment and current ability level of the analyst.

RELATED INFORMATION PROCESSING RESEARCH

Research not dealing directly with qualitative analysis of skill but in related areas of information processing has allowed conjecture on factors that could be important to qualitative analysis. These studies deal with information processing concepts such as topological features, encoding of spatial information, attention and selective attention, and completion.

Topological Features

Topological features are prominent structural components of objects that attract attention. They may affect information processing at the level of filters. Chen (1982) concluded that topological information is a basic factor in perceptual organization. This organization process may direct the flow of information to the correct succeeding filters for further organization and processing. If critical features of a movement can serve as topological features, then focusing attention on those critical features can improve cognitive processing in qualitative analysis.

Encoding of Spatial Information

Information storage is the next major consideration in information processing. This part of perception represents the last part of the sequence. The storage of information, both verbal and imagistic, is the part of memory where stimuli from the environment are matched. An important factor in qualitative analysis is that we appear to encode movement information differently from verbal information (Minas, 1977; Theios and Amarhein, 1989; Simon, 1979). Minas reported a study where subjects were asked to describe a movement in words or copy the movement physically. They did much better at reproducing the movement physically than describing it verbally.

The coding of information in the mind is abstract, neither strictly linguistic nor imagistic. However, information encoded from a visual-spatial source must be reconciled with verbal information. This process tends to take time and can lead to errors due to poor correlations between words and movement information (Theios and Amarhein, 1989). Words and pictures are stored separately, as are the other senses relevant to qualitative analysis. This means that when movement (spatial) information is processed, it must be matched with spatial and movement information stored in memory. Then words must be attached to describe the movement if feedback is desired. Cue words serve a purpose as information storage for the analyst, not just the performer.

Having a good vocabulary or well-defined skill description based on correct language can help not just with feedback but also with information storage. Chunking of information may explain this storage process. Experts appear to be more efficient at information storage than novices.

Attention and Selective Attention

Attention and selective attention are appropriately placed with perception. To some degree, selective attention is demonstrated by the eye-tracking studies previously mentioned (Petrakis, 1986, 1987; Petrakis and Romjue, 1990) and by other eye-tracking investigations (Bard and Fleury, 1976; Bard, Fleury, Carriere, and Halle, 1980). These types of studies show where a person is looking for critical information as a result of her knowledge of movement or information gaps in past observations. The analyst's attention must be driven by the images and verbal information encoded for the matching process.

A good deal of research activity has dealt with attention (Abernathy and Russell, 1987). It has essentially examined factors that make experts more efficient at handling the large amounts of information in skill performances. Differences appear to include the facts that experts chunk information, encode more efficiently, and retrieve information faster. Regardless of what we are doing, our attention is always attracted to certain features in the field of vision. In qualitative analysis, we must use our knowledge base to attend selectively to skill components that will yield valuable information. An inability to direct attention reduces our qualitative analysis potential.

Some skills have so many components, especially skills like those in gymnastics, that it is easy to become distracted and lose track of particular parts of the skill we need to see. Certainly, observation models like the one proposed by Gangstead and Beveridge (1984) can help us direct our attention to the important factors in a skill.

Completion

Williams (1989a, b) demonstrated how partial movement clues could be used to build a complete picture of an activity. His studies demonstrated the pattern-seeking nature of human beings. With only limited movement information, subjects could fill in the missing parts of a skill and name the movements that were presented. These subjects were able to take pieces of information, orient them, match them to information stores in memory, and then successfully describe the movement as it would appear whole. These studies again demonstrate the importance and the potential of the perceptual system. They also explain how some coaches may think they see things that are faster than human vision. Information processing allows their minds to infer what they think happened, even though their senses did not gather direct visual information of the event. Most times the skill is interpreted correctly. However, we can always be fooled. We need to be careful when we are not absolutely sure of the basic information. This is another argument for viewing skills several times, especially in fast movements.

AUTOMATIC AND CONTROLLED PROCESSING

No discussion of information processing would be complete without an examination of the ideas of controlled and automatic processing of information (Naatanen, 1990; Schneider and Shiffrin, 1977). As Schneider and Shiffrin explain it, *automatic processing* involves a sequence of neurons that become active in response to certain stimuli. This activation needs no dynamic control on the part of the subject and is a well-learned sequence. Stimuli are mapped or sent directly to the correct response areas in the brain with limited processing.

Controlled processing is a temporary sequence (not well learned) directly under the control of the subject's active attention. This process has limited information-handling capacity and can be quite slow. Automatic processing has a much greater capacity and is much faster at mapping stimuli to correct responses. Familiarity with the stimuli is a hallmark of automatic processing.

Automatic and controlled processing can be seen in sport situations. A point guard dribbling the ball down the floor to set up a play processes information automatically until unfamiliar stimuli force him into a more controlled mode. The dribbling, the running, and the way the team sets up are all expected stimuli, so processing them is automatic. But if the opposition sets up an unfamiliar defense, then the point guard will have to process the new information in a controlled fashion. Often the team with the ball takes a time-out to solve the unanticipated defense. Many experienced coaches and teachers plan their observation to reduce the potential for unexpected occurrences that would interfere with the smooth operation of the class. This allows them to direct the controlled processing to the analysis of the skill being observed. If anything unexpected occurs in the movement, they can devote their efforts to dealing with it.

In qualitative analysis, most of the visual, auditory, and tactile stimuli are processed automatically until something unexpected or strange occurs. The more familiar the analyst is with the skill, the student, and the environment, the more automatically the information about the performance will be processed. Since automaticity is an indication of learning and requires less effort on the part of the analyst than controlled processing, those interested in improving their qualitative analysis ability should learn all they can about qualitative analysis, the skill to be analyzed, the subjects to be analyzed, the analysis environment, and the possible feedback to a skill performance. This learning will facilitate a greater analysis capacity and greater ease of analysis and should lead to better teaching, as shown in chapter 5. Automatic processing is so quick and effortless that it does not appear to be conscious. But we usually have to learn the process, and we all have different capacities for it.

> **KEY POINT**
>
> *Controlled and automatic processing are important components of qualitative analysis. The more automatic we can make our information processing, the faster and more efficient we will be as analysts.*

A GESTALT

Perhaps the best place to end our brief discussion of information processing is at a place where perception starts—with suggestions to novice teachers and coaches on how to approach the information-gathering process. Different people have varying approaches on how to look for meaning in movement; for example, "Just watch the arms in this skill" or "Watch for the follow-through in this movement." In a conversation with one of the authors, a volleyball coach said she could tell how well a spike was performed by watching the follow-through. While this suggestion may be helpful to some, it may be confusing or ineffective to most.

A good way for most people to begin observing movement for analysis is to build a gestalt representation of the movement to be analyzed (Treisman, 1986; Chen, 1982). A *gestalt* representation is a picture whose totality is greater than the sum of its parts. Gestalt psychologists believe this total picture is built on four basic principles (Anderson, 1990; Yantis, 1992): proximity, simi-

larity, good continuation, and closure. Figure 4.4 from Palmer (1990) demonstrates these organizing principles.

That is, our mind tries to extract information from the stimuli presented by organizing them into patterns that have meaning for us. Recent research and theoretical interpretation of a gestalt have formulated the idea of uniform connectedness as the foundation of information processing. That is, uniform connectedness (regions of homogeneous properties, such as lightness, color, or texture) is the first perceptual factor in a gestalt (Palmer and Rock, 1994). After uniform connectedness come proximity, similarity, continuation, and closure.

Although no qualitative analysis studies have directly addressed grouping, Petrakis (1986, 1987; Petrakis and Romjue, 1990) may have indirectly demonstrated grouping of stimuli by uniform connectedness as a factor in qualitative analysis. Her research examined eye-tracking patterns to see if experienced observers looked at skills differently from inexperienced observers; she found that this was the case. The research further showed that the experts' visual search patterns were more systematic than the novices' and may have been based on the uniform connectedness of sections of the body. The experts tended to look for information concerning the movement being examined from the same regions of the body, while the novices searched wildly over the body for meaningful information. The experts seemed to group information by areas that appeared to be connected in a uniform fashion; novices did not.

> **KEY POINT**
>
> *The idea of a gestalt is important to anyone interested in qualitative analysis. It provides one approach to gathering information in observation.*

Instead of watching for one specific aspect of a skill, qualitative analysts should base their initial response on an overall impression or feeling about the quality of the performance. Since we often get to see several repetitions of a skill performance when we are teaching or coaching, we can go back and look for specific skill components after making an overall decision about the quality of the performance. Then we can focus on the critical features that are organized (grouped) by knowledge and experience, or on the previous

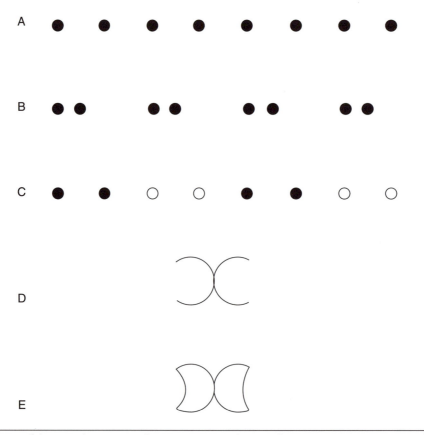

Figure 4.4 Illustrations of the gestalt concepts of proximity (A and B), similarity (C), continuity (D), and closure (E). Reprinted, by permission, from S.E. Palmer, 1992, "Common region: A new principle of perceptual grouping," *Cognitive Psychology*, 24: 437.

observations. Even if we do not get to see several performances of the skill, our short-term memory (Simon, 1979) may allow us to reformulate the performance in our minds so that we remember the individual parts of the skill.

Information processing is a very complex area of study. It can, at best, be hypothesized by indirect measures of brain function and observed behaviors. Although we do not have extensive hard evidence on how perceptual processes occur, perception is crucial to the qualitative analysis of movement and needs to be examined and understood if progress is going to continue in this area of our discipline.

SUMMARY

Perhaps now it is a little easier to understand how much information the skaters have to deal with and how they deal with it. Channels, filters, and

possible responses are all linked together to produce good motor performances. Similar processes are used by spectators, coaches, and judges to determine the quality of the performance. The spectators might respond with applause, the coaches might provide corrective feedback, and the judges would be able to put qualitative analysis to work and score the performance accurately. The complexities of information processing do indeed need to be understood in order to allow the potential analyst to optimize his/her skills.

DISCUSSION QUESTIONS

1. How are the senses and information processing related? Is it possible to see something and not understand it? Think of some optical illusions you have encountered.

2. Where in the information processing model is sensory information organized?

3. What is the difference between controlled and automatic processing? In selected skills (such as pairs skating or gymnasts executing floor routines), what parts of processing would be controlled and which would be automatic? Can these processes change? (That is, can automatic processing be changed to controlled and then changed back to automatic?)

4. What types of research have been done that relate to information processing for qualitative analysis?

5. What does the term gestalt mean? How is this approach useful for people involved in qualitative analysis? Will the ideas of proximity, grouping, and continuation work in movement situations?

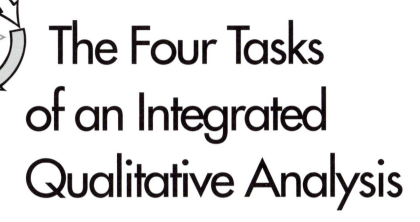

PART TWO

The Four Tasks of an Integrated Qualitative Analysis

The many disciplinary views of qualitative analysis in kinesiological literature suggest that there are four important tasks that make up qualitative analysis. The tasks of preparation, observation, evaluation/diagnosis, and intervention form the essence of our integrated model of qualitative analysis. Chapter 5 outlines the important information that must be gathered in the preparation of a qualitative analysis. The second task, the systematic observation of movement, is covered in chapter 6. The third task may be the most difficult and has two parts, evaluation and diagnosis. Evaluation/diagnosis are reviewed in chapter 7. Part II concludes with a review of the many kinds of intervention that can be used to improve human movement in chapter 8.

Preparation: The First Task of Qualitative Analysis

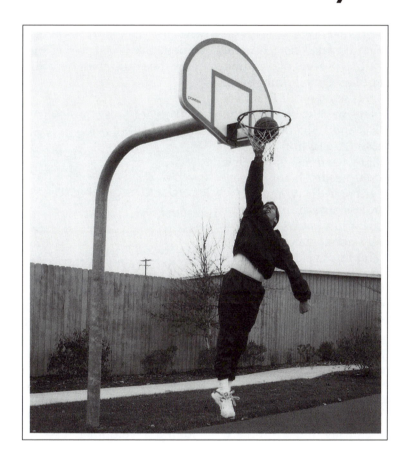

PREVIEW

The booster club just asked you to judge the slam-dunk contest at a regional basketball tournament. Since you are a local movement expert, the boosters want you to develop a rating scale and give the other judges a training session before the contest. What are the key elements of a dunk in basketball? What aspects of a dunk should the judges look for and rate? Should the judges consider the height the hand gets above the rim or the height the athlete must jump? What is the range of correctness for a successful dunk? Could the judges make a fair and consistent rating without knowing the physical requirements and key elements of difficult dunks? How would you qualitatively analyze the dunk pictured?

═══════════════ Chapter Objectives ═══════════════

1. Identify areas of prerequisite knowledge that are important in the preparation task of qualitative analysis.
2. Define critical features and explain how they are identified in the preparation task of qualitative analysis.
3. Explain how preparation in qualitative analysis is related to effective teaching and systematic observation.

The first task in the qualitative analysis of human movement is the continuous process of building a prerequisite knowledge base. In our integrated model of qualitative analysis, we call this task *preparation*. Other scholars have called this the preplanning step (Philipp and Wilkerson, 1990), the preobservation phase (Arend and Higgins, 1976; McPherson, 1990), or have just noted that prerequisite information is needed before observation and analysis can begin (Hay and Reid, 1988). We believe that professionals must continually read and research to build a knowledge base and must think critically about the practice of their profession. For example, physical educators should keep up with current research in the sport sciences and pedagogy, while physical therapists should keep up with research on the qualitative analysis of gait and other everyday movements.

This chapter will review important areas of prerequisite knowledge that professionals interested in human movement should be aware of in preparing for effective qualitative analysis. Good preparation involves weighing evidence from many subdisciplines of kinesiology. The four major areas of this prerequisite information are knowledge about the activity or movement, knowledge about the performer(s), knowledge about effective instruction, and knowledge to develop a systematic observational strategy.

The philosophy of this approach to qualitative analysis is that knowledge is transient. Our state of knowledge and the standards of professional practice are dynamic. Professionals must realize that their career is a neverending search for the latest knowledge, the best approximation of the truth. For a qualitative analysis of human movement to be most effective, the analyst needs to maintain an up-to-date knowledge base. Otherwise, analyses may be based on erroneous or invalid information. For example, a coach who is unaware of the rapid changes in sports equipment may be teaching inappropriate technique for the equipment his athletes are using.

> *The first task of qualitative analysis is preparation, the gathering of knowledge of the activity and performers. Professionals should continuously gather detailed prerequisite knowledge in order to be good qualitative analyzers of movement.*
>
> **KEY POINT**

KNOWLEDGE OF THE ACTIVITY

An extensive knowledge base about an activity is essential to a good qualitative analysis of it. The knowledge base for any activity comes from all the subdisciplines of kinesiology (Vickers, 1989). An elementary physical education teacher needs current motor development information on motor skills and the fundamental movement patterns related to those skills. This includes validated developmental sequences, ages of typical stages, rate of advancement, and outcome measures. The subdiscipline of motor learning contains important knowledge on practice schedules and stages of motor learning that affect all kinesiology professions attempting to teach someone a new movement. Professionals must seek out the information they need from a variety of sources.

In secondary physical education, teachers and coaches need to know about the skills, strategy, and physical requirements of their sport. They should update detailed knowledge of the individual skills and techniques. The goal or purpose of each sport skill needs to be determined (Gentile, 1972; James and Dufek, 1993). If the goal of a skill can be precisely defined, then the technique factors that lead to success in that skill can be more clearly identified for qualitative analysis. Remember that several of the biomechanical qualitative analysis systems reviewed in chapter 2 began by defining the purpose of the movement (Arend and Higgins, 1976; Broer, 1960; Hoffman, 1983; Hay and Reid, 1982; McPherson, 1990).

A good example of a situational or strategic change in the goal of a movement is in the tennis serve. The first serve generally emphasizes placement, speed, or spin in order to put the opponent at a disadvantage, while the second serve's primary goal tends to be accuracy to prevent a double fault. Kinesiology professionals must maintain an up-to-date knowledge base about the movements they analyze qualitatively.

Sources of Information

Three main sources of information contribute to the prerequisite knowledge of an activity: experience, expert opinion, and scientific research. All three are important sources to consider in developing a prerequisite knowledge base for qualitative analysis. There are two difficulties that confront kinesiology professionals in this area: gathering the information from sometimes fragmented sources and weighing the evidence from each source.

Experience

Experience in any profession is invaluable, as evidenced by improvements in employability and salary with increasing years of experience. Most professionals develop positions on issues based on experiences with several patients or clients. This professional experience has the advantage of being population specific and environmentally relevant. Thoughtful coaches are likely to make valid generalizations from experience if their players are relatively homogeneous.

The weaknesses of experience as a source of valid information are that it is anecdotal and can be influenced by a personal bias. Also, experience cannot control all the factors that may affect a particular issue, so professionals should search other sources to verify or refute their own conclusions.

Expert Opinion

The opinions of experts carry a lot of weight in many professions. People with a wealth of experience deserve the attention of their peers. The places to seek out this expert opinion are professional periodicals and professional meetings. In physical education, journals like *Strategies* and the *JOPERD* carry articles written for professional practice. There are also magazines and newsletters that publish teaching tips and expert opinions, like *Physical Education Digest, Peak Performance* (NASPE, AAHPERD), and *The Clipboard* (NASPE, AAHPERD). Coaches should monitor sport-specific publications (for example, *Tennis* or *Golf Digest*), which often interview successful coaches or analysts. Professionals can seek out these expert opinions personally at professional meetings or over the Internet. Professionals should consistently attend professional meetings and conferences, where experts are often invited speakers.

The weaknesses of expert opinions are that they may conflict (figure 5.1) and that opinions often change. Teaching motor skills is often

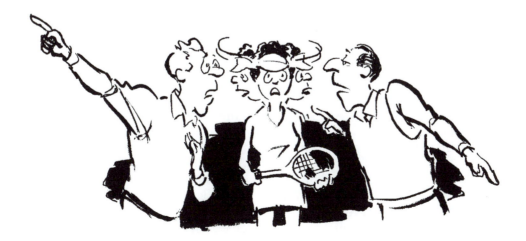

Figure 5.1 Expert advice is often conflicting. This makes the task of building correct prerequisite information for qualitative analysis difficult.

affected by the technique of a current champion or the agenda of the most prominent expert at that particular point in time (Hay and Reid, 1982). The latest rehab protocol may be an improvement over the last protocol, but it may still be far from the ideal.

Both expert coaches and athletes have held opinions about performance in a particular skill that research has shown to be false. The history of sports is full of examples of incorrect notions about key points in many skills. Interested readers can find examples from track and field (Hay, 1993; Hay and Reid, 1982) and golf (Torrey, 1985). Skilled performers commonly have mistaken ideas about what is going on when they are performing. It is very important to remember that championship athletic performance does not require expert knowledge about the kinesiology or qualitative analysis of the athlete's sport. The hallmark of a champion is to perform consistently and effectively, with little conscious thought about the process.

Scientific Research

Another source of prerequisite information for qualitative analysis is scientific research. Research in all the subdisciplines of kinesiology provides the most valid and accurate information available for basing decisions in qualitative analysis. Examples of research are descriptive studies of injury rates for various populations of athletes or for modes of training. Experimental research on different styles of teaching or teacher feedback on learning also provides relevant information to professionals planning qualitative analysis.

But the controls needed in experimental research often limit its real-world application. It is also difficult for practitioners to gather relevant information from research for many reasons. Often research is published in technical journals with difficult vernacular. Reading and interpreting research may be difficult because of the abstract nature of the topics, the technical demands of some measurements, and the complex experimental or statistical designs. Advanced degrees and constant updating may be needed to fully interpret research.

Some periodicals have the mission of bridging the gap between research and practice (Boyer, 1990). One of the first publications to attempt this was *Motor Skills: Theory into Practice*, but it ceased publication in 1985. Examples of good periodicals with scholarly research-based articles for practitioners are *Sports Coach, Track and Field Quar-*

terly Review, JOPERD, Strategies, and *Strength and Conditioning.* In physical therapy, the *Journal of Orthopedic and Sports Physical Therapy* has a reputation for readable and practitioner-friendly research. There are also many newsletters associated with professional organizations or interest groups that provide current information. Examples are *Physical Activity Today* (Research Consortium, AAHPERD), *Physical Activity and Fitness Research Digest* (President's Council on Physical Fitness and Sports), *Sports Science Periodical on Research and Technology in Sport* (Coaching Association of Canada), *Sports Sciences* (National Collegiate Athletic Association), *Fitness FACTS* (American Association for Active Lifestyles and Fitness), and *Olympic Coach* (USOC Division of Coaching Development).

Research also has the problem of accessibility for many professionals, although the advent of powerful computers, data storage, and communication technology has begun to make it easier to acquire sport science information easier. This access increases the impact of good information, but unfortunately it also increases the impact of poor research and incorrect expert advice. Computer-compiled databases of articles and abstracts are available in print, can be searched online, and are stored on CD-ROM. Some of the best databases are the Sport and Leisure Index, SPORT (Sport Information Resource Center (SIRC), Ottawa, Canada), and ERIC (from the U.S. Department of Education). The CD-ROM version of SPORT, SPORT Discus (Institute for Scientific Information, Philadelphia, PA) is now available in many university libraries. Excellent published versions of computer-compiled sources are available in the PE Index (Ben Oak Publishing Co., Cape Girardeau, MO), Sport Bibliography (SIRC), and Physical Fitness/Sports Medicine (President's Council on Physical Fitness and Sports). The explosion of *hypertext* on the internet, specifically on the World Wide Web (WWW), will also make access to information on human movement faster and easier.

Professionals in human movement must weigh the evidence based on their own experience, expert opinion, and research to establish the most valid background information for qualitative analysis. Scientific research should be given the greatest weighting because of the control, greater objectivity, and validity of the observations. The most important issue is to think critically about professional practice and the various sources of information.

Terminology

One approach to studying and organizing knowledge of an activity is to compare the movements to those of similar activities. Although the terminology varies among authors and disciplines, many experts suggest that the study of human movement be based on classifications usually called fundamental movement patterns (Broer, 1960; Cooper and Glassow, 1963; Daniels, 1984; Philipp and Wilkerson, 1990; Wickstrom, 1983). We will use the terminology in figure 5.2 for this book.

Fundamental movement patterns are broad categories of movements for a general purpose. Examples are walk, run, throw, kick, jump, catch, strike, or carry. Fundamental movement patterns can be adapted for specific purposes or combined with other fundamental movement patterns to complete a specific task. Some experts break movements into even smaller categories. A motor *skill* is an adapted fundamental movement pattern for a specific activity or goal. Typically these are related to specific sports. Some skills related to throwing and kicking are football passing, baseball pitching, punting, and place kicking.

Techniques are kinds of skills that have even more specific purposes. The selection of what technique is appropriate often varies with the situation. A banana shot in soccer (a kind of place kick) is an example of a technique. The skill of long jumping has the hang and hitch-kick techniques for flight into the pit. Techniques are further divided into variations in *style*. Style aspects of movement are personal differences, idiosyncrasies, or actions related to a specific performer. At this level, qualitative analysis is very difficult because the analyst must decide whether minor variations in the movement detract from performance.

Whatever the level of analysis, critical features of the movement can be specified. An integrated qualitative analysis uses critical features as the standards for observing, analyzing, and improving movement. The term this book uses for short-term or long-term improvement in a motor skill is *performance*. In the subdiscipline of motor learning, performance often refers to short-term changes in motor skills; long-term or permanent improvements are called *learning* (Shea, Shebilske, and Worchel, 1993). This distinction between short- and long-term changes in a motor skill is important. Motor learning research has shown that long-term improvement often results from practice conditions that challenge the performer, often making practice execution (short-term results) look worse (Schmidt, 1991; Shea, Shebilske, and Worchel, 1993).

Critical Features

One of the most important areas of knowledge about an activity is establishment of its *critical features*. Critical features have been defined many ways. Arend and Higgins (1976) define them as parts of a movement that can be least modified to be successful. Critical features have also been defined as important aspects of performance that are related to the efficiency and effectiveness of the movement (Jones-Morton, 1990a). McPherson (1990) defined critical features as statements describing specific body movements that are observable and that are then used to evaluate whether the key mechanical factors of the movement have been performed ideally. Critical features are sometimes called critical elements or critical performance elements.

We believe that critical features should be viewed as *key features of a movement that are necessary for optimal performance*. They are aspects of movement that are the most invariant across performers and are the least adaptable if the goal of the movement is to be achieved safely and efficiently. Critical features are the points defining good form that are used in teaching and should also be used to help determine the teacher's focus in the qualitative analysis of the skill. For example, the knee angle at deepest knee flexion (an indicator of the countermovement) in a standing

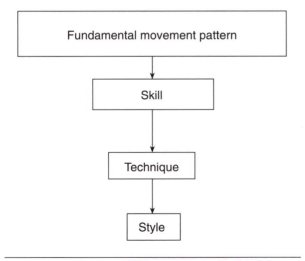

Figure 5.2 Hierarchy of terminology for describing human movement.

vertical jump may be anywhere from 90 to 115 degrees because of range of motion, leverage, and muscle mechanical properties. Critical features for a conditioning exercise like the squat are knee angle, trunk lean, and neutral lumbar lordosis and are strongly related to training effects on muscle and risk of injury.

In other words, critical features are the most important aspects of a movement; they need to be performed in a certain way in order to be successful. We will see that it is useful for the analyst to establish a range of correctness for the critical features and decide which are most important to performance. Integral to critical features is the idea of correct sequence. It does little good to have the correct critical features but the wrong sequence. Imagine a softball batter starting the forward swing of the bat before the stride. Chapter 8 will discuss skill feedback decisions, such as the priority of information. One suggested format is based on where in the movement sequence the error occurs.

Although it is helpful to express critical features in behavioral terms that can easily be visually evaluated, this may not always be possible. Some critical features of human movement are constructs or other abstract ideas rather than clearly defined biomechanical parameters. A teacher/coach may believe strongly in these ideas and may be struggling to find cues or ways to affect this aspect of performance. A good example

related to several sports, among them baseball batting and pole vaulting, is fear. There are many ways coaches try to evaluate the attitude and confidence of athletes where fear of injury has a dramatic impact (no pun intended) on performance.

Three issues can be used to justify the identification of critical features or desirable technique: *safety* or risk of injury to the performer, *effectiveness* in accomplishing the goal of the movement, and *efficiency* of goal attainment. Biomechanics is the primary sport science involved in identifying the quantitative underpinnings for the critical features of a movement. Biomechanical research provides kinematic (range of motion, body angles, length) information on elite and other performers. This kind of research can be of practical use because teachers/coaches may be able to observe some of these variables (Hudson, 1990a and c).

Another branch of biomechanical research is kinetics, the study of how forces create the movement. Kinetic data determine which technique effectively applies force or provides smaller loads to tissues and may have a lower risk of injury. Biomechanical research on the effectiveness of force application in cycling has found that about 76% of pedal forces are used in propelling the bike (Lafortune and Cavanagh, 1983). Figure 5.3 illustrates the total force on the pedal and the effective (rotary) force on the pedal. The shaded

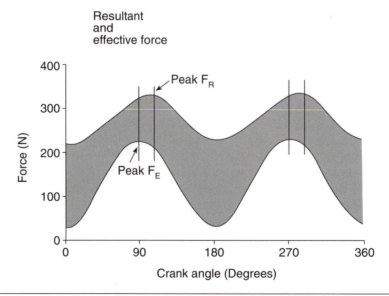

Figure 5.3 Mean resultant force and effective force applied to the pedals of a bicycle. The shaded region shows the amount of unused force within the pedal rotation.
Reprinted, by permission, from M.A. Lafortune and P.R. Cavanagh, 1983, Effectiveness and efficiency during bicycle riding. In *Biomechanics VIII-B*, edited by H. Matsui and K. Kobayshi (Champaign, IL: Human Kinetics), 933.

region shows the forces applied to the pedal that are not effective in creating rotation.

Safety Rationale

A professional must decide if a particular action or technique is safe. Does it have a low probability of acute or chronic injury? These safety decisions depend on many factors, such as the age of the performer, his/her level of conditioning, injury status, previous activity, and rest. For example, how much follow-through in pitching is desirable to help prevent shoulder injury? How much knee flexion in landing from the vertical jump? Greater knee flexion clearly decreases the peak force from the ground on the body in landing, but as knee flexion increases, the shearing forces on the knee increase. So desirable knee flexion to cushion landings could vary among individuals with knee injuries.

> **KEY POINT**
>
> *All human movements have critical features, the key factors that are necessary for optimal performance. Critical features are based on the safety, effectiveness, and efficiency of the movement. Their exact sequence or coordination is also very important.*

Effectiveness Rationale

Each human movement has an associated goal or outcome. The appropriateness of a person's form can be judged based on its effectiveness in achieving the movement goal. Principles of biomechanics can be used to evaluate whether a particular movement pattern or form is optimally effective in achieving a particular outcome. Does a particular body posture in a motor skill allow for desirable stability or the application of force in the direction of the target?

Many striking or throwing techniques employ weight shifts and linear motion that flatten the arc of the hand/implement toward the target, making the athlete more accurate. The linear momentum of the weight shift is transferred to the rotary motions (angular momentum) of the upper body. This weight shift is very important for the effectiveness of these skills.

Efficiency Rationale

The appropriateness of a movement technique can also be evaluated on its efficiency, or the economical use of energy in achieving the goal. Some inefficiencies may be easy to spot. A large pause or hitch in a movement or the excessive up-and-down movement of a distance runner may be easily identified as wasted energy. However, some small variations in technique may be exceedingly difficult to evaluate in terms of which is more efficient. Biomechanists have had difficulty establishing how to document the mechanical energy used to create a movement (Cavanagh, 1990; Cavanagh and Kram, 1985).

The Rationales in Action

Human movement is highly dependent on the environment or context, so the importance of safety, effectiveness, and efficiency can vary within and between techniques. For example, during preseason workouts, a cross-country coach noticed that an athlete appeared to have excessive rear foot pronation as he ran. Inspection of the athlete's shoes tended to confirm this diagnosis. The coach encouraged the athlete to change to shoes with more medial support and frequently changed training routes to minimize the influence of a consistent slope of the terrain and streets he ran on during training.

The safety rationale, or reducing the risk of injury, was deemed most important in this case. The athlete may have felt that he was a better runner (more effective) with his old shoes, but the coach's knowledge of the rear foot motion and the deterioration of running shoes provided a powerful rationale for changing the athlete's equipment.

Another example involving safety is changes in walking gait in icy conditions. Even non-athletes shorten their stride lengths considerably to make up for the loss of horizontal friction forces on ice.

The Range of Correctness for Critical Features

Critical features in a skill should be defined as precisely as possible, bearing in mind that a *range of correctness* is needed to accommodate the variations inherent in people. Schleihauf (1983) suggested that the range of effective movement solutions varies with the nature of the movement. For example, the weight shifts are very different for a golf swing and a fencing lunge. Knowing the range of correctness of critical features makes evaluation and diagnostic decisions easier in qualitative analysis. Good examples are differences in stance and weight shift in throwing and striking. Weight shift is a critical feature in many skills because a weight shift followed by hip and trunk rotation is an efficient and effective way to generate speed in the upper extremity.

In baseball hitting, the emphasis is on bat accuracy because of the difficulty in hitting an unpredictable pitch. Baseball coaches should be aware that open, square, and closed stances may all be appropriate, but the step of the front foot should be a short distance (3 to 8 inches) toward the pitch. A forceful overarm throw, however, should have a square stance with a longer leg drive. The range of correctness that can be observed for qualitative analysis of high-speed throwing may be a forward step from half of standing height (Roberton and Halverson, 1984) to 90% of standing height, typical in baseball pitchers (Atwater, 1979; Hay, 1993). If research can establish desirable ranges of correctness that are observable, the reliability of qualitative analysis of the movement will improve.

Problems in defining the range of correctness are conflict between expert opinions and conflict between biomechanical theory and research. The field of biomechanics has only recently begun to attempt to define what is optimal performance in a particular task for a given environment. There have been major limitations to the development of theories of optimal human movement. The complexity of the neuromuscular and musculoskeletal system, experimental technique, computing power, optimization theory, psychological factors, and theoretical research have all limited the answers to the question of what is good form. Biomechanists may disagree on what determines optimal form and how the musculoskeletal system is creating the movement.

Biomechanical research has shown that many optimization criteria (minimizing energy expenditure, muscle stress, or acceleration) can predict the overall patterns of EMG and movement kinematics exhibited by subjects. Indeed, some would argue that the inherent variability of the body and its physical abilities make it impossible to establish one ideal form for a particular movement (Duck, 1986; Gentile, 1972; Hay and Reid, 1982; Norman, 1975; Spaeth, 1972). What might be possible with biomechanical research is the documentation of a range of desirable form suited to human and environmental constraints (Schleihauf, 1983).

Most of the examples of critical features used so far have related to the movement of the body itself. We will see in chapter 8 that the motor learning research calls this *knowledge of perfor-*

> **Qualitative analysis will be easier and more reliable if the analyst can establish a range of correctness for the critical features and technique points of a movement.**
>
> KEY POINT

mance (KP). It is important to understand, however, that critical features can also be related to the outcome of the movement. This is called *knowledge of results* (KR). The initial trajectory of a typical basketball shot is between 49 and 55 degrees above the horizontal (Knudson, 1993). This angle of release is KR and may be a critical feature of shooting that coaches and teachers should plan to observe. These angles of release provide a range of correctness for the shot because they offer a good compromise between the angle of entry and the speed needed to reach the basket (Knudson, 1993). Many activities have distinct outcomes that may give an athlete an advantage and consequently should be evaluated in a qualitative analysis of the activity.

Critical features and their sequence can be complex ideas, subtle points, common knowledge, professional jargon, or precise values based on modeling or research. Whatever the source or type of critical feature, the analyst needs to gather teaching cues that correspond to it. Teaching cues translate critical features (usually expressed very technically) into easily understood or very descriptive language. For the analyst to communicate effectively with the performer, critical features should be expressed in behavioral terms. This process involves the collection and organization of a wide variety of cue words and phrases. The analyst now has a repertoire of cues to help communicate a point. This flexibility is important because people often interpret cues in different ways. Chapter 8 will review the important points in providing appropriate intervention to improve performance.

Some of the most important prerequisite information that an analyst needs are the critical features of the movements. The range of correctness of critical features may be related to motor development milestones of related fundamental movement patterns. This motor development information is useful in knowing what to look for in analyzing the early stages of learning movements. Remember that some adult learners, unfortunately, have not reached a mature level of many fundamental movements. Motor development knowledge that points to critical features and common errors gives the analyst targets for observation.

Taxonomies and Common Errors

The physical education literature contains many books that provide basic skill information for teaching sport skills. Some books provide an overview of key skills for many sports; others provide detailed analysis of the skills of a particular sport (for example, Human Kinetics' *Steps to Success* Activity Series). In AAHPERD and the related district and state organizations, there are groups interested in basic instruction in physical activities.

However, despite all this literature and interest, there is still a need for *taxonomies* of critical features of fundamental movement patterns and sport skills (Hoffman, 1974). It would be most desirable to get experts from specific sports together with scholars from many subdisciplines of physical education interested in that sport to create taxonomies of critical features for the skills and fundamental movement patterns of the sport. These taxonomies should also include common errors and an exhaustive list of cue words or phrases.

Qualitative analysis of novices is bound to be more effective if analysts are knowledgeable about the most *common errors* of the skills they teach. Analysts can also provide a variety of feedback if they are familiar with several of the most effective cue words or phrases for each critical feature and the associated common errors. In analyzing softball batting, for example, it would be desirable for experts from teaching, coaching, and softball research to get together and identify the critical features of batting, the common errors, and the best teaching cues.

KNOWLEDGE OF THE PERFORMERS

Extensive background knowledge about your students, athletes, dancers, or clients is also needed to prepare for qualitative analysis. Performers come to an activity with a wide variety of abilities based on genetics, anthropometrics, age, gender, experience, training, and skill-related fitness components. The more knowledge the coach can gather about their mental and physical abilities, the better the coach can analyze and evaluate performance.

For example, knowledge about the upper-extremity strength limitations of young basketball players could be used to prescribe additional strength training, establish strength guidelines for initiating certain shooting techniques, or justify the purchase of different basketball equipment. The areas of motor development, anthropometrics, and kinanthropometrics all contribute valuable information on typical changes in the characteristics of humans in motion. For example, the girl hitting the soccer ball in figure 5.4 would be safer with either a smaller or a softer ball.

Knowledge about performers can serve as the basis for equipment and facility modifications that speed up the development of correct

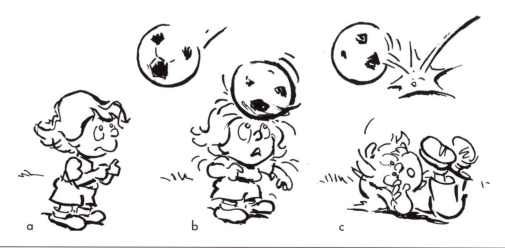

Figure 5.4 Physical limitations of performers and appropriate equipment are important sources of information in qualitative analysis.

technique. Physical educators can select age-appropriate balls, while physical therapists with precise information on typical strength or flexibility of patients with a specific injury can select appropriate rehabilitative aids. Better knowledge of these functional capacities at various stages of rehabilitation can be used to improve diagnostic decisions in treatment. Potential sources of this information about clients include testing, professional literature, clinic records, and communication with professional organizations or peers.

There are many good examples of dramatic changes in people as a result of normal development. The cognitive development of children in early primary grades does not typically allow them to grasp and use abstract strategic information. So in the first few years of school, a teacher should probably not try to provide feedback related to a complex team tactic that fulfills a strategic game plan. One of the most dramatic changes in a short period of time is puberty. Over the course of a few months, an adolescent may find it harder to coordinate his or her longer and larger body segments. One adolescent may experience a minor improvement in strength, while another may have substantial increases in strength and stamina.

The science of motor development has begun to study components of movement (rate controllers) that influence the development and coordination of movements. Rate controllers may be the slowest-changing components in children, while aging adults may lose them more rapidly than other components of movement (Haywood, 1993). Analysts must also adjust the kind of feedback they give and the practice they prescribe relative to each client's stage of motor development. Clearly, analysts of movement must be knowledgeable about the physical characteristics of the people they work with because physical status can dramatically affect the level of performance that can be achieved.

PRACTICAL APPLICATION

In the preparation task of qualitative analysis, coaches must maintain up-to-date knowledge of the performers they coach. In youth sports, this means a good working knowledge of motor development and exercise physiology. Imagine you are the coach watching a child swinging a bat that is obviously too large and heavy for her. Is the child's bent arm swing a technique problem, an immature developmental level of performance, or a strength problem?

The science of motor development describes the typical stages and changes in the development of motor skills. Arm striking patterns tend to develop from an overarm to a sidearm pattern. Are you familiar with the three major stages of sidearm striking proposed by Wickstrom (1983)? Does the performance look as if it was created by an arm-dominated action, a simultaneous body action, or a sequential strike? Motor development literature is very important to the understanding of the status of a person's movement, common actions, and typical changes with development.

When this motor development knowledge is combined with an understanding of movement energy systems and training (exercise physiology), the youth coach has powerful tools to understand the physical limitations of children and how to overcome them. The cramped swing could occur because of poor technique in the readiness and preparatory phases of the movement. Is this performer old enough to have developed the visual perceptual skills (Nelson, 1991) needed to track a moving ball?

If the problem is strength, there are several intervention strategies that could be effective. The child could choke up on the bat, use a lighter bat, and work on increasing upper-body strength. Do you know about developmental changes in strength (Malina and Bouchard, 1991; Nelson, 1991; Roemmich and Rogol, 1995)? Did you know that prepubescent strength training results in strength gains related to neural factors rather than muscle hypertrophy (Wilmore and Costill, 1994)? If you know the child is strong enough, how should you try to change the technique? Should intervention focus on achieving the next developmental level or should the child try to emulate adult form? The practical application of qualitative analysis is clearly an interdisciplinary process that must integrate many perspectives affecting a particular performer and performance. Consistent review of professional literature is essential to the preparation task of an integrated qualitative analysis.

KNOWLEDGE OF EFFECTIVE INSTRUCTION

All kinesiology professions involve some teaching of human movement. Teachers of motor skills need to be aware of pedagogical and motor learning research on appropriate and effective presentation of information. There is a natural connection between presenting movement information and giving similar information as feedback that will be effective intervention. To communicate effectively, the analyst and the performer must share a common vocabulary. To build this vocabulary and teach the movement skills, analysts must follow good instructional procedures. The two major factors in this teaching process are presenting appropriate information and presenting it effectively.

Presenting Appropriate Information

An essential task in presenting motor skill information for initial instruction and as feedback is *translating the critical features into teaching cues*. The teacher/coach must look for the most appropriate language to communicate the critical features. The performer's age, experience, and interest level may affect the choice of cue words or cue phrases to communicate skill information. Good qualitative analysts collect and update a variety of teaching cue words and phrases to get through to the performers they are helping. It is helpful to be able to provide the same correction several different ways, because people make different inferences about words. A good cue phrase for the preparatory weight shift in golf is "shift your weight to your rear foot." "Straight" is a cue word a golfer could use to remember to keep his upper arm comfortably straight during the swing.

Authoritative taxonomies of cue words for sport skills would be invaluable in physical education and coaching. Good sources of information about teaching cues include Dunham, Reeve, and Morrison (1989), Fronske (1997), Fronske and Dunn (1992), Kovar et al. (1992), Landin (1994), and Masser (1985, 1993).

Teaching cues are among the best forms of communication and feedback for performers. One key word, usually a verb (coil, step, opposition) can communicate the essence of a critical feature. A cue phrase describes the critical feature in *behavioral* terms. A figurative or descriptive phrase ("Arch your back as you block on the horse") is often better than a literal description of the action. Most diving coaches know that "wrap your arms" is a better cue phrase for a twisting dive than "decrease your transverse plane moment of inertia," even though the latter is more accurate. Another example is the figurative cue to "scratch your back" with the tennis racquet when you serve. Skilled tennis players do not literally scratch their back with the racquet, but they do drop the racquet head behind their backs to make it easier to create shoulder rotation. Remember that cues need to be relevant to the performer. Small children relate better to "reach into the cookie jar" than "follow through high" as a cue for the follow-through in a basketball shot.

Good cue phrases communicate the essence of a critical feature or technique point concisely so the performer can remember them during practice. Try to keep these behavioral descriptions less than six words, the limit of most people's short-term memory. Remember that you can attach more information to the cue later and add finer points or details to build on the essentials. It is ironic that children can often teach each other a game or movement and get into action much faster than many physical education teachers or coaches. Really good teaching/coaching introduces the critical features of a skill quickly and in terms the performers can understand and relate to.

Housner and Griffey (1994) suggest that learning cues can be categorized based on verbal, visual, and kinesthetic/tactile information. These categories can help instructors select the most appropriate information for the needs of a specific learner. Verbal information presented too metaphorically may confuse a young person but can be very helpful to adults. Tactile information and visual demonstrations may help young children more than verbal skill instruction. As we believe auditory information is important in qualitative analysis, we also believe that auditory information can help the performer. Information on the rhythm of a movement may be an important addition to helping students understand movement, along with the more traditional verbal or visual cues.

Using cues or simple word labels as substitutes for a more complex description of a movement is called *verbal pretraining* (Christina and Corcos, 1988). The phrases "hit and step" in baseball and "right left" for a basketball lay-up carry a great deal of information. Verbal pretraining is important for conveying complex information about human movement. The use of cue words or phrases in instruction can be helpful later in the qualitative analysis process.

Some authors have begun to address miscues, or common teaching cues that are incorrect or can be easily misinterpreted (Adrian and House, 1987a, b). This is a very tricky subject. One method of intervention is to exaggerate or overcorrect a problem area of performance, which often brings about the smaller, desirable change in the person's technique. It is clear that some cues, although less than the truth, have a history of success with performers. Two classic examples are "run on your toes" and "throw by your ear." More research is needed to determine how age, skill level, and aspects of cues interact to foster communication of movement information and aid learning of motor skills.

A variety of cues is also needed because of cognitive and perceptual style differences among performers of different ages. If a qualitative analysis of a novice in elementary school and an adult revealed the same problem, the cues that would best communicate to each learner would most likely be different. The small child with a short attention span would probably respond well to a figurative cue like "open a window when you toss the ball." The adult might respond equally well to a literal cue if she could attach the desired meaning to it. Until more research is done to identify the most effective cues, professionals should strive to develop and refine cues and to share them with others.

Among the best methods of writing cue phrases may be the one proposed by Morrison and Reeve (1993), based on Vickers' (1989) method of writing technical or qualitative objectives. The Morrison and Reeve approach uses the four parts of Vickers' behavior objectives: action, content, qualifications, and special conditions. The *action* is a verb that describes the desirable motion. The *content* is a short description of what is doing the action. *Qualifications* is a short description of how success can be gauged. And *special conditions* can be added to the teaching cues if more information is needed to evaluate the performance. This structure is illustrated in line four of figure 5.5: *swing* indicates the action, *arm* indicates the content, *forward* is a qualification of the action, and *level to ground* is a special condition defining the movement.

Relevant cues for movements can be created for each phase of a movement (preparation, execution, and follow-through), with variations for performers of different ages and levels of expertise (Vickers, 1989). This identification of special cues for various ability levels has also been emphasized by Strand (1988) and Abendroth-Smith, Kras, and Strand (1996). Future research should help professionals develop a variety of effective and developmentally appropriate cues.

If cues are highly effective as teaching and intervention tools, how can cues be integrated into effective instruction? Qualitative analysis would improve if the analyst can plan instruction

> **KEY POINT**
>
> *Cue words and phrases are effective ways to present information to performers. Cues need to be concise, accurate, and appropriate to the age and ability level of the performer.*

Turn side to target

Step on opposite foot/transfer weight

Rotate hips and trunk

Swing arm forward level to ground

Snap wrist

Follow through to target

Figure 5.5 Six behavioral teaching cues for overarm throwing based on the Morrison and Reeve (1993) method.
Reprinted, by permission, from C. Morrison and J. Reeve, 1993, "A framework for writing and evaluating critical performance cues and instructional materials for physical education," *The Physical Educator*, 50(3): 132.

to support later qualitative analysis of clients. One relevant approach is the format for preparing teaching information in motor skills proposed by Dunham (1986, 1994). This format breaks movements into two phases, anatomical and motor, rather than the traditional three phases of preparation, execution, and follow-through. The anatomical phase occurs just as the skill performance starts. The motor phase describes the major actions and the follow-through. Teaching cues used in the motor phase can be phrased behaviorally, as suggested by Morrison and Reeve (1993), to create a task sheet. Figure 5.6 shows a task sheet for the overhand throw. Task sheets in teaching and examples from many activities have been published (Dunham, Reeve, and Morrison, 1989).

Task sheets tell performers exactly what to do to execute a movement. Additional details can be added to the teaching cues as they become necessary. The preparation of task sheets can be evaluated using a process proposed by Morrison and Reeve (1993). Figure 5.7 illustrates the components of effective movement instruction materials. The two most important content factors (be-

havioral cues and their sequence) are weighted the most. The score sheet has been separated from the explanation of each section because the score sheet needs to be short and concise. Once the instructor has used the score sheet a few times, he/she will not need to explain the scoring. In fact, instructors may modify the score sheet to suit their teaching situation.

It is important to have clear teaching cues for instruction. Not only do they aid the learner in acquiring the skill, but they also serve as the criteria against which the teacher judges the skill and the performer interprets feedback. Any discrepancy between what the analyst teaches and the feedback can confuse the student. An example is the tennis instructor who taught his class the forehand. But he forgot to tell them to keep the wrist stiff during the swing. His first correction was keep the wrist stiff. How was the class to know this critical feature was important if they were not taught it?

This poor preparation for instruction illustrates the connection between instruction and qualitative analysis. An explicit method of information preparation and presentation would have avoided or minimized the forehand problem and allowed for greater learning. Also, a method of checking information presentation could have caught the omission. If the skill or task sheet for the forehand had been prepared properly, then the process of instruction and qualitative analysis would have proceeded more smoothly. How does an analyst take appropriate skill information and plan effective instruction? Although this is not a teaching methods text, we will summarize the actual presentation of skill information to performers, since it relates to qualitative analysis.

Overhand throw

Anatomical phase

Body orientation: Non-throwing side to target
Feet: Shoulder width apart
Knees: Slightly bent
Hips: Slightly bent
Trunk: Back straight
Shoulders: Non-throwing shoulder to target
Arms: Throwing arm extended back at shoulder height
Hands/fingers: Three middle fingers on top of ball
Head: Eyes on target

Motor phase

1. *Step and point* with foot closest to target
2. *Rotate* hips then trunk
3. *Elbow comes through first*, staying high
4. *Follow through*—bring throwing hand close to floor

Figure 5.6 Sample overarm throw task sheet for teaching the overarm throw.
Reprinted, by permission, from C. Morrison and J. Reeve, 1993, "A framework for writing and evaluating critical performance cues and instructional materials for physical education," *The Physical Educator*, 50(3): 133.

Effective Presentation of Information

Once appropriate instructional information is identified, the analyst needs to present that information effectively. Pedagogical research has shown that highly effective teachers generally present information to students more efficiently than less effective teachers (Siedentop, 1991; Werner and Rink, 1987). The starting point for effective presentations is the preparation of teaching materials. If the skills to be taught can be organized in a systematic way and presented consistently, students can learn under one of a variety of teaching styles (Mosston and Ashworth, 1986; Siedentop, 1991).

Analytic scale

Reader _____ Author _____

1. Content and sequence

	Low		Middle		High
a. Keys/cues/critical features	2	4	6	8	10
b. Sequence	2	4	6	8	10

Total _____

2. Appropriately presented

a. Concise description phrases	1	2	3	4	5
b. Accurate language	1	2	3	4	5
c. Consistency of terms	1	2	3	4	5
d. Extraneous information	1	2	3	4	5
e. Repetition	1	2	3	4	5

Total _____

Grand total _____

Scoring: Higher score means better content.

1. a. Keys/cues/critical features—Are the major parts of the skill all included? Are only the most important selected (5 to 6)?
   b. Sequence—Are the keys/cues/critical features presented in the correct order, beginning to end?
2. a. Concise—Is the information presented as briefly as possible?
   b. Accurate language—Does the word selection describe what happens?
   c. Consistency of terms—If technical/description terms are used (flexed/extended, abducted/adducted) are they used throughout the presentation?
   d. Extraneous information—Are thoughts and ideas included that do not really apply to skill?
   e. Repetition—Is information presented in ways that are unnecessary and redundant?

Figure 5.7 Analytic scale developed by Morrison and Reeve to help instructors evaluate their skill instruction. Reprinted, by permission, from C. Morrison and J. Reeve, 1993, "A framework for writing and evaluating critical performance cues and instructional materials for physical education," *The Physical Educator*, 50(3): 133.

This organization of information about motor skills for instruction is very important because poorly taught skills will not be learned and will require greater qualitative analysis. Intervention will also become more difficult. Research on information presentation shows that certain components of instruction are essential for effective teaching. Most good teachers provide a good demonstration of the skill, explicit verbal explanation, summary cues, direction of student attention to important factors, and a way to check for student understanding (Graham, 1988; Graham, Hussey, Taylor, and Werner, 1993; Kwak, 1993; Masser, 1985, 1993).

Many pedagogy experts see the effective presentation of motor skill information and qualitative analysis as part of what can be called effective teaching or coaching. Graham (1988) tied the idea of good teaching presentation to the use of appropriate feedback and organization of the teaching environment. Kwak (1993) emphasized the importance of cognition in learning. Cognition is a cornerstone of understanding and using qualitative feedback. Masser (1985, 1993) provided evidence for the use of refining in skill acquisition. This refining process relates instruction directly to suitable feedback. Finally, Reynolds (1992) describes monitoring, the process of following students carefully during class time so that feedback on performance can be tied directly to instruction. Teachers and coaches can likely improve the effectiveness of qualitative analysis by planning for effective presentation of skill information. All kinesiology professionals can improve their qualitative analysis of motor skills by studying pedagogical research on the effective presentation of motor skill information.

KNOWLEDGE TO DEVELOP A SYSTEMATIC OBSERVATIONAL STRATEGY

The preparation task must also focus on knowledge about the observation of human movement, because that is the next task in qualitative analysis. A key component of observation in qualitative analysis is the use of a systematic observational strategy (SOS), a plan to gather relevant information about a movement. Information from many subdisciplines of kinesiology affects the selection of the best SOS for a particular movement. Good preparation for qualitative analysis involves locating information related to the movements to be observed and identifying the SOS that is most appropriate for that movement.

In planning how to observe the movement, the kinesiology professional may review literature on the phases of the skill, appropriate vantage points, visual limitations, or the number of observations needed. The analyst may choose aids to observation, like visual models, checklists or rating scales, or videotape replay. If the movement is fast and complicated, an analyst may practice the anticipated SOS to improve her qualitative analysis on the job. This practice may help to create positive visual habits in the actual observation of live movement. Unfortunately, Kretchmar, Sherman, and Mooney's (1949) question, what are the best visual habits for observing human movement, is still not answered. The next chapter provides a detailed review of important factors in the second task of qualitative analysis, observation.

SUMMARY

The first of the four tasks of qualitative analysis is preparation. Kinesiology professionals preparing for qualitative analysis must weigh evidence from many subdisciplines about four areas: the activity or movement, the performers, effective instruction, and an appropriate systematic observational strategy. They should review experience, research, and expert opinion in preparing for qualitative analysis. Analysts must continuously update their knowledge of the critical features (elements of a movement that are essential to optimal performance) to be analyzed. Since qualitative analysis is often part of the larger process of teaching motor skills, analysts must keep their knowledge about appropriate and effective presentation of information up to date. They must also prepare for the observation of human movement, the next task of qualitative analysis.

DISCUSSION QUESTIONS

1. In preparing for qualitative analysis, what factors should you weigh in evaluating the importance of various sources of information on human movement?

2. What factors are most important in selecting the critical features of a movement?

3. What subdisciplines of kinesiology are most important in selecting critical features of movements?

4. What factors are most important in establishing the range of correctness for the critical features of a movement?

5. In a world of rapidly changing knowledge and technology, how important are specialized publications that bridge the gap or summarize the application potential of scholarly research?

CHAPTER 6

Observation: Developing a Systematic Observational Strategy

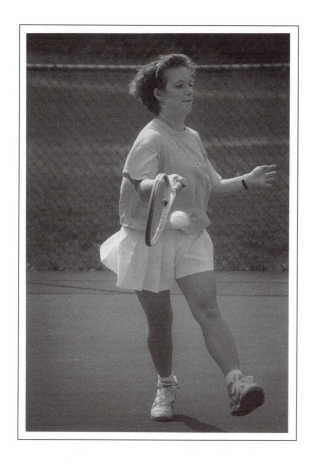

PREVIEW

A friend has asked you to videotape her tennis match in the finals of a local tournament. What key strokes, player movements, and ball motions would be useful to a tennis player? Should both players be in the field of view? What vantage points would provide the best view of the action, and what actions would be missed from those vantage points? These are some important questions to think about in planning to observe human movement. The videotape images, like the visual information coaches collect in qualitative analysis, must be carefully selected to get as much important information as possible.

Chapter Objectives

1. Explain how to compensate for perceptual limitations by planning a systematic observational strategy.
2. Identify the key elements of a systematic observational strategy.
3. Identify several effective systematic observational strategies.
4. Explain how all the senses can be integrated to improve observation.

"You can observe a lot just by watchin'."

—Yogi Berra

The observation of human movement is the second task of an integrated qualitative analysis. The quote from Yogi Berra implies that movement observation is an easy, natural task. We disagree; this is untrue about visual observation and leaves out the other senses that can contribute to the task of qualitative analysis. Once analysts have organized prerequisite information in the preparation task of qualitative analysis, they use this information to plan a *systematic observational strategy* (SOS). An SOS is a plan to gather all the relevant information about a human movement. This chapter will review several proposals for observational strategies, identify key elements of an SOS, and discuss the integration of all the senses that contribute to the task of observation in qualitative analysis.

An SOS is needed in qualitative analysis for many reasons. First, large amounts of information about the movement from many subdisciplines must be condensed into critical features that will be the targets of observation. Second, the sensory and information processing limitations discussed in chapters 3 and 4 must be considered. Third, the knowledge and expectations of the observer strongly influence what is observed. Edgar Dale (1984:58) pointed out the importance of prerequisite knowledge in observation by saying: "We can only see in a picture what our experience permits us to see." In other words, the analyst must be smart enough to know what to look for. A good SOS will allow the analyst to gather appropriate and unbiased multisensory information on a person's performance of a motor skill.

The goal of an SOS is to provide a platform to gather relevant information on the status of a person's movement performance. All kinds of information must be attended to and apprehended. Remember that observation includes all sensory information a teacher/coach can garner about human movement. In the past, the predominant thinking has limited observation to identifying errors in performance based on some "good form" model envisioned by the teacher/coach. We believe that the task of observation should be broad enough to encompass many modes of sensory perception but limited to the collection of this multifaceted information. The observation task of qualitative analysis is focused on collecting information, not evaluating or diagnosing it.

We have chosen to separate the information-gathering task (observation) from the diagnostic task (evaluation and diagnosis in our model) to emphasize the two different processes. Radford (1989) reviewed the research on observation in kinesiology and concluded that observation and the decision making that follows it must be conceptualized as separate. (This is the view expressed by the information processing model used in this text.) Some scholars argue that these two tasks are related and can occur at the same time (Pinheiro and Simon, 1992). But we define observation as the process of gathering, organizing, and giving meaning to sensory information about human motor performances. Most information processing models consider this process separate even if they use direct mapping from the perceptual components to the decision areas.

A simple view of observation of human movement essentially involves two main decisions:

The second task of qualitative analysis is observation. In this task, analysts gather information from all the senses about a movement with a systematic observational strategy (SOS). There are several ways to organize an SOS for the qualitative analysis of human movement.

KEY POINT

what (focus) to observe and *how* (a plan to observe). The preparation task of qualitative analysis identified the critical features of the movement. These critical features are the focus of the SOS, so observing them is crucial to gathering useful information. The next section summarizes key proposals from the kinesiology literature on how to observe human movement. The how of an SOS is more complicated and may be different for different analysts.

PROPOSALS FOR OBSERVATIONAL STRATEGIES

Several scholars have proposed guidelines for developing skill in observing human movement. They offer different approaches for an SOS. Observation is only one task within qualitative analysis, and several observational strategies are effective. Different plans of observation may even be needed to accommodate the perceptual differences among observers.

Barrett's System

Barrett (1977) identified three key tasks in the development of observational skill in physical education: analysis, planning, and positioning. She suggested that the lack of professional preparation for observational skill may be due to trends in education that emphasized the importance of reliability and outcome scores rather than process variables. Barrett (1979b) later published a review paper on the growing body of literature that addresses the task of observation within the qualitative analysis process.

Her ideas on how to apply this research in planning observations were nicely summarized in other publications (Barrett 1979a, c). According to Barrett, three components are needed in planning an observational strategy: deciding *what* to observe, planning *how* to observe it, and knowing what factors influence the *ability* to observe. In 1983, Barrett presented a model of observation as a key skill in teaching motor skills. A recent paper based on her work suggested that the first task, deciding what performance variables to observe, is the most important in planning movement observation (Allison, 1985b).

Radford's System

A paper by Radford (1989) reviewed the literature on observation in kinesiology and proposed

a theoretical framework for movement observation. Observation was seen as three independent subprocesses: attention, template formation, and motivation. *Attention* is the process of limiting sensory information and can be controlled from the top down or the bottom up. For example, viewing the overall action draws attention to extraneous movements (bottom-up processing), while top-down processing is a conscious decision to direct observation. Viewing the overall performance would develop a gestalt of the skill, while an observational model such as the one presented by Gangstead and Beveridge (1984) on page 18 could be used for bottom-up processing.

Template formation (analogous to deciding on critical features and their acceptable ranges) is the cognitive, abstract, symbolic representation of a model of human movement. Templates of human movement are multilayered, plastic (shapable), and generalizable to many performers. A template is not an image of an ideal movement, but a generalized paradigm that accommodates differences within a definable range. The last subprocess, *motivation*, is involved throughout the whole process because good observation requires "persistence, effort, practice, and the subsequent elaboration of movement templates" (Radford, 1989:23).

James and Dufek's System

Recently, James and Dufek (1993) proposed seven steps for the observation of movement. The focus of their paper is similar to what this book calls qualitative analysis. The steps in their observational strategy are to classify the skills to be analyzed, divide the movement into phases, observe several times in order to evaluate each phase critically, and focus attention on four major areas.

They call the first step, classifying the fundamental movement pattern or the mechanical objective that is the focus of the skill, important to planning observation. Knowing the number and location of phases of the movement may assist in planning observations to see the important events in each phase. The last two steps are the guidelines for planning observation by focusing attention on either phases or four different areas. The authors suggest that the plan for observation should first focus on the total body (the rhythm or continuity of the whole body). Next, focus on the pelvis and trunk (the center of gravity) and the large muscles, which initiate most movements. The third focus is the base of support and how it changes, because it is often the source of balance and reaction forces that drive the movement. Fourth, the observer should focus on specific actions of the extremities. These movements are often fast and difficult to see, so they advocate focusing on joint actions rather than specific segments. This model starts with a gestalt and concludes with an organized system of observation advocated by other authors (Beveridge and Gangstead, 1984, 1988; Gangstead, 1984; Gangstead and Beveridge, 1984).

KEY ELEMENTS IN A SYSTEMATIC OBSERVATIONAL STRATEGY

Our review of the observation literature in kinesiology leads us to propose that there are five major areas that professionals should consider in developing an SOS. They should plan to *focus* attention on critical features to aid in the analysis. They should exercise as much control over the observational *situation* (teaching, coaching, therapy environments) as possible. They should plan the angle of view, or *vantage points*, from which to view the performance and the *number of observations* they expect to need. Finally, they

may need to include plans for *extended observation*. The primary sense involved is often vision, although the other senses will also be used to gather information about the movement.

> **KEY POINT**
>
> *A good systematic observational strategy should include what critical features to focus attention on, how to control the situation, the vantage points of observation, the number of observations needed, and a decision on whether extended observation will be needed.*

Focus of Observation

The first task of qualitative analysis outlined the critical features of the movement to be analyzed. These critical features and any other variables that may be related to the performer and the situation become focal points for the systematic observational strategy to follow. Barrett (1979c) calls this idea of planning focuses of attention in observation a *scanning strategy*. A scanning strategy is a plan to define what to look for, when, and how long to look. Planning for a gestalt or observing with an observational model can achieve the goal of a scanning strategy.

PRACTICAL APPLICATION

The stolen-base leader in the conference is taking a big lead off first base. You are the field umpire of a two-person umpire crew. You crouch into position, anticipating the pitch and the runner's break to second base. Out of the stretch, the pitcher rockets a throw to the first baseman, who applies the tag as the runner dives back to the base. What's the call?

Your qualitative analysis of this situation strongly depends on your attention and your ability to get into the correct position and systematically observe the movement of the ball and the runner. Were you attending to the pitcher at the time of release? Were your body, head, and eyes positioned at a 90-degree angle to the path of the runner to the base? How close were you to the action? Where did you focus your eyes during the flight of the ball and when the tag was applied? Did your observation focus on the determining factor in the judgment of whether the runner was out or safe? Did the defense have to qualitatively prove the runner out, or did the runner have to prove he was safe? What level of perception (detection, discrimination, recognition, or identification) was used in this situation?

A baseball umpire's systematic observation is similar to observation within other qualitative analyses of human movement. Choosing what to focus attention on prepares the analyst for observation, but it may bias the observer to see some events and be less sensitive to others. How can analysts prepare to observe systematically to increase their accuracy, yet limit the effect of observer expectations in biasing information gathering for qualitative analysis?

Besides critical features, there are many variables an analyst may need to observe in qualitative analysis. Aspects of the movement that relate to the rules of the sport need to be observed. For example, a badminton coach will need to focus on the racquet head in some serves because the shuttle must be contacted below the waist. Other variables to plan to observe might be environmental factors that constrain the appropriate technique in open motor skills, deviations in movement rhythm, extraneous motions, and cues that fatigue or psychological stress is affecting the performer. For example, a beginning swimmer's fear may prevent proper execution of swimming skills.

With all these aspects of performance to observe, how does one organize the scanning strategy? The qualitative analysis literature has proposed four approaches. Observation can be organized to follow the phases of the movement, balance, the most important features, and the path from general impressions to specific actions.

Observation by Phases of the Movement

The most common scanning strategy in qualitative analysis may be to observe critical features within the normal order or phases of the movement (Gangstead and Beveridge, 1984; James and Dufek, 1993; Philipp and Wilkerson, 1990; Pinheiro, 1994). This observational strategy de-

creases the perceptual overload by focusing attention on the three primary phases of most movements: preparation, execution, and follow-through. However, it is often not clear what phase should be evaluated first, although it is assumed that observation follows the sequence of the movement. This observational strategy may be most appropriate in open motor skills. Since open skills are highly dependent on the environment, a strategy to observe the environment and how preparatory actions match the environment is very important.

This observational strategy is exemplified in the work of Gangstead and Beveridge (Beveridge and Gangstead, 1984, 1988; Gangstead, 1984; Gangstead and Beveridge, 1984). Chapter 2 introduced this observational model of qualitative analysis where the focus is primarily on knowledge of performance for various parts of the body during three phases of the movement (figure 6.1). The movement itself is of primary concern, although it is important to remember that knowledge of results can be relevant to improving performance.

If this observational strategy is used without a gestalt, then a body component of interest is observed through the temporal phases of the movement. For example, the path of the hub (belt buckle or slowest moving part) is observed in the preparation, action, and follow-through phases.

Body components	Temporal phasing		
	Preparation	Action	Follow through
Path of hub	Over base of support	Shift forward to target	Continue movement to target
Body weight	Over base of support	Shift forward to target	On front foot closest to target
Trunk action	Non-throwing side to target	Rotate open to target	Follow arm to target
Head action	Face target	Eyes on target	Eyes on target
Leg action	Apart, weight on back leg	Step to target with closest leg	Bring back leg up to front leg
Arm action	Throwing arm extended back	Bring throwing arm forward	Throwing arm across body
Impact/release		Snap wrist	

Figure 6.1 Observational model proposed by Gangstead and Beveridge with overarm throwing cues filled in. An example of observation by phases of the movement.
Adapted, by permission, from S.K. Gangstead & S. Beveridge, 1984, "The implementation and evaluation of a methodological approach to qualitative sport skill analysis instruction." *Journal of Teaching in Physical Education*, 3 (Winter): 62.

Any other body components are observed in a serial fashion. Descriptive phrases, like the throwing ones illustrated in figure 6.1, can be inserted in the observational model to help guide the analyst.

If an analyst uses a gestalt observational strategy, the Gangstead and Beveridge model will be of use in focusing on specific aspects of performance. In a gestalt the analyst observes for an overall impression of the movement. If she suspects a problem in a particular part of the movement, the observational model will help the analyst find a specific weakness in performance.

Observation of Balance

There is a saying in construction that you can't build a cathedral on the foundation of a house. The second way to organize an observational strategy is rooted in this philosophy. A scanning strategy can be based on the concept of balance and the origins of the movement. Many coaches like to focus on the base of support and the initial movements of the lower extremities for some skills because they believe that balance and the actions of the legs (or arms) strongly affect the actions of subsequent segments. Observing movement from the base of support and initial movements is especially appropriate for gymnastics and any other activity where balance and base of support can dramatically affect subsequent actions. Movement in many sports requiring great accuracy, like baseball pitching, is strongly affected by variations in balance. DeRenne and House (1987) call balance one of the four most important aspects of baseball pitching.

Observation Based on Importance

The third type of organization of observational strategy is based on a ranking of the importance of the critical features identified earlier. This approach is favored in research by Morrison (Morrison and Harrison, 1985; Morrison and Reeve, 1986, 1988, 1989, 1992; Morrison, 1994). This approach evolved from an earlier study by Harrison (1973). Obviously, if an analyst believes that a particular critical feature is most important for safe movement, that feature should be observed first. The logic behind this observational strategy is similar to the origins of movement approach, because some critical features may influence other aspects of the movement.

Generally, the sequence aspect of this approach drives this system of observation. A professional who has thoroughly researched a movement and reflected on his/her practice to identify critical features may have definite opinions on what aspects of the movement deserve the most attention. Biomechanical models of qualitative analysis tend to emphasize this approach by selecting variables for analysis that are related to the goal or primary mechanical purpose of the movement.

Observation From General to Specific

The fourth approach is to move from the general to the specific. It has been proposed by several authors (Brown, 1982; Hay and Reid, 1982; James and Dufek, 1993; McPherson, 1990). It is what Radford (1989) called bottom-up attentional processing and chapter 2 referred to as a gestalt observational model (Dunham, 1986, 1994). This approach is also similar to the gestalt talked about in chapter 4, in which the analyst considers all the parts of a movement and develops an overall impression of the quality of the movement. The whole, complete skill is greater than the sum of its parts. If the analyst feels that there is something wrong in the skill, he can pinpoint the deficiencies by looking at the phases of the movement or individual body parts or a combination of phases and body parts.

Whatever the approach used to organize the observational strategy, some experts advocate written plans for observation. Examples may take the form of checklists (Adrian and Cooper, 1989; Bayless, 1981; Davis, 1980; Frederick, 1977; Hoffman, 1977b; McPherson, 1990; Pinheiro, 1994), diagrams (McPherson, 1990), task sheets (Dunham 1986, 1994; Reeve and Morrison, 1986; Morrison and Reeve, 1993; Klesius and Bowers, 1990), or rating scales (Hensley, 1983; Hensley, Morrow, and East, 1990; Rose, Heath, and Megale, 1990).

Situation for Observation

The exact nature of the movement task and the environment in which the task is performed should be controlled as much as possible by the analyst. Yet the task performance must be as realistic as possible for the qualitative analysis to be most effective. The Balan and Davis (1993) model (chapter 2) could provide an answer to the problem of how to teach in a way that improves qualitative analysis while successfully structuring an environment that is friendly to both analysis and practice. Unfortunately, qualitative analyses are most often performed in situations where the lack of environmental control either minimizes or exaggerates relevant technique problems. The environment should be carefully planned so that modifying for speed, competition, distractions, or psychological pressure will elicit realistic performances.

For example, most qualitative analyses of tennis groundstrokes should be conducted during normal play, practice rallies, or with a ball machine that can project balls in an inconsistent fashion. A player's forehand or backhand strokes are often dramatically affected by the environment. At the advanced level of open motor skills, the athlete's movement and tactics may be of primary interest. Coaches need to plan situations for their observations of *open skills* that mimic the competitive environment—for example, a point guard dribbling the ball up the floor who must adjust his dribbling to the defense.

Since *closed skills* are performed in a relatively stable environment, they do not need adjustment as they proceed. But even they can be made more realistic with psychological pressure. An excellent situation for the qualitative analysis of free-throw shooting in basketball is a free-throw competition at the end of practice. The combination of fatigue and psychological pressure to perform (to win or avoid penalty) creates a situation in which the coach can evaluate good and bad habits that may affect the outcome of a game. Remember, the very fact that the instructor or coach is watching has an effect on performers. Some thrive on the attention and pressure; others perform worse. Analysts must take this factor into account when setting up observations and later when evaluating and diagnosing performance.

The speed and timing of movements for observation should be matched as closely as possible to the situation in which the movement occurs in competition or public performance. For example, a novice tennis player usually encounters slower groundstrokes from opponents and should not consistently be observed in a time-stressed position of returning shots with great speed or spin. Early skill practice and systematic observation by instructors should take place in closed environments. Unfortunately, practice routines in sports are often organized for convenience rather than for effective qualitative analysis. For example, coaching or teaching a movement with players in a shuttle position (fielding a ground ball, throwing to first, and returning to the back of the line) does not allow the analyst to observe several trials. And multiple observations are essential to evaluation and diagnosis.

Once the play/movement situation is as realistic as possible, the analyst may have control over the background from the vantage points to be used (Brown, 1982). An effort should be made to set up the subject's movement to allow for a stable background.

Vantage Points for Observation

The analyst should specify the optimal positions for observation for a particular movement. A specific vantage point may be crucial to seeing the critical features identified for the qualitative analysis. In most cases, the best vantage point for observing a particular movement or critical feature is at right angles to the plane of motion. This often means that a movement needs several vantage points. Figure 6.2 illustrates split-screen video images of the address position of a beginning golfer. What different aspects of his technique are observable from the different vantage points?

Because most human movement involves important motions in all three cardinal planes, observation often requires several vantage points to obtain undistorted views of key actions. An example is the apparent excessive elbow flexion in preparing to throw a ball illustrated in figure 9.11 (frame d, p. 145). The knowledgeable analyst knows that this rear view can exaggerate the appearance of elbow flexion due to the extreme external rotation of the shoulder in this phase of the throw.

Brown (1982) suggested that vantage points should have stable backgrounds, without distractions or moving objects. A uniform background with a contrasting color relative to the subject would be ideal. Horizontal or vertical references in the background make the visual estimation of motion and angles easier. The practical matter of getting to and from desirable vantage points may affect the fine tuning of what to observe in the SOS.

The observer's distance from the movement is also an important factor in selecting vantage points for observation. It is clear from the research on vision (chapter 3) that this distance affects the angular motion of the analyst's eyes as they track the movement. Therefore, the distance from the movement should be as large as possible while still allowing for observation of important details. Sufficient distance provides a background on which to have the movement superimposed and reduces the tracking demand on the eyes.

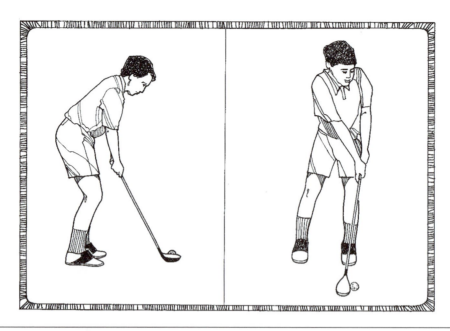

Figure 6.2 Split-screen video images from two vantage points of the address position of a beginning golfer. Which aspects of performance are visible from only one vantage point?

How much distance should there be between the observer and the movement? There is no universal answer because the speed and complexity of human movement varies, the critical features of interest vary, and the environment may limit the selection of a viewing distance. The faster the movement, the greater the viewing distance should be to limit the demands on the observer's eyes. Hay and Reid (1982) advocated viewing distances of 10 to 15 meters for movements that have limited over-ground speed or take place in small areas and 20 to 40 meters for movements that are fast or cover a large distance.

But viewing distances beyond 10 meters are much larger than many physical therapists or physical educators can use. The lab or gym space may not allow these large distances. They would also require the observer to travel to the performer to provide feedback or intervention. We suggest that *5 to 10 meters* is a good rule of thumb for the minimum distance for observation of most human movements. The analyst may want to observe from closer vantage points if the movement or event is very small and slow so the observer can consistently see the action of interest. For example, a golf coach may not be getting enough information on ball spin from the flight of the ball and may choose to stand close to the golfer to examine the location of divots. This provides a clue about the path of the club and consequently the spin on the ball.

The evidence suggests that the best rule when using visual observation is to observe from as far away as pragmatically possible. However, if the distance is too great, it may limit the gathering of auditory, tactile, and kinesthetic information. Particularly when using the latter senses, the observer must be closer to the performer.

Peripheral vision should also be taken into account as part of the vantage point. If clothing (hats, visors, etc.), people, or objects limit peripheral vision, understanding of skill performance may be inhibited. Remember, peripheral vision is important in the development of cognitive maps.

Number of Observations

The analyst needs to plan the number of observations that should be necessary to gather enough information for diagnosis and intervention. Clients need to repeat the movement because of the analyst's perceptual limitations and because the *consistency* of correct or incorrect technique points is an important issue in diagnosis and intervention. Clark, Stamm, and Urquia (1979) found that the observation of six trials of a balancing task for children was sufficient to provide a reliable relative estimate of performance.

The problem is that many teaching, coaching, or clinical situations do not allow for large blocks of time for individual attention and observation of many trials. Unlike the elite level, where most coaching is one on one, at more typical levels most coaches must divide their attention among several athletes. Therefore, they must compromise between gathering enough information for a good evaluation and diagnosis of the performance and bowing to the time constraints of the situation.

There are few guidelines for planning the number of observations needed for a qualitative analysis. The exact number is probably best determined by the individual doing the analysis for a particular situation. It can also vary between observers, depending on the complexity of the skill and the ease of observation. Logan and McKinney (1970) recommended observing a minimum of eight trials, while Hay and Reid (1982) suggested 15 trials as a guideline. Based on qualitative analysis instruction studies by Morrison (Morrison and Harrison, 1985; Morrison and Reeve, 1989, 1992), some sport skills require only five repetitions for consistent qualitative analysis.

In Morrison's original videotape skill analysis test, the children performed each skill five times in sequence, and then that sequence was repeated. The latter two studies cited here did not use the second set of performances because those viewing the test analysis tapes (in intervening projects) felt they had decided the merits of the performances during the first sequence. Initial scores on the latter studies with similar subjects were in the same range as scores for the original study. Reliability studies (Mosher and Schutz, 1983; Painter, 1990; Ulrich, Ulrich, and Branta, 1988) also suggest that five observations are usually enough.

Clearly, it is best if multiple trials are observed systematically before any intervention is decided on. Based on this discussion and the reliability studies reviewed in chapter 2, a reasonable rule of thumb for the number of trials observed systematically in most qualitative analysis situations is *between five and eight observations*. Although some simple and slow body actions can be reliably observed in one trial, it is important to observe more because of the variability of performance. More observations also let the observer focus on information from all the senses. Unfortunately, sports officials and gymnastics judges must base their judgments on the observation of a single event.

Perceptual limitations and the variability of human performance suggest that multiple trials are needed in qualitative analysis. It is not appropriate to correct a performer after observing only one attempt (unless it is a situation or competition with only one observable performance). The consistency of a performer's strengths and weaknesses are key issues in the evaluation/diagnosis task of qualitative analysis (chapter 7). The number of trials observed may also vary according to the skill of the performer, the skill of the analyst, and other aspects of the situation. For example, novices to a motor skill often exhibit inconsistent performance and errors, so they should be observed more times than skilled performers.

Extended Observation

Extended observation is a plan for gathering more information on a movement than is usually observable. Good examples of extended observation are recording performance on videotape, using multiple senses, and using multiple observers. Observational power using videotape is enhanced by the freeze-frame, frame advance, and slow-motion replay of the images. A detailed discussion of using videotape to assist in qualitative analysis is presented in chapter 11. The use of other senses besides vision is also an example of extended observation. A coach or therapist may use the sounds created by a performer to gather information on the rhythm or identify a weak phase of a movement.

If a critical feature of interest in a qualitative analysis is difficult to see, extended observation is called for. For example, a gymnastics coach who thinks the athlete has enough height on a stunt but still fails to rotate enough for consistently good landings may choose to spot several attempts. The sense of touch during spotting gives the coach a feel for the level of performance and what intervention should work best.

If videotape is unavailable and the analyst's senses are not enough, Hay and Reid (1982) suggest a visual trick that may help the analyst get a look at fast movements. They suggest the eye-close technique, in which the analyst closes her eyes at the instant of an important event of the movement to fix a temporary image of it. This trick relies on the short-term sensory memory and/or short-term memory described by Pinheiro and Simon (1992). The idea can be transferred to other senses as long as no competing stimuli are allowed to compromise the most recently gathered information.

THE INTEGRATED USE OF ALL SENSES

How can analysts extend their observational power by using all the relevant senses? Several authors have suggested that all the senses work together in the observation task of qualitative analysis (Hay and Reid, 1982; Hoffman, 1983; Radford, 1989). Hay and Reid stated that aural, tactile, and kinesthetic observation can supplement visual information. Chapters 3 and 4 support this holistic view of observation.

Many sports generate distinct sounds that can be used to provide information on the movement itself or on an outcome. The sounds of preparatory footwork in the tennis forehand or the rhythm of the final steps in the long jump supply valuable information about how the athlete performed the skill. The sound produced by the slice technique in tennis is quite different from that of the flat serve. These sounds of impact provide important cues on the amounts of spin and speed applied to the ball.

The sense of touch can also be used to increase observational power in qualitative analysis. Teachers who spot gymnastic, diving, or other skills can sense the athlete's ability to generate the forces or torques required. Teachers or coaches with good physical skills may compete with performers to simulate various styles of play, which provides a great deal of information on the strengths and weaknesses of an athlete. Smart coaches who use their sense of touch can quickly check the appropriateness of equipment or the strength of a performer.

Hay and Reid (1982) use the term *kinesthetic observation* to describe the assessment of performers' sensations of movement. They suggest that good qualitative analysis is a cooperative effort between the performer and the analyst. As performers increase their skill level, they usually develop a greater kinesthetic sense and feel for their performance. Skilled athletes can often tell the coach exactly what position their body was in or what mistake they made in a particular trial. Wise coaches and teachers of skilled performers use the performers' observations to supplement their qualitative analysis. Baseball batters or tennis players may be asked whether they hit the "sweet spot" on particular trials. Players can assist the coach and learn to evaluate shots by the sound of the impact and vibration they feel. Good

communication with performers is essential and may help motivate them to implement the corrections prescribed.

SUMMARY

The second task of qualitative analysis is observation. Good observation of human movement is based on a systematic observational strategy (SOS) to gather information about the critical features of a movement. An SOS can be organized based on the phases or sequence of the movement, by balance or base of support, by the importance of critical features, or from a general impression to specific aspects of performance. The key elements of an SOS are to focus attention, control the situation, plan vantage points, plan the number of observations, and extend observational power if needed. Analysts can extend observational power by getting information from all their senses, using more observers, or recording the performances on videotape. The information gleaned from observation will be used in the next task of qualitative analysis, the evaluation and diagnosis of performance.

A review of important points in an SOS follows:

- Observation is based on knowledge of the activity, the performer, effective instruction, and a systematic observational strategy.

- Observation is based on a variety of sensory information and the interaction of all the senses, not just vision.

- Attention is an important component of observation, so be ready to focus your attention with an SOS.

- An SOS can be organized by the phases of the movement, by balance, by ranking of critical features, or from the general to the specific.

- Control the situation to optimize observation and the subject's performance.

- Select appropriate vantage points, viewing distances, and numbers of observations.

- Integrate your observations with the performer's perceptions.

- Use techniques like video replay to extend your observational powers.

DISCUSSION QUESTIONS

1. What factors make the use of a systematic observational strategy necessary in qualitative analysis?

2. How do differences in analysts' psychological and cognitive styles affect the choice of observational strategy?

3. What kinds of motor skills are best suited for visual observation? Auditory observation? Tactile observation?

4. Does specific knowledge about the critical features of a movement and about a performer's *physical limitations* bias the observation?

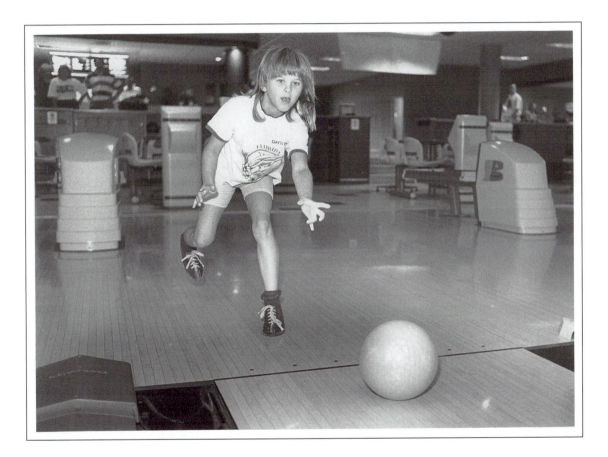

Evaluation and Diagnosis: The Third Task of Qualitative Analysis

PREVIEW

A young girl who has several obvious faults in her bowling technique asks for your help. After viewing a few performances, you decide that there are four major flaws. This bowler has a bounding and inconsistent approach, a limited backswing, and an inside-out downswing. This youngster has asked you, "What can I do to knock down more pins?" How would you respond? This question has put your qualitative analysis of the situation to an important test. How do you know which fault is most strongly related to pin count? How will you select the intervention that will help the bowler the most? What is more important, short-term or long-term improvement in her score?

Chapter Objectives

1. Explain why evaluation of performance errors is necessary for qualitative analysis.
2. Discuss several strategies for prioritizing weaknesses in critical features.
3. Identify relevant subdisciplines of kinesiology that contribute to the evaluation and diagnosis of performance in qualitative analysis.

After observing a performance, the analyst must identify desirable and undesirable aspects of that performance. A critical evaluation of these aspects and a diagnosis of the performance lead to a ranking of priority for the corrections the analyst will give the performer. Evaluation and diagnosis are the two parts of the third task of an integrated qualitative analysis. This chapter will review the various rationales for prioritizing possible intervention in improving performance. Because of the many interrelated factors involved in human movement, the evaluation and diagnosis of performance may be the most difficult task in qualitative analysis.

The systematic observation of human movement results in a large amount of information about a person's performance. This information must be processed in the analyst's mind. Essential skills in this third task of qualitative analysis are the ability to *evaluate* the strengths and weaknesses of performance and to *diagnose* performance. Diagnosis of performance identifies the errors that directly limit performance so that they can be corrected in the intervention task of qualitative analysis. Not all "errors" or differences in movement technique are related to performance, and providing too much or incorrect intervention will have a negative effect on performance.

In evaluating and diagnosing, the analyst essentially becomes a human movement detective or physician. The analytical tasks of deciding "whatdunit?" or "what caused the problem?" are difficult and may have far-reaching consequences, because the intervention selected could do harm rather than good. An analyst who focuses the performer's attention on minor or symptomatic errors at the expense of more important problems may indirectly contribute to an injury. A coach who focuses practice on errors symptomatic of another problem is wasting valuable practice time. Evaluation of performance is the important first step in making sense out of the information gathered in the systematic observation of human movement.

EVALUATION

The terms *evaluation* and *diagnosis* are used to emphasize the essential processes in the third task of qualitative analysis. Evaluation typically refers to a judgment of quality, to ascertaining the value or amount of something. This is important because the analyst often must establish the good points of the performance as well as the errors or weaknesses.

Much of the research has focused only on errors or faults in performance. Early in its development, qualitative analysis of movement was often referred to as error detection. This is understandable since the primary method of qualitative analysis involves comparing a model of correct form to the observed performance, with the goal of identifying differences or errors. But some motor development scholars argue that it makes little sense to judge performance as right or wrong; movement should be interpreted in reference to a continuum of development (Painter, 1990).

Performing an integrated qualitative analysis accomplishes more than simply identifying errors. Our evaluation of the performance's strengths will affect our diagnosis of the weaknesses and how we choose to provide feedback to the performer. A good evaluation may ask: Are the critical features of the movement within a desirable range? What are the strengths of the performance? What are the weaknesses or errors? The Arend and Higgins (1976) model of qualitative analysis used the term *evaluation of performance*, suggesting that evaluation should focus on the efficiency of the movement and its appropriateness to the environment.

KEY POINT

The third task of an integrated qualitative analysis has two distinct processes: the evaluation of the strengths and weakness of performance and the diagnosis to select the most appropriate intervention to improve performance.

The Process of Evaluation

It has often been assumed that professional experience and knowledge allow analysts to observe and evaluate human movement. There has been little research on the process of evaluation in qualitative analysis, and only a few authors have hypothesized as to what occurs in this process. It is likely that several cognitive methods are used to identify strengths and weaknesses of critical features.

The kinesiology literature about qualitative analysis suggests there are two distinct ways the evaluation of performance can occur. Hay and Reid (1988) call them the sequential and the mechanical method. The *sequential* method involves comparing mental images of body positions throughout each phase of the movement. Most coaches use this mind's-eye image of the desirable actions and phases of a movement to compare with the actual performance. Figure 7.1 illustrates how this visual comparison might look in

the evaluation of a volleyball bump or pass. This focusing on the difference between a model of good form and the actual movement has been hypothesized to be the primary method of evaluation in qualitative analysis (Arend and Higgins, 1976; Hoffman, 1983; Pinheiro and Simon, 1992). This is likely how the emphasis on error detection developed.

The *mechanical* method, which was illustrated in figure 2.1, uses a model of the mechanical factors that affect performance. The evaluation task of qualitative analysis then becomes a process of deciding to what extent each mechanical variable was achieved. Qualitative analysis models based on this approach suggest that knowledge of a few biomechanical principles can be used to evaluate a variety of motor skills and that these principles are directly related to corrections that can improve performance (Hay and Reid, 1988; Norman, 1975). Like different observational strategies, different approaches to evaluation can be effective in the qualitative analysis of human movement.

We propose that the process of evaluation within an integrated qualitative analysis can benefit from using both the sequential and the mechanical methods. Most people will be comfortable using mental images of desirable form for critical features of the movements they analyze qualitatively. To keep the task manageable, evaluation of performance should be based on a

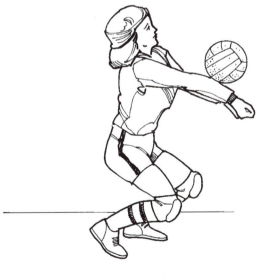

a Incorrect technique

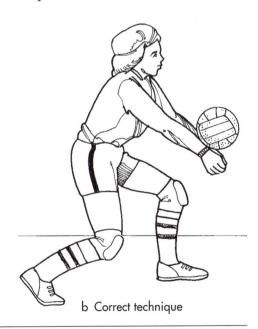

b Correct technique

Figure 7.1   The evaluation of performance in qualitative analysis typically compares the observed performance (a) with a mental image of desired performance (b). Evaluation is more than just identifying errors but also identifying strengths.

few (about four to eight) critical features. So the quality of the critical features of the movement becomes the focus of the evaluation task. This evaluation is not viewed as dualistic; the performer's technique is not judged either correct or incorrect (error).

If a performer consistently exhibits technique outside the range of correctness for a critical feature, this must be evaluated as a weakness or performance error. These errors should eventually be corrected because of their negative effect on performance or risk of injury. This is why it is important to specify as completely as possible in the preparation task the range of correctness of all critical features of a movement to be evaluated. The range of correctness can be defined or quantified in the analyst's mind (for example, step with the left foot 3 to 7 inches [7.62 to 17.78 cm]), but it is usually expressed behaviorally to the performers. "Step over the bat" is a good cue to achieve the small, controlled weight shift that helps control the swing of the baseball bat. Examples of critical features using mechanical principles are the concepts of sequential coordination and summing segmental velocities.

The evaluation of critical features in an integrated qualitative analysis should result in an unbiased, accurate assessment of the critical features relevant to performance. A simple evaluation process that is reliable, accurate, and leads the analyst to appropriate intervention is desirable. We advocate rating evaluation of performance of critical features at one of three levels: *inadequate, within the desirable range,* or *excessive.* This provides three levels of ordinal data, increasing reliability and making available enough categories for diagnostic decisions.

> **KEY POINT**
>
> *Evaluation in qualitative analysis is concerned with identifying the strengths and weaknesses of performance. A useful approach is to rate critical features into one of three categories: inadequate, within the desirable range, or excessive.*

Difficulties in Evaluation

There may also be deviations from prototypic form that are difficult to judge as in or out of the range of correctness of critical features or

desirable form. The variety of environmental constraints and differences in performer anatomy and physiology may lead to differences in technique that cannot easily be identified as errors or incorrect technique. Some important difficulties in evaluating performance are variability, kinds of errors, differences between critical features and ideal form, and analyst bias.

Performance Variability

A major problem in establishing whether a critical feature is within the desirable range of correctness or is a weakness is the issue of performance consistency or *variability*. This is why the systematic observational strategy should include at least five to eight observations. The analyst should evaluate an inadequate level of a critical feature differently if it occurs once as opposed to consistently occurring across several trials. Early in motor development, performers exhibit a wide variety of errors, and an error in one trial may not be significant. The more advanced the performer, the more consistent performance becomes. Strengths and weaknesses are more subtle but tend to be more consistent over repeated trials. Whatever the performer's ability, use repeated observations to help you evaluate the consistency of critical features of a movement.

Unfortunately, movement consistency is not the only problem in the evaluation of performance. Other problems are finding agreement on the critical features, their range of correctness, and their order of importance to performance. Chapter 5 discussed some of the areas of disagreement on what is important to performance. This is a problem since there is no universal agreement about which features are critical for a movement—much less which critical features are more important than others. Since interdisciplinary task forces for each sport are not likely to spring up and write position papers and research grants to address this issue in the near future, each analyst must use his or her own knowledge and experience to establish critical features and ranges of correctness.

Kinds of Movement Errors

Even if evaluation were limited to error detection from an agreed upon set of critical features, it would still not be a simple task. Several authors have discussed how problems or errors in performance can have several sources. Hoffman (1983) proposed that errors can be related to critical abilities, skill performance, or psychosocial factors. A schematic of these classifications of

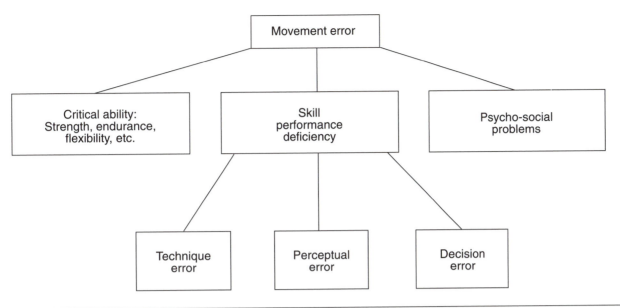

Figure 7.2 The kinds of performance errors that form the basis of Hoffman's diagnostic problem-solving approach to qualitative analysis (1983).

errors is presented in figure 7.2. Note that even when errors are isolated as skill-related, they may still have three different causes: technique, perception, or decision.

A similar approach was proposed by Philipp and Wilkerson (1990), who classified errors as biomechanical, physiological, perceptual, or psychological. Biomechanical errors relate to technique problems in body position or timing. Physiological errors are deficiencies in physical capacities such as strength, endurance, or flexibility. Perceptual errors are misunderstandings of technique or mistakes in evaluating environmental cues. Psychological errors are motivational and attitude problems that interfere with performance. These error classifications are built into the Philipp and Wilkerson model of qualitative analysis and are linked to specific interventions to improve performance. The problem with this approach is that a performance problem may be due to the interaction of several of these errors, and there is no diagnosis process to select the best intervention to improve performance.

All these factors may arise from a particular deviation in prototypical performance, making the tasks of evaluation and diagnosis of performance difficult. For example, an analyst would want to determine whether a volleyball player is missing passes to the setter because of bumping technique, fatigue, or perceptual problems in tracking the serve.

Critical Features Versus Ideal Form

The underlying assumption in the teaching of most motor skills is that the teacher knows what is the best or most appropriate movement response. The belief that a certain technique or form is best has been at the core of motor skills instruction for years. The quote by Brown (1982:21) illustrates this belief: "While some performers may compensate for the lack of 'good form' through excessive practice, strength, and speed of movement, improper form usually limits the ultimate level of performance." Most motor skill instructors would agree with this premise, but most have also had experiences similar to the expert opinion disagreement illustrated in figure 5.1 (page 69). There is a large difference between maintaining current knowledge to refine critical features and knowing what optimal form is for a specific person and situation.

If optimal form and the critical features for a movement are easy to establish, why have some skills undergone radical changes in technique independent of changes in equipment or rules? Why do many sports go through cyclic changes in predominant technique based on the best-known athlete or teacher at a given time? Why do experts in biomechanics disagree on the causes of particular movements? Why do some scholars argue that it is inappropriate to assume that the teacher can specify one ideal form that would help all learners succeed (Gentile, 1972)?

Clearly, the evaluation of human movement is a difficult task complicated by a lack of consensus and of knowledge about how humans move. Imagine two different approaches to a basketball free throw, the underhanded technique of Rick Barry or the technique used by Michael Jordan. Is there an ideal form for a free throw? Even if there was, the free throw is a closed motor skill, while shooting in game conditions is an open motor skill. Skills in closed environments are more likely to have a tighter range of correctness, approaching the idea of ideal form. Skills in an open environment require greater flexibility to accomplish the goal and will have less restrictions on effective technique.

The critical features of any skill are dynamic and interact with a multitude of other factors that affect performance. This interaction of critical features, performer traits, movement environment, and other factors makes it very difficult to establish one ideal form for a particular movement. Kinesiology professionals should make a concerted effort to summarize the body of literature by inviting scholars from many subdisciplines and practitioners to begin to develop taxonomies and position papers on motor skills. Defining the critical features of motor skills and their range of correctness would make the evaluation of performance in qualitative analysis easier.

Analyst Bias

Whatever the approach to evaluation, an unconscious tendency or *bias* may creep into evaluation in qualitative analysis. The reliability study by Ulrich et al. (1988) discussed in chapter 2 found statistically significant interactions between observers and performers. The age of the performer tended to color the analysts' evaluations. Young performers' skill levels tended to be underrated, while older performers tended to be overrated. Remember that observational assessments of human movement have not been as reliable as quantitative analyses. Some scholars believe that the strong measurement and reliability emphasis of the physical education profession has hurt the development of qualitative analysis (Barrett, 1977). The difficulty of achieving consistent, unbiased evaluation of human movement is not an argument against using qualitative analysis. Qualitative analysis can be reliable and unbiased when analysts plan and conduct their analyses carefully.

The more specific the range of correctness of a critical feature can be made, the less sensitive the observer will be to any unconscious tendency to rate a performer differently from the standards. Too much specificity, however, reduces reliability by decreasing the potential agreement among different analysts. A 10-point rating scale for the critical features of a movement may go beyond the analyst's ability to discriminate true levels of performance.

Evaluating human movement within qualitative analysis involves judging the strengths and weaknesses of a person's performance. Critical features should be evaluated only after an adequate systematic observation has been performed to gather relevant information. A few (four to eight) critical features should be evaluated to one of three levels: inadequate, within the desirable range, or excessive. This evaluation process is not too complicated and points logically to the correction appropriate for that critical feature. In the following section, we will see that diagnosing the strengths and weaknesses identified in evaluation is also a difficult process.

DIAGNOSIS

Once the characteristics of performance have been evaluated, the analyst must diagnose the situation to establish what specific intervention is best for the performer. *Diagnosis* usually refers to critical scrutiny and judgment in differentiating a problem from its symptoms. The many subdisciplines of kinesiology have often used other terminology for these steps or included them within the process of observation. It is not surprising that several subdisciplines have slightly different names or definitions for this process.

What is surprising is that with well over 100 years of history in kinesiology in the United States, there is no consistent rationale for the diagnosis of movement errors. This is analogous to medical schools teaching anatomy, physiology, and the variability of these parameters but forgoing courses in the diagnosis of symptoms and the clinical rotations used to teach this skill. What would a patient think of a doctor who had no basis for diagnosing disease and prescribing a remedy? Doctor to nurse: "I'm not sure what's wrong with Mrs. Smith. She's the fifth patient today with a sore throat. Have her take a sample of medication X home. I'm not sure why or if it will work, but it's what my old doctor (insert "coach" to make this story more familiar) always used."

One problem that may account for the lack of a theoretical basis for diagnosing movement is the difficulty of establishing critical features discussed in chapter 5 and the previous section of this chapter. Another potential barrier to the development of a theoretical basis of diagnosis is the erroneous belief that qualitative analysis is easy and teachers/coaches will develop a talent for it with experience alone. Remember that in the early stages of motor learning/development, errors are often obvious deviations from correct form. The difficulty is in the frequency and *variability* of these errors. Despite these controversies, one aspect of diagnosis appears to be agreed upon. It should narrow down the strengths and weaknesses in performance to focus the performer and analyst on the single most important intervention (Arend and Higgins, 1976; Hay and Reid, 1982; Hoffman, 1983; McPherson, 1990).

Prioritizing Intervention

Focusing on one intervention in qualitative analysis is important because the research in psychology and motor learning suggests that most learners can focus on only one correction at a time during practice (Christina and Corcos, 1988; Schmidt, 1991). To prevent paralysis by analysis, the teacher/coach must *prioritize intervention* and select one solution as the best (Arend and Higgins, 1976; Hay and Reid, 1982; Hoffman, 1983; McPherson, 1990). We believe that this is *not* an easy task because there is a lack of guidelines for the diagnosis of performance to select the best intervention and because the cause of a particular problem may be far removed from its observable effect(s) (Hay, 1993; Luttgens and Wells, 1982).

The subdiscipline of kinesiology traditionally associated with diagnosis of motor skills is biomechanics. Hoffman (1974:6) stated: "Diagnosis appears to rely on the observer's ability to use biomechanical concepts to accurately interpret the visual data at hand. The nature of the task suggests that a thorough understanding of principles in biomechanics, including the structural and functional relationships of joints and skeletal segments, is a prerequisite for diagnosis." Biomechanics is the science of how forces and torques move the human body.

The best diagnosis of performance, however, should use knowledge *integrated* from many subdisciplines of human movement (Hoffman, 1983). Even if an optimal form could be established for a task, the analyst would have to decide whether the performer was flexible and strong enough to use that form. If a performer is several developmental stages from desirable or mature form, is it wise to try to emulate this form if it is beyond his or her physical abilities? Biomechanics, motor development, exercise physiology, motor learning, pedagogy, and psychology all affect the answer to this question.

Does kinesiology research support any theories or guidelines for prioritizing movement errors into appropriate intervention? Do we know what is the best feedback or intervention to help a person move from, say, an immature level of throwing to a mature overarm throwing pattern? Unfortunately, the answer to both questions is no. There has been limited research to test which kinds of diagnostic decisions result in faster short-term and long-term improvement.

The kinesiology literature has only begun to stress that diagnosis is a critical task in qualitative analysis (Hoffman, 1974, 1983; Hay and Reid, 1982; McPherson, 1990; Pinheiro and Simon, 1992). Pinheiro and Simon (1992) proposed a three-stage model of motor skill diagnosis based on their research on novice and expert analysts of the shot put and medical diagnosis literature. They found that expert analysts were better at the observation task of qualitative analysis, called *cue acquisition* in their diagnosis model. The second stage was the *interpretation of cues*, or making connections between the cues and the cognitive representation (schema) of the skill. We call this finding of meaning in the information observed the process of evaluation. The last stage of the model was considering the causes of the errors observed and making a *decision*. Pinheiro and Simon suggest that experts in qualitative analysis are *simultaneously* using these three stages in their thinking when they analyze movement.

Few qualitative analysis scholars have tried to hypothesize about how the diagnosis process occurs. The papers by Hoffman (1983) and Pinheiro and Simon (1992) are among the few that have addressed this problem. Most qualitative analysis models do not elaborate on how the diagnosis of performance occurs. Since there has been little systematic research to examine which approaches to prioritizing corrections result in faster and longer-term improvement, we can only review some logical approaches and discuss their merits based on research that has been focused on other kinesiology issues.

Rationales for Prioritizing Intervention

In prioritizing possible intervention, it is very important to keep in mind the goal or purpose of the movement being analyzed. Just as a physician's diagnosis is based on knowledge of many possible outcomes of a disease, diagnosis within qualitative analysis must be based on knowledge of the possible outcomes of intervention. The diagnosis of a person's overarm throw would differ depending on its purpose. The purposes of a throw from the outfield, from the catcher to second base, and from the pitcher home are all different. Clearly, the analyst must understand the goal or purpose of the movement and the goals of the performer. This knowledge of goals and outcomes will shape the priorities of corrections.

A review of the kinesiology literature on diagnosis within qualitative analysis supports the view that prioritizing possible intervention or corrections is important. Christina and Corcos (1988) warn analysts against rushing to provide feedback if they are uncertain about the diagnosis, because inappropriate feedback may frustrate the performer and damage the analyst's credibility.

In reviewing the variety of qualitative analysis literature, we found six logical rationales that scholars have proposed for prioritizing intervention in the diagnosis of performance. These rationales may be summed up by the following phrases: relationship to previous actions, maximizing improvement, order of difficulty, correct sequence, base of support, and critical features first.

Teachers or coaches may unconsciously be using one or more of these criteria when they select specific feedback or corrections over other possible interventions. Other coaches may just have strong opinions on what types of movement errors must be corrected first. No one rationale for prioritizing feedback or corrections should be considered the best because research has not directly compared the various rationales and the best rationale may be *specific to the person or the motor skill*. For gymnastics skills that are strongly determined by balance, corrections could likely be prioritized from the base of support up. A coach's experience and reading may lead her to emphasize execution phase actions over preparatory or follow-through actions in a particular sport skill. The variety of successful approaches is like the different strategies for the systematic observation of movement, which

can all be used to gather information about performance.

Relationship to Previous Actions

The first rationale for prioritizing intervention is to *relate actions to previous actions* in a movement (Hay and Reid, 1982, 1988). It may be possible to identify errors or weaknesses that are only symptoms because they are caused by another problem. This rationale is similar to Hoffman's (1983) idea of primary and secondary errors. Some deviations from the desirable form, or other style differences, may be less important or mere symptoms of more important problems. If a missed ball (secondary error) can be related to a previous action (primary error) like improper preparation, vision, or directed attention, it would be foolish to correct the swing mechanics that are symptomatic of the real problem.

Knowledge needed to relate an action to a previous action comes from biomechanical principles, research, and practical experience in qualitative analysis. For example, if the goal of an overarm throw is distance, it is important to know the critical features of throwing that relate to the ball's height, angle, and speed of release. These three factors determine the distance of the throw. The throwing actions that relate to these parameters will help the analyst diagnose throwing performance. This is one of the strengths of qualitative analysis models based on the principles of biomechanics. The evaluation and diagnosis of performance are focused on key movement issues that lead directly to potential intervention (Norman, 1975).

> **KEY POINT**
>
> *Diagnosis within qualitative analysis involves a judgment that identifies the underlying causes of poor performance from the observed strengths and weaknesses. Diagnosis is used to set priorities for possible intervention. There are six different logical rationales for prioritizing corrections to select the best intervention.*

Teachers, coaches, and athletes often have good hunches or opinions on what action relates to another. If the majority of coaches and professional athletes in a sport have the same opinion, it is most likely correct. It should not be assumed, however, that the opinions of athletes and coaches are always correct; there have been many instances where they have been wrong. Researchers have a difficult time relating actions to previous actions even in controlled biomechanical research and computer modeling. The two biggest problems in relating biomechanical actions to other biomechanical actions are the interaction of the segments and the effects of muscle actions at joints they do not even cross (Zajac and Gordon, 1989). These and other biomechanical research issues make it very difficult to establish exactly what actions are related to what other actions.

Good examples of relating an action to an earlier action can be found in both open and closed motor skills. Suppose a gymnast over-rotates in a vault and stumbles in landing. Biomechanics tells the coach that two things can result in too much rotation: conditions at take-off that determine angular momentum or the timing and changes of body position that manipulate the resistance to rotation (moment of inertia). If the analyst's evaluation of the take-off was good (trying to relate to a previous action), he may focus corrective efforts to the flight phase of the vault.

An open motor skill like baseball batting might have several factors related to an awkward action in the follow-through of the swing. The pitch may have been in a bad position, the batter may have been fooled by the pitch, or a loss of balance could have accounted for the poor follow-through.

Another example relevant to many overarm patterns involves sequential coordination. The powerful trunk rotation in an overarm pattern (throw, spike, tennis serve) results in the arm lagging behind because of its inertia. This humeral horizontal abduction and external rotation create an eccentric stretch of important muscles (pectoralis major, subscapularis) that contribute to the acceleration in the last 50 milliseconds of the movement. For performers to have advanced arm actions in overarm patterns, they must have good leg drive and trunk rotation. Cues to keep the arm back will not lead directly to the coordination and timing needed in high-level overarm skills.

Attentional, psychological, or motivational factors may create performance errors. The awkward baseball swing could be related to nervousness or just a lack of attention and concentrated effort. An analyst may notice that one performer is rarely enthusiastic and is very attentive to other students' reactions to his performance. If this performer has confidence and self-esteem problems, the best diagnosis may be to emphasize success and praise. Future work with this performer could get him to focus more on the movement and less on the result. Relating actions to previous actions in the diagnosis of motor skills must be based on principles from all the subdisciplines of kinesiology.

The science of biomechanics studies how muscles and external forces create motion of the human body. Biomechanical research on throwing technique and exercise will provide information on which you can base your diagnosis of the throwing problem of the baseball player. What muscle groups would you emphasize in weight training or conditioning exercises to help improve his throwing? Most professionals would likely say the triceps. It might surprise you to find that biomechanical research suggests that one of the most important joint actions is humerus internal rotation (Adrian and Cooper, 1995). The high angular velocities of elbow extension appear to be related to the coordination and interaction of the arm segments (Atwater, 1979). Roberts (1971) reported on a study by Dobbins that paralyzed the triceps with a radial nerve block. The subject could create about 82% of initial throwing velocity after several practice trials. Triceps do appear

PRACTICAL APPLICATION

One of your best infielders is having trouble creating speed on her overarm throw. Fast batters and long throws to first base will be problems unless you can improve the speed of her release. This player has good technique on the major critical features of the overarm throw. This leads you to believe that improvement will be difficult and will require improved coordination or conditioning. (See chapter 9 for the critical features of the overarm throw.) How do you decide if conditioning or throwing technique should be the focus of intervention?

to contribute to overarm throwing speed, but probably not to the extent that many coaches expect. Coaches should review recent research on testing and conditioning for overarm throwing (DeRenne, Ho, and Blitzblau, 1990; Janda, and Loubert, 1991; Jones, 1987) to optimize performance and, more importantly, to minimize the risk of overuse injuries.

If you already have a good conditioning program, this athlete may improve if you prescribe appropriate practice to improve the sequential coordination of the throw. Unfortunately, biomechanical research is not conclusive on why sequential coordination is best in overarm throwing. Biomechanists have not even agreed on a way to define coordination using biomechanical variables. There are various approaches to documenting the kinetics or mechanical causes of movement. The biomechanical research on the kinetic chain/link principle, commonly seen in a proximal-to-distal sequential coordination of high-speed movements like the overarm throw, is not conclusive. It is not clear whether the slowing proximal segment speeds up the distal segment or the acceleration of the distal segment slows the proximal segment (Feltner, 1989; Phillips, Roberts, and Huang, 1983; Putnam, 1991). Currently, biomechanics research is not in a position to provide a great deal of guidance for coaches trying to improve coordination in throwing.

Maximizing Improvement

Another rationale for prioritizing intervention is to select intervention that can be expected to *maximize improvement* (Hay and Reid, 1982, 1988). In 1988, Hay and Reid proposed that diagnosing performance is a two-step process of excluding faults that appear to be effects of other faults and prioritizing the faults that are left based on the improvement that can be expected in the time available. On the surface, this seems like a logical approach to selecting corrections. The problem, however, is that it is not clear *how* to judge which correction leads to the most improvement and what time frame should be used.

Prioritizing to maximize improvement is probably a good approach, but more research is needed to determine what factors are most significant in both short-term and long-term improvement. One technique change could create a lot of initial improvement but in the long run make it difficult to achieve advanced levels of performance. On the other hand, motor learning

research has shown that more randomly assigned practice conditions (high contextual interference) create lower initial performance but better long-term performance (Schmidt, 1991).

In Order of Difficulty

Research in psychology, pedagogy, and motor learning has shown the importance of positive reinforcement and success in motivating practice and the learning of motor skills. These disciplines tend to recommend that the *easiest corrections be made first* if movement errors seem unrelated and cannot be ranked in importance (Christina and Corcos, 1988). The explanation is logical, since easy technique changes lead to the performer's perceived success, improvement, and greater motivation to continue practice. Selecting intervention in order of difficulty may produce small but consistent increases in skill. The question, however, is what is the best way to prioritize intervention to get the most improvement. A correction that is easy to communicate to a performer may not lead to improvement, especially if the action in question is related to another action. Like the rationale for prioritizing intervention, selecting intervention in order of difficulty for the performer is logical, but there is no clear research showing that it is most effective in improving performance.

Correct Sequence

Another approach for prioritizing intervention is to *correct in sequence*, or provide intervention in the sequence of the actions in the motor skill. Correcting actions in the preparation phase of a movement first may have effects on the execution and follow-through phases. This approach has been used by Morrison and Harrison (1985) in teaching qualitative analysis to classroom teachers with no background in kinesiology. This order of priority may also be implied by the many qualitative analysis models that break the movement into the preparatory, execution, and follow-through phases.

There is little scientific evidence to support this domino theory of technique. It is logical that some skills could be highly sequential; actions in preparation might strongly influence later actions. The correct-in-sequence rationale may be a good approach for making tough decisions between two very similar corrections, or for analysts without a strong background in biomechanics and other subdisciplines. A volunteer youth sport coach or early childhood specialist at a day-care center might be able to help children improve a variety of motor skills by providing corrections in sequence. Fast sport skills in open environments are highly dependent on preparatory movements and might benefit from prioritizing intervention in sequence.

Base of Support

In many activities, coaches choose to provide intervention to improve performance *from the base of support up*. For activities requiring balance or the control of large forces generated by the strong muscles of the lower extremities, this approach may be logical. One author knows a golf pro who bases teaching and qualitative analysis of the golf swing (a closed motor skill) from the stance (base of support) up. This PGA professional, who has a master's degree in kinesiology, has come to the conclusion that most errors later in the golf swing are a result of actions in the setup and backswing. The golf swing requires great precision to strike the ball with the correct clubhead speed and path for a specific shot.

A target shooting analogy illustrates the importance of stance and balance in accuracy sports. Tell performers to compare the accuracy and stability of an Olympic marksman to the accuracy they can expect with their current lower-extremity technique in an accuracy skill. As with the other approaches to diagnosis, research is needed to see whether balance or precision motor skills improve the most with intervention directed to the base of support and balance compared to other kinds of intervention.

Critical Features First

The last rationale for prioritizing intervention is to *improve critical features first*, before other minor variations in performance. The kinesiology literature is full of professional articles offering opinions on the most important aspects of motor skills. This is *not* what we mean. By definition, critical features are the most important factors in determining the success of a movement. They are established by rigorous review of professional experience and research. If the right critical features have been established, correcting them before addressing other general points of correct form or style should help the performer achieve the movement goal faster.

The problem with this approach to diagnosis is that most movements have several critical features, and we have seen that it is difficult to establish which are the most important. An analyst may have strong convictions about several critical features but may have only educated guesses or beliefs regarding their relative importance.

Sport-specific research and experience can lead a professional believe that the sequence of a skill is very important. That professional may then diagnose performance based on the sequence of the critical features of a movement. A therapist may prioritize intervention in gait analysis by relating actions to previous actions and maximizing improvement. The definition of maximum improvement may change as the goals of therapy change from safe or pain-free gait to a more cosmetically normal gait. The best diagnosis of performance may use information from all relevant subdisciplines of kinesiology to try to relate actions to previous actions in combination with another prioritization rationale relevant to that motor skill.

SUMMARY

The third task of qualitative analysis of human movement requires skill in two processes, the evaluation and the diagnosis of performance. This may be the most difficult task of an integrated qualitative analysis. The analyst must evaluate the strengths and weaknesses of the movement's critical features, which were identified in the observation task. The process of diagnosis involves prioritizing these strengths and weaknesses so that one intervention can be selected to improve performance. There are six rationales that may be used to prioritize intervention: relating actions to previous actions, maximizing improvement, making the easiest corrections first (working in order of difficulty), correcting in sequence, moving upward from the base of support, and fixing critical features first.

In the absence of kinesiology research to show what kind of intervention creates the most improvement in performance, *it's up to the professional to decide what rationale or combination of rationales to use*. One good way to diagnosis performance is to combine the rationale of relating actions to previous actions and another rationale relevant to the movement being analyzed. Once a critical feature has been selected as most likely to improve performance, the analyst is ready for the fourth task of qualitative analysis, intervention.

DISCUSSION QUESTIONS

1. How do the processes of evaluation and diagnosis differ?

2. What factors in the evaluation of performance affect accuracy, reliability, and potential bias of the qualitative analysis?

3. What subdisciplines of kinesiology contribute knowledge necessary for prioritizing strengths and weaknesses identified by the evaluation of performance?

4. What important research questions need to be answered to improve the diagnoses of performance in qualitative analysis?

Intervention: Strategies for Improving Performance

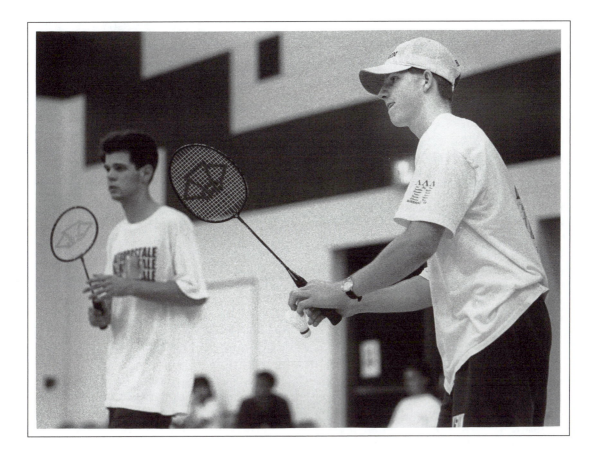

PREVIEW

This badminton player is having difficulty getting the desirable speed and downward trajectory of the smash. Your observation of several trials suggests that the player positions himself poorly, letting the shuttle get over or behind his head. Your feedback to the player is to "stay back a little" before hitting the shot. Since the player has been learning the smash with his body turned at a right angle to the net, your cue is misunderstood to mean that he should move back toward the sideline. Clearly, feedback must be phrased carefully to be effective. What other intervention would help this player? Would general feedback to "hustle" be effective, or should a more specific cue relevant to this performer be used?

Chapter Objectives

1. Identify the variety of intervention strategies used in qualitative analysis to improve performance.
2. Identify research-supported guidelines for the provision of augmented verbal feedback.
3. List the functions of feedback used as intervention in qualitative analysis.
4. Describe how to develop appropriate cue words and phrases.
5. Identify situations where the intervention of exaggeration, modification of practice, manual or mechanical guidance, or conditioning would be appropriate to improve performance.

Once a systematic observation has been conducted and the strengths and weaknesses of the movement have been evaluated and diagnosed, the last task of qualitative analysis is intervention. *Intervention* is the analyst's administration of feedback, corrections, or other changes in the environment to improve performance. This is a critical step in the qualitative analysis process where the instructor communicates with the learner about the desired change that will lead to improvement. Intervention requires the integrated use of knowledge from all the subdisciplines of kinesiology. Improper intervention can result in decreased performance.

In other models of qualitative analysis, the task of intervention has been given a variety of names. Some scholars use the term *feedback* (Arend and Higgins, 1976), while others have used *remediation* (McPherson, 1990; Knudson and Morrison, 1996) or *instructions to performers* (Hay and Reid, 1988). The integrated model of qualitative analysis uses the more general term of intervention because it encompasses all the possible actions a kinesiology professional can take. Intervention is not limited to the various forms of feedback, instruction, or error-correction approaches of previous qualitative analysis models. Instructors can choose to give verbal feedback, positively reinforce good aspects of performance (technique or effort), use modeling, provide physical guidance, modify practice, prescribe training, adjust competition or equipment, or choose not to intervene at all. This chapter will discuss how to optimize the intervention to improve performance.

> *The fourth task of qualitative analysis is intervention, which may involve providing feedback to performers, making technique corrections, or other prescriptions in order to improve performance.*
>
> **KEY POINT**

FEEDBACK

The predominant mode of intervention in teaching motor skills is verbal feedback from the teacher. Whenever a person executes a movement, information about the outcome is available immediately. This information is *intrinsic feedback*. The physical sensations of walking in deep sand, the kinesthetics of carrying a heavy object, and visual information on the path of a thrown ball are examples of intrinsic feedback.

The other major kind of feedback is *extrinsic* or *augmented feedback*. It comes from an external source after the movement has been completed. Augmented feedback is the primary mode of intervention in most qualitative analyses in kinesiology. Examples of augmented feedback are praise, corrective directions, and specific information about the completed movement. This section will focus on how analysts can use feedback as intervention to improve performance. A great deal of research has been conducted on feedback in learning motor skills. Before we summarize the research, providing principles for using feedback as intervention, the next two sections will review the various classifications of feedback and the functions they serve in learning movements.

Functions of Feedback

Movement feedback has three major functions in helping people improve their performance: *guidance*, *reinforcement*, and *motivation* (Sage, 1984). Each function of feedback can be used as a target of intervention in the qualitative analysis process. Arguably, the most important function of augmented feedback is guidance, or information about how to perform the next practice trial. The guidance function of feedback is also often called the information function.

Guidance Function of Feedback

Guidance is the information that feedback provides to correct movement errors. Performers use the guidance function to plan the next movement response in the process of practicing and learning the movement. A therapist who wants to improve the safety of a patient's gait with a cane can use feedback to teach the patient how to position the cane relative to the injured leg.

The primary power of good augmented feedback is the guidance it gives in shaping future responses. The motor learning scholar Dr. Charles Shea illustrates this idea by describing feedback as "cognitive training wheels" for performers. Correct feedback provides the most appropriate mental images that help the person shape the next response, similar to bicycle training wheels set to an appropriate height. For example, a dance instructor might ask a dancer to keep his trunk more upright or vertical during a particular move.

> **KEY POINT**
> *Feedback used as intervention in qualitative analysis has three major functions: guidance, reinforcement, or motivation. These functions of feedback are what help the performer improve.*

A classic example of failure to use the guidance function of feedback occurs when a coach provides poor feedback, often in frustration as a performer repeats the same error over and over. Teachers or coaches may get caught in a correction complex that is sometimes manifested by a stream of *don'ts*. "Johnny, don't step in the bucket, son." "You did it again, don't lift your head!" Feedback with a *don't* message does not directly guide performers in what they *should* do. It also communicates a negative, discouraging message. More effective intervention would be to provide

feedback that helps the performer get the idea of what to do. For example, the teacher could say: "Johnny, remember to take a small step toward first base for outside pitches." Or "Remember to step about the width of a bat, Johnny."

A common error of novice golfers is to lift their head during the swing, which often affects the trunk and the plane of the swing. It would be poor feedback to say to such a student, "Don't lift your head!" A more creative coach might use the guidance function of feedback and say, "I would like you to really focus on the ball and only pick your head up away from the ball when I say lift!" The student takes his practice swing, concentrating on "head down, eyes on the ball," and executes a nice shot. "Hey! You didn't say lift," he says. The nice shot and the silence have made the coach's point.

Reinforcement Function of Feedback

The second function of feedback is reinforcement, which can be either positive to help encourage correct technique or negative to diminish the frequency of undesirable actions. Readers may remember Thorndike's law of effect (1927). When applied to learning motor skills, Thorndike's law would say that people tend to repeat responses that are rewarded and avoid responses that are punished. Feedback to a performer should begin with reinforcement of a strength of performance that the evaluation within qualitative analysis has identified. A therapist might tell a patient, "Great job! I know that was hard, but those were your smoothest, most even steps so far!" A strength coach might tell an athlete, "Nice job, Sheila! You kept your back straight for some very heavy squats!"

It is sometimes appropriate to provide negative feedback. Behavior that is inappropriate or dangerous may warrant a swift, negative response from the instructor. But this type of feedback should be used only sparingly and only in the right circumstances. Relying on negative feedback can result in an adversarial relationship with clients, which is neither productive nor pleasant. Psychologists also say that several positive reinforcers are needed to compensate for *one* negative reinforcement or criticism. Emphasizing positive reinforcement of appropriate behavior tends to decrease inappropriate behavior.

Motivation Function of Feedback

The third function of feedback is similar to reinforcement, but it focuses on providing motivation to practice. Indeed, many psychologists argue that this type of feedback is of primary importance. Teachers and coaches should provide positive feedback that rewards consistent effort and tends to create a positive attitude and climate. For example, elementary physical educators should carefully provide positive feedback that reinforces in each child the attitude, "I can do it." Pedagogy research has shown that good teachers provide a great deal of praise and positive feedback (Siedentop, 1991).

A recent study showed that specific, corrective feedback in a volleyball unit increased the number of successful practice trials in a junior high school physical education unit (Pellett et al., 1994). Clearly, a good intervention approach is to provide feedback that lets the performer know what to do next. This feedback should be expressed in a positive, encouraging manner. In coaching athletics or other high levels of performance, the coach is responsible for motivating the intense practice and training needed to prepare for competition.

The higher the skill level of the performer, the more important the motivation function of feedback becomes as intervention. The muscle memory that is the hallmark of skilled performance becomes a problem when an analyst tries to correct a weakness in performance. Intermediate and advanced performers often resist the intervention (Langley, 1993). They are often not motivated to make these difficult technique adjustments unless performance improves immediately, but performance usually suffers until the new motor pattern is learned.

Langley (1993) makes some useful suggestions for overcoming learners' resistance to intervention. Individual attention that focuses on the performance limitations of a technique problem and personal motivation to make changes help improve performance in these performers. The next sections summarize the research on how to select feedback that is effective in improving performance.

Classifications of Feedback: KR and KP

The two major classifications of feedback used in motor learning research are important to understand so that the analyst may select appropriate feedback as intervention. Feedback can be classified as either *knowledge of results* (KR) or *knowledge of performance* (KP). KR is information about the outcome of the movement or the extent to which the goal of the movement was achieved. KR is easily observable in some activities, like when a ball misses the basket or an arrow hits the bull's-eye. Other times KR may be unknown or less obvious to the performer. A sprinter may believe she won the race, but the photo and times it generates will provide more precise KR.

KP is information about the movement process, the actual execution or movements of the body. For example, a basketball student shooting a free throw receives KP from a physical education teacher who comments on her good wrist action at release. KP feedback in softball hitting might be "Keep more weight on your back foot at the beginning of the swing."

In some human movements, the outcome or goal is to move the body in a "perfect" or "stylistic" way. Judges at dance, diving, or gymnastic competitions have the difficult task of analyzing movement qualitatively. Coaches and teachers must realize that KP and KR are one and the same in these situations. The outcome of interest is the actual movement of the body. But usually these two classifications of feedback are different and provide unique information to performers when used as feedback during qualitative analysis. However, when providing augmented feedback as intervention in qualitative analysis, analysts should remember that KP is often more powerful in most situations.

Since the main function of feedback is to guide the learner in the next practice response, information on the actual movement and how it should be changed is often more valuable than the outcome or result of the movement. Several studies have examined motor learning when giving KP as feedback. A classic study that provided both KR and KP showed the power of KP feedback (Hatze, 1976). A 10-kilogram mass was attached to the foot of a subject, who attempted to minimize movement time in a leg-raising task. For the first 120 practice trials the subject received KR as movement time, producing the classic negatively accelerating learning curve (figure 8.1). With the effects of KR at a plateau, KP was provided as velocity-time curves of the optimal and subject's movement. A second learning curve occurred that approached the optimal movement.

Studies have shown the superiority of KP over KR if KP is provided as a continuous graph of the performance (Howell, 1956; Newell et al.,

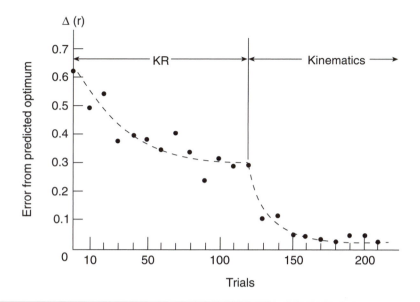

Figure 8.1 The guidance power of KP over KR in a kicking task.
Reprinted, by permission, from H. Hatze, 1976, Biomechanical aspects of a successful motion optimization. In *Biomechanics VB*, edited by P.V. Komi (Baltimore: University Park Press), 10.

1983; Newell, Sparrow, and Quinn, 1985). Recent biomechanical studies have shown how graphic presentation of KP can improve performance in cycling (Broker, Gregor, and Schmidt, 1989; Sanderson and Cavanagh, 1990). Research has shown that allowing the learner to control when the instructor provides KP results in greater learning than other fixed schedules of KP feedback (Janelle, Kim, and Singer, 1995). But don't let all this evidence give you the impression that KP is always the most effective form of feedback; in many of these studies, the goal of the movement can be easily defined in biomechanical terms.

In the real world of a clinic or gymnasium, much of this carefully controlled research is hard to apply. Gentile (1972) argues that too much emphasis can be placed on KP feedback in teaching motor skills. She proposes that KP is most appropriate when the movement itself is the goal of interest, as in a dive or a gymnastics routine. She also hypothesizes that undue emphasis on KP, when the goal of the movement is some other outcome, could interfere with motor learning. Gentile emphasizes that kinesiology professionals may direct the learner's focus to form and teacher feedback, limiting attention on the outcome (KR) of the movement. In these more open-environment movements, skill is essentially the ability to achieve the goal by reacting to changes in the environment.

Knowledge of results, therefore, is also an important and powerful feedback. Remember that

critical features can be related to the movement itself (KP) or a different outcome (KR). The trajectory of a basketball shot and the break of a baseball pitch are crucial aspects of performance and provide important information to the performer.

Another promising line of research involves the combined use of KP and KR feedback (McCullagh and Caird, 1990; McCullagh and Little, 1990). Kinesiology professionals performing an integrated qualitative analysis should select the mode of feedback that matches the movement and environment. When the analyst is confident that a critical feature related to body motion needs improvement, the research suggests that KP feedback is more effective. Let's look at some principles for providing feedback that have been supported by kinesiology research.

Principles for Providing Augmented Feedback

To summarize the kinesiology research on augmented feedback, we propose seven guidelines that will help the analyst shape the intervention chosen after the diagnosis phase. The feedback guidelines are based on the general consensus of the literature and are not meant to be a scholarly review of the subject. There are several good review articles dealing with movement feedback (Annett, 1993; Bilodeau, 1969; Lee, Keh, and Magill, 1993; Magill, 1993, 1994; Newell, 1976;

Newell, Morris, and Scully, 1985). There are also good professional articles on providing feedback (Sharpe, 1993; Tobey, 1992). Tobey suggested that the three main issues are that feedback be specific, immediate, and positive.

Neither are the guidelines intended to define an optimal approach to feedback. Kinesiology research has just begun to study what kinds of observational models (correct form, incorrect form, developing/learning form) given as feedback create the most learning (Martens, Burwitz, and Zuckerman, 1976; McCullagh and Caird, 1990; McCullagh, Stiehl, and Weiss, 1990). Other studies have tried to identify what modeling and critical cues improve performance best in children (Fronske, Abendroth-Smith, and Blakemore, 1995; Masser, 1993; Weiss, 1982). More such studies are needed. The best intervention for short-term versus long-term performance, for open or closed skills, and for the different stages of motor learning (Gentile, 1972) or motor development must also be determined. The best we can offer at this time are some guidelines that have consistent support within the kinesiology literature.

- Don't give too much feedback.
- Be specific.
- Don't delay feedback.
- Keep it positive.
- Provide frequent feedback, especially for novices.
- Use cue words or phrases.
- Use a variety of approaches.

Don't Give Too Much Feedback

A common mistake that many professionals, especially novices, make is to provide *too much feedback* to performers. Even if they understand the feedback, performers are often overloaded with several corrections, making it impossible for them to plan future executions to practice the movement. Coaches with a correction complex often rifle off a stream of corrections and feedback. This creates information overload (figure 8.2) for the performer and leads to paralysis by analysis. Remember that this problem is the reason there is an evaluation and diagnosis step in qualitative analysis. Diagnosis of performance results in the selection of *one* intervention to help the performer improve (Arend and Higgins, 1976; Hay and Reid, 1982; Hoffman, 1983; McPherson, 1990). Any feedback selected should also be directed at only one aspect of performance.

Practice and game performance can suffer from the psychological pressure of keeping too many things in mind. Too much information can be worse than no information. This overanalysis and extra feedback can create greater problems during competition. Psychological research has shown that in sports competition, the brain of a skilled right-handed performer has a very active right hemisphere (visual, spatial functions) and the left hemisphere (analytical functions) is essentially turned off (Torrey, 1985). The phenomenon is similar for left-handed players. When an athlete is so confident, focused, and relaxed that peak performance is achieved, this is called playing "in the zone." This experience may be accompanied by altered perception of effort, time, and

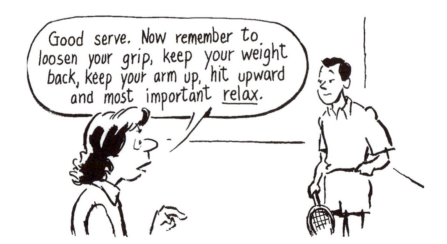

Figure 8.2 Too much augmented feedback as intervention can cause paralysis by analysis in performers. The subtle irony is that the important message of relaxation (essential in high-speed movements) is negated by the excessive corrections.

pain. A coach who provides too much information, forcing the athlete to overanalyze what she is doing, may hinder performance.

Be Specific

For feedback to guide the performer's next practice trial, it should be as specific as possible. Specific feedback focuses on the exact element and how it needs to be changed (Christina and Corcos, 1988). The feedback should also be specific to the motor skill and at the student's level of understanding (Lee et al., 1993).

A good example of specific feedback is a coach helping a Little League hitter. Using the word "step" to remind players to stride in the direction of the throw could be too vague. It would be more helpful for the athlete if the coach said, "Sally, remember to step toward the target at least two feet (60.96 cm)." The cue "step" could then be used as reinforcement for continued batting practice. In teaching and analyzing weight training, saying "Take a wider grip on the bar" is less useful than saying "Line up your hands on the hash marks right here."

An excellent way to make feedback specific and motivational is to tailor the feedback to each individual. Many factors interact to determine what will be effective feedback for a particular person and situation. The performer's stress level, age, and personality are all factors in the choice of feedback. A good coach or therapist tailors the exact mode of feedback, cue used, and tone of voice to the individual. To do this, the professional needs a feel for the person's attitude, body language, and interaction with others.

Research in pedagogy has demonstrated that the pattern of instruction in physical education usually results in initial general feedback regarding a common error of many students (Siedentop, 1991). Later the teacher begins to provide more specific feedback focused on the individual. Unfortunately, the majority of feedback in physical education is general rather than specific (Siedentop, 1991). How can analysts create specific, individualized feedback as intervention?

Considerable research from psychology on personality and learning styles is helpful in individualizing feedback. In general, learners tend to be visual, auditory, or kinesthetic. Visual learners respond well to pictures or diagrams, so demonstrations or videotape replays are effective for them. Auditory learners tend to relate to and remember the words used by an instructor, so cues are very helpful for them. Kinesthetic learners tend to use their bodies to help them learn. They could benefit, though, from manual guidance or limited verbal feedback intended to focus their attention on a specific aspect of their movement during practice trials.

Perceptive analysts use their insights about their clients' or students' learning styles to devise specific feedback for each individual. An analyst might choose to use a cue emphasizing proper technique with a verbally oriented novice to help him get the basic coordination or *motor program*. For visual or kinesthetic learners, the analyst would supplement traditional verbal feedback with other kinds of intervention like illustrations, diagrams, and *manual guidance*.

Don't Delay Feedback

Coaches' corrections and augmented feedback should be provided as soon as possible after the performance or trial because they will be used to plan the next practice trial (Lee et al., 1993). Immediate feedback, after observing several trials, helps learners make connections between that feedback and their kinesthetic sense and proprioceptive information (intrinsic KP) from the trial. The kinesthetic sense, proprioceptive information, and muscle memory of the movement are essential to learning motor skills.

The performer must focus on how the movement felt and relate this feeling to a judgment of its correctness. It takes time to think about the feedback and its association with the person's intrinsic KP. If feedback is immediate (within a few seconds), the performer has time to compare it with the experience. At least five seconds should also be allowed for the performer to process and integrate these two sources of information before further practice (Schmidt, 1991).

Research suggests that feedback need not be instantaneous and that summary feedback is effective in learning motor skills (Schmidt, 1991). Analysts can provide effective feedback that summarizes the performance of a block of several trials, though the potential link of the feedback with the performer's perceptions will be weaker. Many real-world settings are not like research settings, where feedback can be given very quickly. Creating ideal feedback conditions may not be possible in most clinical and field situations.

Keeping feedback close to the actual performance is another reason why the evaluation and diagnosis step of qualitative analysis is very difficult. The analyst must not only evaluate and diagnose the performance effectively but attempt to do it immediately. Certainly the validity of the judgment is most important, but it is also desirable to maximize the guidance function of the feedback by responding as quickly as possible.

Keep It Positive

To be most effective, augmented feedback should be worded to instruct the performer with a positive connotation (Christina and Corcos, 1988; Lee et al., 1993). Unfortunately, some teachers of motor skills have not followed this advice. Since motor skill teachers typically use visual models to identify "errors" in performance, their feedback may lapse into a series of *don'ts*. But selecting cues that are positive still tells the performer what to do, without sending a negative message.

Research in typical physical education settings has shown that the majority of feedback is negative (Siedentop, 1991). Negative feedback is sometimes appropriate, but it should not be the primary mode of feedback. There is a big psychological difference between the message, "Let's work on this" and "You still haven't done this right!"

In short, feedback should convey the message that the analyst believes in the performer so the performer is more likely to think "I can do it." When performers have self-confidence and self-concept problems, positive feedback is very important. Feedback should encourage the student and paint a positive picture of his or her potential (Ziegler, 1987).

James and Dufek (1993) suggest that intervention in qualitative analysis should refine strengths before correcting weaknesses in performance. Reinforcing or rewarding good performance characteristics helps athletes learn that part of the performance and may also help motivate continued practice. This is a good intervention strategy to make sure the feedback has a positive tone. A coach should say, "Great shot! Now step with your left foot over the blue line" rather than "You stepped with the wrong foot, Chet!"

So far we have focused on the tone of verbal feedback, but nonverbal communication should also be positive. Gestures, facial expressions, and other body language can strongly communicate positive or negative messages to performers. Analysts need to choose their intervention carefully and make sure their nonverbal communication is consistent with their positive verbal feedback. Patients and athletes will begin to doubt your credibility when they read differences between what you say and what your body language says.

Provide Frequent Feedback, Especially for Novices

Early in motor learning it is important for the teacher to provide frequent feedback to guide the learner's subsequent practice trials. To help prevent paralysis, provide some time for young learners to mentally process the feedback. In large classes teachers do not usually have a chance to provide too much feedback to any one student, so pedagogy research suggests that feedback rates should be high enough that every individual receives some feedback. In situations where there is more one-on-one qualitative analysis, intervention should follow the motor learning principle of intermittent reinforcement: Feedback is provided not with every trial, but almost randomly (in conjunction with a trial related to the feedback). The frequency of this intermittent feedback should decrease as the skill level of the performer increases.

As learners become more skilled, they need to rely more on their kinesthetic and proprioceptive intrinsic feedback than on the augmented feedback from the teacher. This is why analysts need to decrease the frequency of their feedback as performers become more skilled. In the advanced stages of motor skill, the kinesiology professional may question performers about what they feel were the good and bad points of their performance. Enlisting the athlete's help in the diagnosis can focus attention on the occasional correction.

PRACTICAL APPLICATION

Imagine you are a physical education teacher in a typical gym with 50 fifth graders. Your basketball unit is under way and you have the class at eight stations practicing shooting and ball-handling skills. Research in sport pedagogy suggests that to be effective, the teacher should move randomly throughout the gym, actively supervising practice, providing positive feedback to motivate students, and qualitatively analyzing their performances. Motor learning research has shown that the many novice subjects in this class require frequent augmented feedback to improve. How are you going to work it all in?

Your attention is drawn to Hugo, who is having difficulty hitting the spot on the wall for the chest pass. Observation and evaluation/diagnosis suggest that his step is correct, but his arms do not appear to propel the ball with enough speed. How do you select appropriate intervention when you focus on one performer to qualitatively analyze shooting? Your mind flies. "Quick! Hugo's throw, shooting, and push-up score are above average. Hugo is a great little person who always tries his best. I bet he needs a little more pronation and coordination with the extending arm." Your voice and smile turn on. "Nice pass, Hugo!" "I bet you could pass like Jason Kidd if you used your hands more." "Give me that upside-down five (hand slap) on this next pass." "Great!"

Moving on to the next performer, you give another general prompt/hustle to the whole class in your gym voice. "Squad four looks great! Kim and Hugo almost knocked the targets off the wall!" Looking over to squad five, you think, "Bobby looks like he needs some praise. Let's see what looks good in his shot." In 15 seconds, you have weighed information from many subdisciplines of kinesiology. Pedagogy and psychology considerations made it important for you to praise the effort and good aspects of the children's performance. Knowledge of the children made diagnosis and intervention of their basketball skills more accurate. You were also sensitive to the body language of a child who might need a little attention and praise to feel good about his shooting ability. The intervention you used for Hugo included augmented verbal feedback about the forearm action of the pass. You linked the feedback to a previous cue (upside-down five) and used some manual guidance by putting your hand in the follow-through position for Hugo's next pass.

Use Cue Words or Phrases

Kinesiology professionals have known for years that performers can remember and use information in practice better if it is presented in concise cue words or phrases (Masser, 1993). Many books are available that provide cues for teaching the skills of specific sports. There are also articles that suggest cues for teaching motor skills (e.g., Fronske, Wilson, and Dunn, 1992; Kovar, Mathews, Ermler, and Mehrhof, 1992). Fronske (1997) has compiled a book of cues for teaching many sports.

Good dance instructors are highly effective in their use of cues. Dance exercise instructors must carefully time their cues to the music, use as few words as possible, and combine nonverbal cues to lead the group effectively (Shields, 1995). Simple words like *grapevine, box, cross*, and *plyo* can carry a great deal of information to a performer that has been taught these movements. For example, the cue *plyo* can communicate to a step aerobics performer that a certain rebound move is to be executed next. A way to translate critical features into cue words or phrases was discussed in chapter 5.

Use a Variety of Approaches

A dictionary may lead a tourist to believe that words in a foreign language have multiple, but

> *In general, verbal augmented feedback should be specific and expressed positively with cue words or phrases appropriate to the performer.*
>
> **KEY POINT**

stable, meanings. Teachers who have written test questions or experimented with various cue words know that words have a variety of meanings and the changes in those meanings may be quite dynamic. This is why kinesiology professionals should collect cue words or phrases for each critical feature of the motor skills they teach. They will then be able to provide several cues to communicate the essential idea of each critical feature they evaluate.

Professionals should also try to have a variety of modes to communicate these cues as feedback. Some performers respond best to a verbal cue, others to a visual one, and still others to a kinesthetic one. Cues for the last step in a basketball lay-up might be verbal ("Long step and jump"), visual (footprints on the floor), or kinesthetic ("Make it feel like stepping over a beach ball").

Analysts need to use age-appropriate cues when teaching small children and cues using current slang when teaching in elementary and secondary schools. Most veteran physical educators or coaches will have had an experience similar to that of Jeanne Jones, who was teaching a basketball unit to junior high students. A particular student was having trouble shooting along the appropriate trajectory. Ms. Jones had worked with this student over several class periods, providing cues like "shoot with a high arch" and "shoot upwards" to help correct the angle of release. Finally, she used a cue that clicked with the student by saying, "shoot up through the top of a phone booth." The student began shooting better and said, "Why didn't you tell me this before!" Ms. Jones smiled, even though she wanted to say, "I've been telling you for the past week!" Jeanne Jones knew that she needed a variety of cues that she could use to communicate to the diverse group of people she taught.

To check to see if different feedback is needed, question students or clients on what feedback was given. A dance teacher could ask, "John, what were we working on with your waltz last time?" If the student is not making the changes you want, feedback should be repeated or rephrased. Questioning is a good technique for when you can't tell whether the performer understands what specifically you want her to work on (Christina and Corcos, 1988).

There are some tricks of the trade beyond traditional augmented verbal feedback for providing intervention to improve motor skills. They include using visual models, exaggeration, task modification, manual or mechanical guidance, and conditioning. While some of these could be viewed as some kind of feedback, others are clearly not feedback. Unfortunately, a narrow view of intervention may have limited the effectiveness of some professionals' qualitative analyses. These nonfeedback forms of intervention have not been studied from an interdisciplinary perspective to determine which are the most effective. The following sections describe some of these methods; analysts must make their own decisions about which methods are most appropriate.

VISUAL MODELS

There are several ways to provide visual feedback on the status of performance or a desirable correction to a performer. *Demonstrations* by the instructor may be effective because the majority of people have a visual learning style. Years of motor learning research have shown that modeling or observational learning is one of the most effective ways to convey information to people who are learning a new pattern of coordination or are establishing coordination in the early stages of learning a skill (McCullagh and Caird, 1990; Messier and Cirillo, 1989; Wood, Gallagher, Martino, and Ross, 1992). In *observational learning*, the analyst provides visual information like a picture or demonstration to a learner.

Posters of key body positions in exercise are highly effective in the weight room. The walls of elementary school gyms could have key cues and corresponding pictures for teachers to use as intervention. Such visual aids are excellent for improving the atmosphere of the gym and decreasing the stress on a teacher's body caused by demonstrating for many classes every day of the week. Figure 8.3 illustrates how a golf instructor can use a hoop to create a visual model of the swing plane of the golf swing.

Several scholarly reviews of modeling or observational learning research can assist the qualitative analyst in using this form of intervention (Gould and Roberts, 1982; McCullagh, Weiss, and Ross, 1989). Wiese-Bjornstal (1993) recently summarized the research in observational learning for practitioners to propose guidelines for providing good demonstrations. Multiple trials should be presented by a skilled model similar to the performers (McCullagh, 1986, 1987; Wiese-Bjornstal,

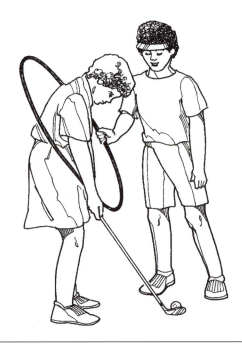

Figure 8.3 An instructor can use the visual image of a hoop to illustrate the desirable swing plane of the golf swing.

1993). The demonstration should also be presented from the performers' perspective (Ishikura and Inomata, 1995).

It is important, however, for analysts to understand that there are two situations where observational learning has not been shown to be superior to other types of feedback as intervention. Observational learning is not very effective in creating improvement in motor control or refining and customizing a movement to situational constraints. For example, watching a pitching coach demonstrate a pitching technique is not likely to help a high school pitcher improve his or her control or pitch location.

Another common form of visual intervention is the *videotape replay*. There has been a great deal of research on the effectiveness of motion pictures, loop films, and video replays in teaching motor skills. A classic review of video replay as intervention in learning motor skills was reported by Rothstein and Arnold (1976). The review examined 52 studies; the majority found no significant difference between video replay and normal teacher feedback. The more recent research on video intervention has supported these results (Emmen et al., 1985; Miller and Gabbard, 1988; van Wieringen et al., 1989). Although there is little scientific evidence that video replay as intervention is superior to traditional teacher feedback, its use for qualitative analysis may be justified. Chapter 11 discusses how to maximize the effectiveness of videotape for all the tasks of qualitative analysis, not just intervention.

EXAGGERATION OR OVERCOMPENSATION

The muscle memory that is necessary for skilled movement is also our biggest obstacle in creating changes in a movement. Because even small changes in technique can be very difficult for players to create, many experienced teachers and coaches exaggerate the desired correction in feedback. Good examples of this are the serve in tennis and shooting in basketball.

The initial trajectory of the ball in the tennis serve of recreational players needs to be nearly horizontal or slightly upward. A common error is to hit downward on the serve and net a lot of serves. Players who have trouble getting the feeling of the upward action of the serve can be encouraged to "try to hit the back fence" with the serve. Often this results in the desired small upward service action and a serve that lands deep in the service box.

Exaggeration or overcompensation can also be used to correct a common error in basketball shooting. Players often shoot on a low trajectory at the rim when they should have a higher angle of release. Telling players with this problem to shoot with a "high arc" is effective in improving shooting, although skilled basketball players do not really shoot with a high trajectory (Hay, 1993). This cue and the qualitative analysis of the jump shot are reviewed in chapter 9.

An analyst using overcompensation as intervention should do so with care. Whether the exaggeration is effective or not, the performer should be informed later that the cue words were not literally the truth. The analyst can explain that the exaggeration was necessary to create the desired change, or just that it is a good description of what the desirable technique *may feel like*. Do not let misconceptions about performance persist in athletes. Eventually the exaggerated technique may develop, or the cue may be passed on to other performers when it is inappropriate. Remember, the performers of today are often the instructors of tomorrow, and they are likely to teach as they have been taught.

> *Some techniques of intervention beyond traditional verbal feedback in qualitative analysis are the use of visual models, exaggeration of corrections, task modification, manual and mechanical guidance, and conditioning.*
>
> KEY POINT

MODIFYING THE TASK OR PRACTICE

An option often overlooked by professionals is to change practice as intervention to improve performance. The kind of practice used varies with the kind of motor skill being learned and the performer's skill level. Analysts must often make the practice easier for novice performers to accommodate strength and skill deficits. Coaches working with advanced athletes should change practice tasks frequently to challenge the athletes and maintain their motivation to practice. Remember that advanced performers require a great deal of practice to improve a small amount.

Fortunately, there is a large body of motor learning research on the effectiveness of various forms of practice and practice schedules. For example, the first (cognitive) stage of motor learning is focused on learning the basic motor program for a particular task. Good intervention for a person having trouble in this stage might be a combination of feedback and *modified practice*. Breaking the task into parts, making it easier, or eliminating attention to outcome could all be effective ways to modify practice to help learning. Schleihauf (1983) demonstrated that a successful way to modify breaststroke swimming practice was exaggerating the glide phase to give the athletes more time to cognitively process the coach's feedback.

The Practice Environment

The large cognitive demands of learning a new motor skill usually require that any change in practice as intervention should be performed in a *closed environment*, in which the conditions of the immediate environment do not change a great deal. The external factors of performance are reasonably consistent. Conversely, in an *open environment*, the conditions (opponents, obstacles, etc.) are changing.

Modifying practice in progression for a beginner learning to dribble a basketball would typically mean moving from a closed to a more open practice environment. The performer would dribble in a small area, dribble moving slowing in one direction, dribble around objects, dribble with others moving randomly, and finally dribble to avoid defensive pressure. In the early stages of learning, cognitive attention is focused on the movement. As the performer learns, attention can progressively be moved from the skill to the environment.

Practice Equipment

Another possible intervention in qualitative analysis is to change the equipment used by performers. Practice with different equipment can improve performance in several ways. Improvement in performance can be dramatic when the right equipment for a performer is identified, like the correct golf club length for a person's height or a children's tennis racket. Equipment that is lighter or heavier than normal may be used in practice to provide an overload or training effect. Training with under- and overweight baseballs has been shown to improve throwing velocity more than normal throwing (DeRenne, Ho, and Blitzblau, 1990). An analyst can modify equipment for practice or long-term use as an intervention strategy to improve movement.

Practice Scheduling

The prescription of practice and practice schedules has been a major area of motor learning research. The classic practice scheme in athletics of repeated practice trials without rest may not be the best way to learn motor skills. The practice of a movement may be organized (practice to rest schedule) along a continuum from massed practice to distributed practice. *Massed practice* employs many practice trials with little or no rest between them, while *distributed practice* schedules longer rest intervals between a variety of tasks.

For discrete motor skills (tennis serve, basketball shot), massed practice does not result in degradation of learning. For continuous motor skills where fatigue can be a factor, massed practice tends to decrease practice trial performance but has a small effect on learning (Schmidt, 1991). When prescribing practice as intervention, carefully evaluate the performer's situation and goals. Modification of practice interacts with many other aspects of physical training and with learning other motor skills.

Planning practice with multiple skills or tasks then becomes a factor in modifying practice as intervention. Practice of several movements can be either blocked or random. *Blocked practice* involves many repetitions or trials of a task in a block before another practice task is introduced. Motor learning research suggests this kind of practice leads to good performance in practice and an exaggerated sense of skill, followed by poorer long-term learning. Early in learning a new movement, blocked practice is effective in helping performers develop a basic motor program. *Random practice* has practice trials alternating rapidly among different movements. This results in poorer practice performance but better long-term motor learning (Schmidt, 1991).

If a complex movement can be broken into phases easily, it might be a good idea to provide intervention by *progression*. Part-whole learning is generally not as meaningful or as easy to put together as whole-part, but it's a good remedial approach for someone who is having a problem. An example is a student having trouble with footwork in the basketball lay-up. It might be good intervention to modify the task by allowing the student to carry the ball and work on the approach footwork in isolation.

The consensus of research suggests that if practice is to be modified to help improve motor learning, the approach should depend on the level of the performer, the kind of movement, and the other movements that are being learned. The quality of practice is very important, and the time spent on a task is less important than was once thought. It is clear that frequent changes in practice conditions, tasks, and repetitions assist in motor learning. A challenging practice session may look worse in execution, but the retention and transfer of skill in the long run is better (Schmidt, 1991).

Frequent changes in task and feedback are important if a performer is working on a difficult correction or change in a movement pattern. A good intervention strategy in situations like this is to change the practice task and then returning to the task of systematic observation. Remember that in the real world, the analyst can move from intervention back to observation. This immediate gathering of new information on performance and on the intervention's effectiveness should speed up the improvement in the client's performance.

The last thing to remember about modifying practice is that competition may be a big help in qualitative analysis. Most coaches know that you cannot look at practice and predict performance in actual competition. Some people thrive on pressure, while others fold in competitive situations.

Motor learning research shows that there is no simple association between practice performance and performance in retention trials (learning). Drills and practice should be changed frequently, with many activities involving competition and gamelike situations. Making practice drills competitive can help nervous performers get used to playing under pressure. In an intermittent activity like tennis, practice can mimic match conditions with short, intense drills followed by a short rest. Coaches can use this intervention and teach relaxation techniques for players to use during these breaks.

MANUAL AND MECHANICAL GUIDANCE

Sometimes a teacher physically moves or holds a performer's body in specific positions to give the athlete a feel for the position or action. This is called manual guidance. Spotting in gymnastics and having an athlete freeze on command so the coach can manually change his body position are examples of manual guidance. Giving the performer this kinesthetic sense of the position or action can be very effective, but the analyst must be careful not to violate people's cultural or personal taboos against being touched. Kinesiology professionals need to be sensitive to these sorts of concerns.

Mechanical guidance involves using some aid or mechanical device to help the performer make the appropriate movements (Lockhart, 1966). Mechanical guidance may be provided by a golf swing aid, a brace, or a strap. The sports of golf and basketball seem to have a continuous stream of mechanical devices being introduced that are supposed to help the player perform a swing or a shot correctly.

The problems with both manual and mechanical guidance are transferring the new feeling into practice movements and unlearning the older muscle memory or faulty motor program. It is very difficult for players to unlearn motor programs, especially if they have been using the movement for some time. Manual guidance should be used carefully; the analyst needs to make sure the performer understands that it will take concentrated effort and a lot of perfect practice to make the change. Manual and mechanical guidance may be most effective when the performer is at a low skill level and is comfortable with instructor contact (Lockhart, 1966).

Analysts also have to be very careful with guidance because it can risk injury. An example of this risk is given by Vic Braden, the famous tennis professional. A tennis pro wanted a player to get the feel of keeping his feet on the court during the serve to correct an early jump in his serve. The pro asked the player to serve with his foot in a shoe that had been fixed to a board that was nailed to the clay tennis court. The player served and got the feeling of an injured ankle! Helping the performer feel the correct movement can be effective, but it must be done with care. A tennis player dragging her toe and a golfer with a weight-shift problem can be made to feel their performance better if they remove their shoe to focus their attention on the foot in question.

CONDITIONING

If the analyst believes that a critical ability is lacking, appropriate intervention may be physical training or conditioning. A student who lacks strength to perform a skill might be helped by several intervention strategies: changing equipment, modifying practice, or prescribing physical training to increase strength. If a performer lacks dynamic flexibility to perform a skill optimally, an integrated qualitative analysis might prescribe a static stretching program in conjunction with modified skill practice to gradually increase range of motion. If a lack of a critical ability poses a risk of injury, intervention should focus exclusively on this issue until safe practice is possible.

Qualitative analysts often try to verify their judgments of physical limitations with physical tests (40-yard dash, vertical jump, three-hop test). Advancements in motor development, exercise physiology, kinanthropometrics, and sports medicine research may help identify key quantitative measurements related to performance and potential injury.

SUMMARY

The fourth task of qualitative analysis is the provision of some intervention to help the performer improve. Intervention is not limited to traditional augmented verbal feedback. It includes other methods to teach and train a person to move better. A rich history of research on feedback suggests that augmented verbal feedback used as intervention should be limited to a cue word or phrase that is as specific as possible and is given with minimum delay. Augmented feedback can be very effective if it is given in positive terms, as knowledge of performance (KP), and in language that is age-appropriate or specific to the individual.

DISCUSSION QUESTIONS

1. What kinds of augmented feedback are best for a novice, an intermediate, and an expert performer? Do these kinds of feedback vary with different sports or activities?

2. What motor skills would benefit from a performer focusing attention on intrinsic feedback as intervention?

3. How does the age of the performer affect selection of the mode of intervention in qualitative analysis?

4. You are a high school soccer coach. What are some hand signals you can use to provide intervention to players who cannot hear you in competition?

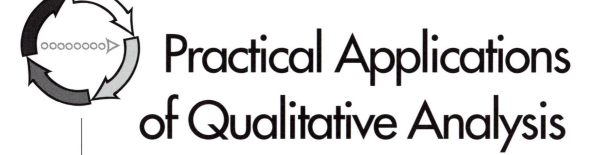

PART THREE

Practical Applications of Qualitative Analysis

Part III is dedicated to the practical application of our integrated model of qualitative analysis. The best way to illustrate an integrated model of qualitative analysis is to describe the process in several examples. Chapter 9 presents selected examples from a variety of human movements that are designed to highlight the interdisciplinary nature of the tasks of qualitative analysis. Video from real movement situations are illustrated for these tutorials in qualitative analysis. Chapter 10 poses hypothetical situations in which qualitative analysis could help solve problems in human movement. These situations put theory into practice and are therefore effective in bringing about discussions of qualitative analysis between professionals in different fields. Chapter 11 provides important technical and practical information on using video technology to enhance qualitative analysis.

CHAPTER

9

Tutorials in Qualitative Analysis
of Human Movement

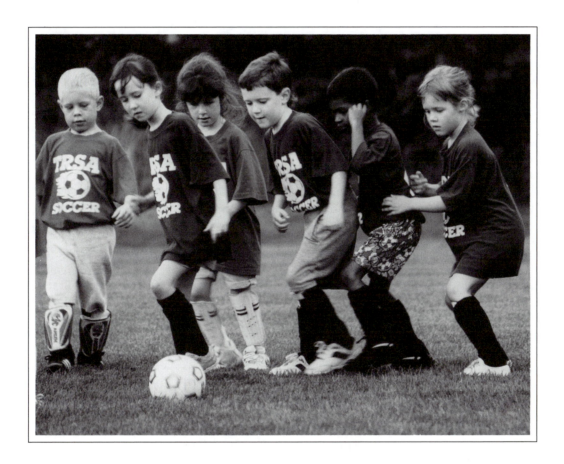

PREVIEW

Like the children in this picture, you may be asking yourself, "When do I get a turn?" This chapter will lead you through selected tutorials or practical examples of the qualitative analysis of six human movements. The skills are illustrated from video images of actual performances. Several different approaches to integrated qualitative analysis are illustrated. Explanations of the critical features, systematic observational strategies, evaluation and diagnosis, and intervention are presented for each movement. It is important to think about the differences in the depth of analysis required for different movements and performers.

Chapter Objectives

1. Illustrate an integrated approach to qualitative analysis of selected motor skills.
2. Discuss how the approaches to qualitative analysis of the presented skills differ.
3. Discuss how similar movement patterns may have different qualitative analysis strategies.

Research has conclusively shown that instruction in qualitative analysis improves ability at qualitative analysis, but this ability tends to be sport- or movement-specific. Qualitative analysis research has also shown that practice with many examples of correct and incorrect performances are necessary for the development of skill in qualitative analysis. This chapter cannot provide enough experience to make a reader a skilled analyst of human movement; it can only present some examples from a variety of human movement activities. Fundamental movement patterns (catching, overarm throwing, walking) and sport skills (place kick, jump shot, tennis serve) are presented to illustrate the process of an integrated qualitative analysis and to emphasize important issues in qualitative analysis.

The critical features and sample teaching cues are identified for each movement. These critical features and cues are based on research and the opinions of the authors. We do not present them as the only right or perfect choices, but simply as examples of an integrated qualitative analysis of human movement. As the performances get more complex, the amount of discussion and potential controversy over the critical features and the diagnosis of the performances will naturally increase.

The figures in this chapter are drawn from selected frames of normal video (30 frames per second) to illustrate critical features of real-world examples as closely as possible to the actual performance. Each subject's size is maximized to make them easier to see and because there is essentially unlimited viewing time. In real-world qualitative analysis, the analyst must be far enough away from the performer to use background objects to judge the motion of the body. The time between images is noted in the figure captions.

For each movement sequence, systematically observe the changes in body position based on the critical features and observational strategies presented. Use as much information from the text, illustrations, background, and figure captions as possible to inform your qualitative analysis. It is very important for professionals interested in developing skill in qualitative analysis to practice various observational strategies and approaches to qualitative analysis using videotaped or live movements.

CATCHING

The fundamental pattern of catching is a good movement to use to illustrate several important points about an integrated qualitative analysis. Qualitative analysis of this movement can be fine-tuned to apply to other specific catching skills. Qualitative analysis of catching is somewhat simplified because the goal or mechanical purpose of catching is clear and easy to evaluate. This, combined with an understanding of the sequential nature of the movement, makes the diagnosis of performance within qualitative analysis easier.

Critical Features

Several authors have reported models for the qualitative analysis of catching (Morrison and Harrison, 1985; Kelly et al., 1989b; Jones-Morton, 1991b). The majority of the technique points mentioned by these authors can be summarized in five critical features of catching in table 9.1, listed roughly in order of their occurrence in catching.

Systematic Observational Strategy

A systematic observational strategy for analyzing live or videotaped catching performances is based on the sequence or phases of the catching movement. Teachers should first observe the performer's state of readiness and attention to

Table 9.1
Critical Features and Cues for Catching

Critical feature	Cues
Readiness	Crouch, arms and legs flexed
Attention	Watch the ball
Intercept	Move to meet the ball; reach for the ball
Hand position	Thumbs in or out, fingers up or down
Ball momentum absorption	Give with the ball; retract hands and arms

the object being caught. Next, observation is focused on the motion of the body and arms to intercept the object. The final two critical features to observe are the position of the hands and how the body, arms, and hands give to dissipate the motion energy of the object. Figure 9.1 (pages 126-127) illustrates the performance of a child catching a bouncing tennis ball. Use the critical features in table 9.1 to perform an integrated qualitative analysis of the movement.

Subject 1

The subject was using a typical immature approach to catching, trapping the ball against her body. It looks as if the performer had her attention focused on the ball, was lined up with the ball, and was bending down with feet apart. Her readiness and preparation are a baseball coach's dream come true. The hands were in correct position, but the arms had limited forward reach to intercept the ball. Intervention could focus on motivational efforts to closely attend to the flight of the ball and anticipate where it will be. Providing feedback about giving with the arms is inappropriate if the person cannot first move the arms forward to intercept the ball in a position to give with the ball. Good intervention might be: "Good job! On the next try, watch the ball closely and move your hands to the ball." Or "Guess where the ball will be and move your hands there first." Is there any additional information that would help you improve the diagnosis and intervention? Would it be useful to observe additional trials?

Figure 9.2 (pages 126-127) shows the same child catching another bouncing ball in the *very next trial*. What intervention would be appropriate if you had just observed these two trials? Is this intervention different from what was suggested by figure 9.1? Why or why not?

The diagnosis of performance after the observation of two trials is easier and may result in different intervention compared to the diagnosis of only one trial. The child can catch correctly in an almost identical trial. Figures 9.1 and 9.2 are typical in teaching catching to young children. Teachers need to expect movement variability and *plan to observe several performances*. The best intervention may be to reinforce good attention and effort and to focus feedback on the critical feature of ball intercept. Good feedback could be: "Great job, remember to reach forward to catch the ball away from your body." The importance of reaching for the ball in catching has been supported by recent research showing that visual information on hand position is used in catching (Donkelaar and Lee, 1994).

Although not evident from figures 9.1 and 9.2, this girl frequently attempted to catch with her arms/hands to one side, with trunk and head motion away from the ball. Fear of the ball is an important issue for young children and may continue into adulthood. A good analyst should be aware of these fears and might change the observational situation to supplement observation. Throws could be faster or more difficult, or a soft foam ball could be introduced to see if the subject changes her approach to catching in different situations. Clearly, the observation of more catching trials would help improve performance diagnosis and intervention. An analyst who takes an integrated approach tries to observe multiple trials and evaluate all relevant factors about the performer and the situation.

Subject 2

Figure 9.3 (pages 126-127) illustrates an attempt to catch a playground ball by a young child playing catch with another child. Perform an integrated qualitative analysis of this performance. (Assume that several trials showed similar strengths and weaknesses.) This person and her partner were being very cooperative by tossing the ball directly to each other from a short distance. What could an analyst do to modify the task to gather additional information on this child's catching ability?

This girl exhibits several common errors that are typical at immature levels of catching motor development. She catches by attempting to trap

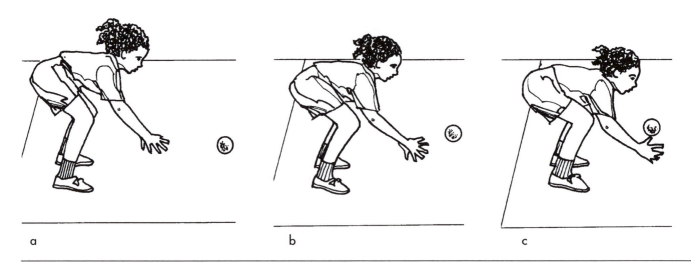

Figure 9.1 Sequence images of a child catching a bouncing tennis ball. What would be the best intervention to help this child improve her catching ability? Time between pictures is 0.07 seconds.

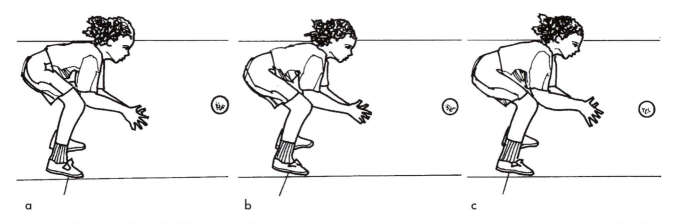

Figure 9.2 Sequence images of the same child catching in the trial immediately after the one illustrated in figure 9.1. What is the appropriate intervention in this case? What does this second observation tell you about the previous feedback? Time between pictures is 0.07 seconds.

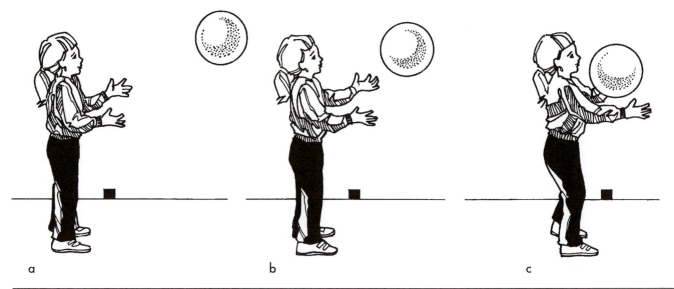

Figure 9.3 Sequence images of a child catching a large playground ball. What is the appropriate intervention in this case? Time between pictures is 0.07 seconds.

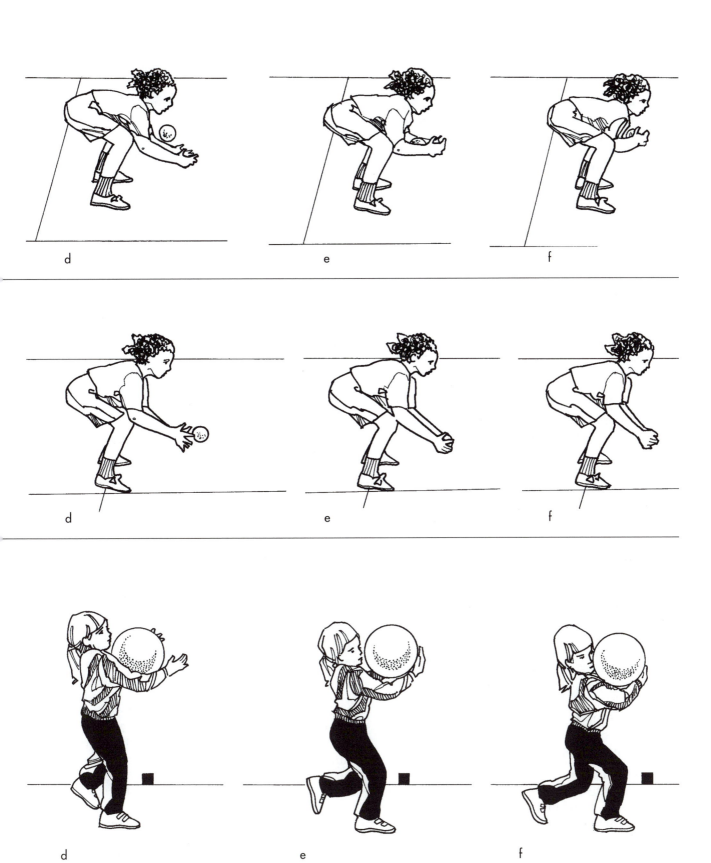

the ball between her forearms and her chest. Her body reacts to the ball after it has struck her body, turning her head to avoid contact with the ball. A good intervention strategy should modify the task to see if she would use more mature catching form if the task were made even easier. The analyst could have the children use a smaller and softer foam ball or could toss the ball to the child himself or herself.

Good feedback to give this performer would be to praise her attention and success at catching the ball. The analyst could use an indirect style of teaching and ask: "Does the ball sometimes bounce out of your grasp?" "What catching cues that the class learned would help you?"

SOCCER INSTEP KICK

Place kicking, or what we will call the soccer instep kick, is an adapted striking pattern involving the lower extremity impacting a stationary or moving ball on the ground. A variety of sports require skill in this movement. How could an American football coach or a soccer coach qualitatively analyze this kick?

Critical Features

High-speed kicking in a variety of sports has been extensively researched. The integrated qualitative analysis we suggest is based on this body of research and several models proposed by previous authors (Jones-Morton, 1990a; Kelly, Reuschlein, and Haubenstricker, 1990; Tant, 1990; Morrison and Reeve, 1986). There are six critical features to be evaluated in a qualitative analysis of the soccer instep kick (table 9.2). These critical features are also presented roughly in the order of occurrence in the movement. Does the movement sequence in kicking correspond to the potential influence of the critical features? If the objective of a placekick changes, do the critical features change in importance?

Systematic Observational Strategy

It is likely that several systematic observational strategies (SOSs) are effective for the qualitative analysis of human movement. It is, however, difficult to actually practice different SOSs with the figures in this chapter. Readers should try three systematic observational strategies when analyzing live or videotaped kicking performances. The most common strategy is to observe according

Table 9.2
Critical Features and Cues for the Soccer Instep Kick

Critical feature	Cues
Eye focus	Head down and watch the ball
Opposition	Turn your side to the target
Plant	Plant your foot next to the ball
Sequential coordination	Rotate your hip and leg
Solid impact	Kick through the center of the ball
Follow-through	Follow through toward the target

to the sequence or phases of the movement. A similar strategy is to observe from the origins of movement (from slower-moving to faster-moving segments). The third observational strategy is the gestalt approach, moving from general impressions to specific. Which observational strategy is easiest or most comfortable? Why do you prefer one over another? In the absence of evidence that a particular rationale for diagnosis is best, should novice soccer coaches observe in sequence and provide intervention according to the sequence of the movement?

The soccer kick is an excellent example of a motor skill involving sequential coordination for generating high speeds of a distal segment. Some soccer kick techniques have minor variations in these critical features to meet situational requirements. The kick will be dramatically different if the purpose is to travel accurately 10 feet to a teammate, versus getting as far from your own goal as possible. For example, the critical feature of solid impact would be less important in the short pass. The analyst would pay closer attention to the foot position at impact, the sound of the kick, and the trajectory of the ball to evaluate the quality of the impact for long kicks.

Slow-speed kicks do not require sequential coordination and may use the side of the foot to push the ball to a target. This leads to a common misconception, that the side of the foot is the desirable striking point for high-speed kicks. In reality, the neutral position of the hip and hard and flat surface of the instep (shoelaces) when the foot is pointed are what make the instep kick proper technique for high-speed placekicking.

Another common error is to minimize opposition by not approaching the ball at an angle. Efficient use of hip rotation and the levers of the lower extremity can be made by an approach angle to the ball between 30 and 60 degrees (Tant, 1990). The other common errors are not focusing attention on the ball, planting the foot behind or in front of the ball at impact, and an exaggerated concern for accuracy that typically results in slow foot speed and a limited follow-through.

Subject 1

Perform an integrated qualitative analysis of the kick illustrated in figure 9.4 (pages 130-131). The subject is kicking a stationary soccer ball toward a target to maximize speed and accuracy. What would be the best intervention in this situation? For figure 9.4 and the rest of the movements illustrated in this chapter, *assume that the performance strengths and weaknesses were consistent across several trials*.

The young person in figure 9.4 essentially achieved the goal of kicking the ball toward the target, and he keeps good eye focus on the soccer ball. There are weaknesses though in the critical features of opposition, foot plant, sequential coordination, and solid impact. Note that the foot position at impact with the ball is not totally clear. This judgment is even more difficult in real-time qualitative analysis of kicking. Is there anything else that can be modified in this situation? It would be quite obvious if the student were trapping, receiving passes, or blocking a shot on goal. If possible, it would be appropriate for the analyst to provide a smaller soccer ball, rather than the full size ball.

Intervention beyond a change in equipment must be focused on one critical feature, even though the player has quite a bit of kicking development ahead. Remember that in kicking development young children have difficulty impacting the ball and therefore typically approach the ball from behind and may even stop before kicking the ball. This player has enough experience to aggressively approach the ball, keep his eyes focused, and impact the ball. Intervention should focus on the foot plant or the opposition (an angled approach), because coordination is related to opposition and the correct foot position is difficult to achieve in a straight approach to the ball. A soccer coach could say either, "That's

a powerful kick Billy. I bet you can get even more power if you remember to *plant your foot next to the ball*," or "That's a great kick Billy. I would like you to try an angled approach to the ball. You can get more power if you *approach from the side* and *turn your side to the ball*." Once these basic techniques have been established the analyst should focus on the correct foot position at impact (toe down and kick with the shoe laces) which will maximize energy transmitted to the ball for a given foot speed. With this kick, a powerful sequential coordination of the hip and leg is most likely the last critical feature to develop.

Subject 2

Try another integrated qualitative analysis, this time of the instep kick illustrated in figure 9.5 (pages 130-131). This subject is also kicking for speed and accuracy in a game of mat ball (kickball with large mats for bases). Select appropriate cues for intervention. Remember the assumption that the strengths and weaknesses illustrated were consistent across several kicking trials. Do you think the subject in figure 9.5 is more or less skilled than the one in figure 9.4? Think about what critical features are most related to this decision.

The performer in figure 9.5 is kicking in a more open environment than placekicking a stationary ball. The smooth motion of the ball prior to the kick suggests that this trial may not be a difficult kick for this person to make. The critical features this player needs to improve are *foot plant, opposition, coordination*, and *solid impact*. Movements that may have caught an observer's eye were an upright trunk early in the approach, the knee quite bent at impact, and the very high and straight follow-through of the leg.

The subject approached the ball straight on and placed the plant foot too far forward for the speed of the ball. The optimal point of impact was passed because the plant foot was ahead of the ball by the time impact occurred. A good evaluation and diagnosis of this situation would likely lead to intervention on the foot plant or the approach angle/opposition. Providing cues on foot plant is helpful only if the person is consistently placing the foot too far forward. In an open environment like mat ball or soccer, the analyst needs many observations to make this evaluation. The ability to coordinate hip rotation and leg actions and to create a solid impact (get the leg, ankle, and foot almost completely extended at impact) are related to the approach and foot plant.

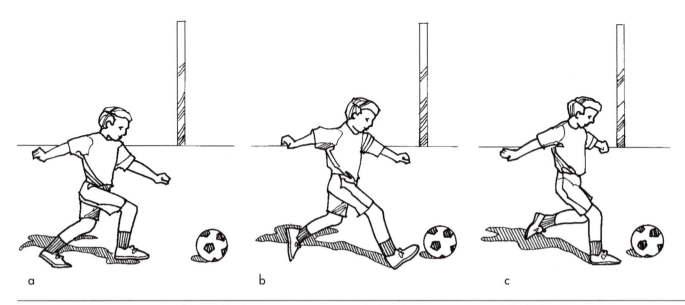

Figure 9.4 Sequence images of a child kicking a stationary soccer ball. What correction would help this player improve the most? Time between pictures is 0.07 seconds.

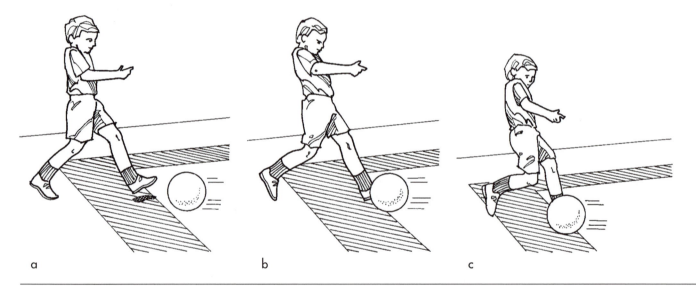

Figure 9.5 Sequence images of a child kicking a moving playground ball in a game of mat ball. What correction would help this player improve the most? Time between pictures is 0.1 seconds.

Providing a cue to work on an effective approach angle would be the best intervention to try. Examples might be "turn your side to the target" or "approach the ball from the side." The teacher might say, "That was a great kick, Cory! I bet you could get more power. Try to approach the ball from the side." The analyst could then repeat the qualitative analysis to monitor how that intervention affected critical features and overall performance.

Subject 3

The person illustrated in figure 9.6 (pages 132-133) is kicking a stationary soccer ball for speed

and accuracy. Perform an integrated qualitative analysis of this kicking performance in order to provide appropriate intervention for this performer.

There are no major weaknesses in the critical features in this performance. Note the performer's strong hurdle, foot plant, kicking foot position before impact, and forward body motion, all of which create a low ball trajectory. Analysts must use care in prescribing technique changes in skilled performers and must avoid the tendency to overcorrect. Because skilled performers have developed great consistency

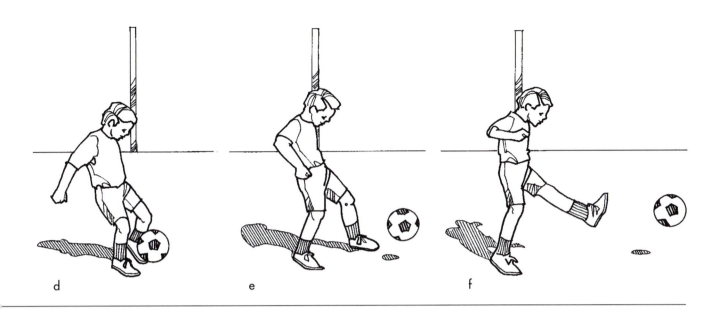

d   e   f

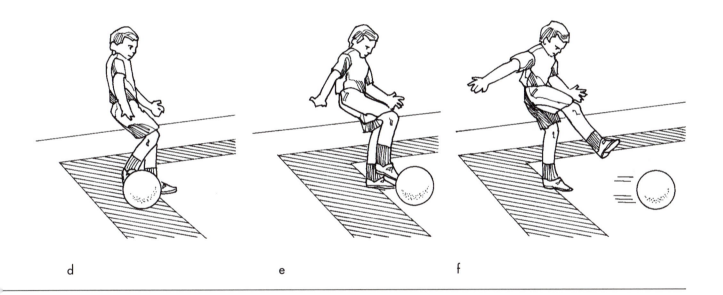

d   e   f

and control, changes in technique will take tremendous effort. Changes in technique should only be prescribed to prevent injury or when other interventions (conditioning, competition, practice, rest) will not produce improved results. Good intervention for this performer should be infrequent reinforcement and praise, followed by frequent modifications of the task. The performer may benefit from greater body lean to the side so that the foot can be angled diagonally across the back of the ball at impact. The main challenges for the analyst are maintaining the variety and intensity of practice.

BASKETBALL JUMP SHOT

Shooting in the game of basketball takes a variety of forms. The most common shot, however, is the jump shot. Jump shots in competition are difficult because of the small margin for error and the uncertainty of the defensive pressure. This section will illustrate the qualitative analysis of jump shooting, paying special attention to physical differences in performers.

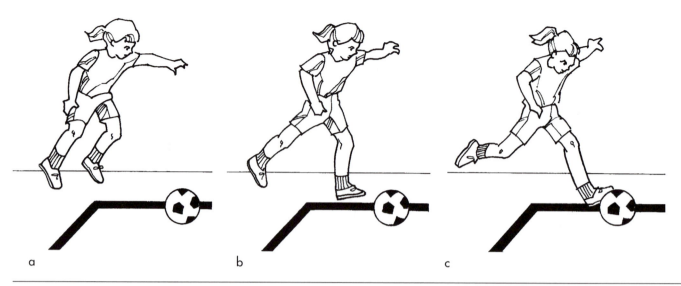

a   b   c

Figure 9.6 Sequence images of a performer kicking a stationary soccer ball. Are there any weaknesses in kicking technique? Time between pictures is 0.1 seconds.

Critical Features

The discussion of critical features for the qualitative analysis of the basketball jump shot is based on the review of the jump shot by Knudson (1993). Teachers and coaches of basketball need to be keenly aware of the open nature of basketball. The uncertainty imposed by the defense, teammates, and the clock can dramatically affect how a player shoots the ball. Factors like the distance of the shot, the age of the shooter, and the release height also affect the optimal release conditions for a shot.

Knudson reviewed the biomechanical research and identified six critical features for typical midrange jump shots (table 9.3). The critical features of the jump shot focus on both the motion of the athlete's body (KP) and the outcome variables of the ball motion (KR). This is an example of selecting critical features based on a consensus of biomechanical research. Performer characteristics like age and strength, or environmental factors (defense, basket height, ball size) are all able to influence the critical features of shooting in a specific situation.

Systematic Observational Strategy

The observational strategies to use with this model include moving from movement origins, moving from general to specific technique points, and rating the importance of the critical features. Carefully review the critical features of the jump shot and determine which are most important to improving shooting success. Are there any other key points of shooting a basketball that are left out? Prioritize the critical features and use them to guide your ob-

Table 9.3
Critical Features and Cues for the Basketball Jump Shot

Critical feature	Cues
Staggered stance and vertical jump	Boxer's stance
Shooting plane	Shooting plane; powerline
Optimized height of release	Release at the top
Angle of release	Golden arch; best path
Cooperation of upper and lower extremities	Smooth; jump and shoot
Ball rotation	Flip the wrist for ball rotation

From "Biomechanics of the basketball jump shot: Six key teaching points" by D. Knudson. Adapted with permission from the *Journal of Physical Education, Recreation & Dance,* February, 1993, 67-73. *JOPERD* is a publication of the American Alliance for Health, Physical Education, Recreation and Dance, 1900 Association Drive, Reston, VA 22091.

servation of the jump shot illustrated in figure 9.7 (pages 134-136). The performer was shooting a small basketball in a game situation toward a lowered (7-foot) hoop. What is the most appropriate intervention for the subject in figure 9.7?

Subject 1

The performance in figure 9.7 illustrates a typical transition period from a set shot to a jump shot.

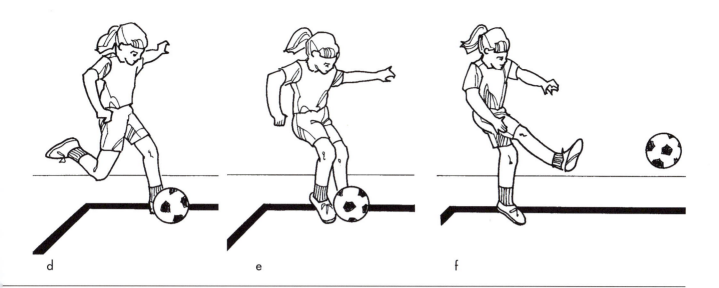

d   e   f

The person is also exhibiting a common error of many basketball players. The key outcome variables of the shot—the speed and *angle of release*—are not optimal for the ball to pass cleanly through the hoop. This weakness of shooting out instead of up may be related to the low *height of release.* Many performers tend to shoot the ball directly toward the rim (low arch and higher-speed shot) rather than up over the rim. These flat shots require greater ball speeds to reach the rim, since gravity makes the ball drop throughout the trajectory of the shot. This is a very important error because the hoop was low enough for the person to use the desirable trajectory.

The other common errors in this performance were jumping toward the basket and shooting *during* the jump. These errors could be related to a lack of strength or could be real technique errors that may have been developed by practice with regulation basketball equipment. The strengths of the performer are good alignment with the basket, cooperation of the arms and legs, and good backspin on the ball.

How does the analyst weigh these many factors in evaluating and diagnosing this performance? How does information from the disciplines of motor development, psychology, and motor learning contribute to the diagnosis? See if you agree with the following diagnosis and intervention.

The best intervention for this situation would be cues to correct the shot's angle of release. The performer has good cooperation of the upper and lower body and has good wrist action in shooting

the ball. A higher angle of release might indirectly improve the height of release; more importantly, it would increase the probability of making a basket. One good approach to intervention would be to use the following augmented feedback: "Excellent release and ball rotation!" Follow up by cues like: "Remember to shoot upward" or "Remember to shoot with a high or golden arc." Another cue using a visual image would be "Shoot up through the top of a phone booth," as if the shooter were standing in a phone booth.

Observation of subsequent shots could focus on the angle of the shot, the height of release, and the direction of the jump. All three of these factors can strongly affect the path of the ball. Cues like "release at the top" to increase the height of release might be helpful. With improvement in release parameters, intervention can focus on a more balanced position and vertical jump. For young basketball players like this, the least important factors to correct are the fine points of arm preparation not related to the shooting plane. As strength develops, the preparatory arm position can be moved up to the forehead from the set shot position in front of the shooting shoulder. The most important critical feature for shot accuracy is the shooting plane. It is easier to build with the strengths of the performer who shoots from a lower position than to make him or her bring the ball above the eyes, jump, and then shoot.

What aspects of performance were difficult to observe in these drawings? What aspects of this person's performance could you not make a decision about because of the lack of information? The

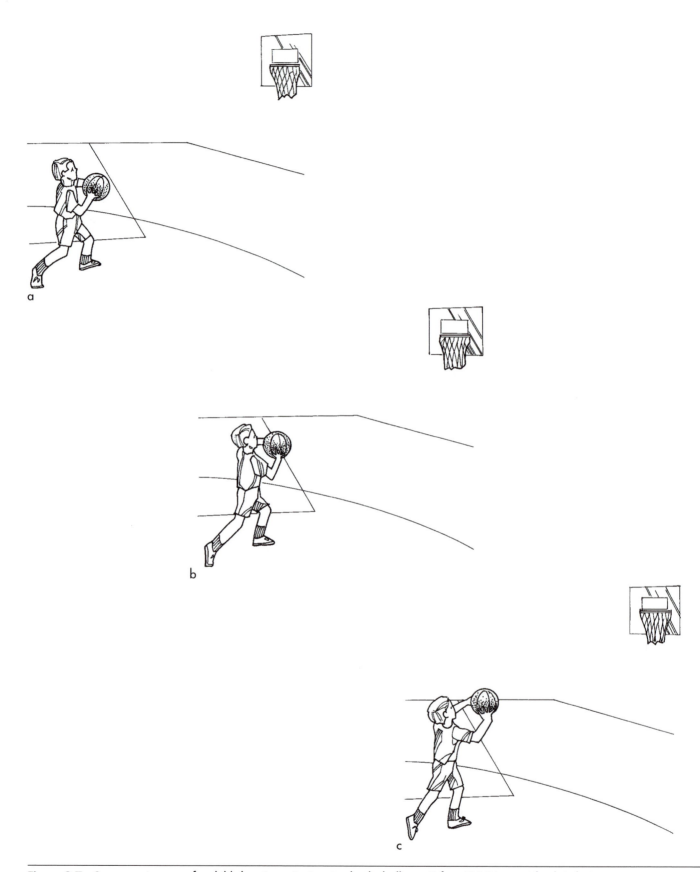

Figure 9.7   Sequence images of a child shooting a junior-size basketball at a 7-foot (2.13 meters) basket during a game. What intervention would be appropriate based on the qualitative analysis model presented? Time between pictures is 0.1 seconds.

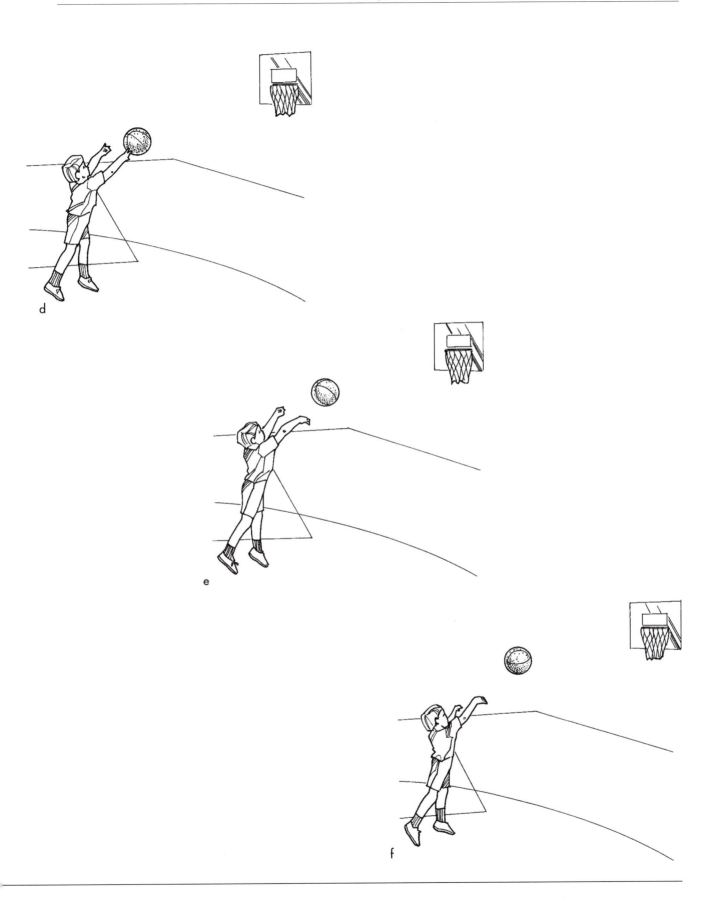

game situation made it difficult to catch the performance from optimal viewing angles. What other views of this performance would you be interested in seeing? Evaluation of the shooting plane and motion of the body would be improved if observations could be made from a rear view. Perform an integrated qualitative analysis of the jump shot of another subject from a different vantage point.

Subject 2

Figure 9.8 (pages 138-139) shows a 10-year-old shooting a junior basketball at an 8-foot basket. The vantage point provides an excellent perspective for most of the critical features except the shooting plane. Many critical features were performed well, with weaknesses in the *staggered stance and jump*, the *height of release*, and possibly the *shooting plane*. Ideally, the analyst would move behind the subject to check his alignment in a shooting plane with the basket. What other vantage points might be of interest?

The subject uses both the upper and lower body well and is just getting strong enough to shoot with correct jump shot form in these conditions. Note that the subject takes the ball back behind the head and coordinates the arms and legs simultaneously. The height of release is limited due to the lack of a jump, not lack of extension of the body or arm. Providing intervention for the stance and jump or the shooting plane will likely help the performer. Unfortunately, these are difficult corrections, and they are related to each other.

The analyst might try this approach to intervention: "Your shot has super arm action, but let's try to get more power from your legs." The analyst might also focus on the jump by saying, "Jump first and then shoot." Providing a cue for the jump might increase the height of release and ball speed enough that the shooter would not have to take the ball behind the head. This may be the best approach to intervention of this situation, since improvement in the jump may affect the weakness of taking the ball back behind the head and maintaining a shooting plane aligned with the basket. As with the previous performer, this switch from a simultaneous push to a jump with a slightly delayed upper-body shot may be difficult to develop and may need to come in time with an increase in strength. An analyst coming to this conclusion could change practice by moving the performer closer to the basket. Many basketball players like to take long shots, well beyond the perimeter of where they can score consistently.

Another approach to diagnosing this performance would be to prioritize the shooting plane as the most important correction. Good feedback would be, "That arm action is almost perfect. Remember to keep your *shooting plane aligned* with the basket," or "Try to keep the ball aligned with your dominant eye." The analyst might later explain the importance of this powerline for shooting accuracy. This correction will also be difficult for the performer to change, so the analyst will need to provide motivation. Correcting the shooting plane is important because of its effect on accuracy. The problems are the difficulty of the change and the potential lack of enough strength to achieve desirable form.

Subject 3

The child illustrated in figure 9.9 (pages 140-141) is shooting a basketball at a 7-foot basket with a technique that is transitional between a set shot and a jump shot. What would doing an integrated qualitative analysis of this situation help the analyst to suggest to help this performer?

The ball size and basket height are appropriate for this performer, but another situational factor is strongly affecting performance. This person is attempting a shot near the limit of her strength, and it is a shot that a coach would not like to see attempted in competition because of its poor chance of success. There are weaknesses in the angle of release, height of release, and vertical direction of the jump, but these might be related to the distance of the shot. There appears to be good cooperation between the legs and arms, and the wrist appears to create the proper ball rotation. This performer appears to align herself with the basket, although this is a bad vantage point from which to make this assessment.

The best intervention would be to have the player shoot several times from positions closer to the basket. If this technique persisted, the analyst should focus on the stance and vertical jump. This might help create a more effective angle of release and improve the height of release. Feedback at this stage could be, "Those shots look very good. On the next few shots, concentrate on jumping straight up." The analyst goes back to the task of observation to see if the performer effectively makes this change and if the ball's angle of release is affected. When actions are related, it is important that the analyst observe practice trials and evaluate and diagnose those trials before intervening any further.

OVERARM THROWING

Overarm throwing is an important fundamental movement pattern in many sports. This section illustrates an integrated qualitative analysis of the overarm throw in conditions with different goals. Like the previous examples, analysts will need to be sensitive to how the goal of the movement may affect the importance of critical features.

Critical Features

The high-speed overarm throw is another movement that has been extensively researched. The classic review by Atwater (1979) summarized early research on the biomechanics of overarm throwing and the related injuries. The extensive motor development research on overarm throwing was summarized in chapter 2 (Roberton and Halverson, 1984; Wickstrom, 1983; Wild, 1938). Jones-Morton (1990b) proposed five critical elements for analyzing the overarm throw: Step with opposition, open up, rotate the trunk fully forward, elbow leads with elbow extension, and weight transfers from the back to the front foot. Kelly et al. (1989b) used five qualitative criteria for the forceful overhand throw of fourth graders: side orientation, near complete arm extension backward in the windup, weight transfer to the opposite foot, marked sequential hip and shoulder rotation, and follow-through beyond ball release.

We summarized this research and professional opinion on overarm throwing in a paper presenting our integrated model of qualitative analysis (Knudson and Morrison, 1996). Since forceful overarm throwing is a vital skill in many sports, this section reviews our six critical features of overarm throwing. These critical features and suggested cues are presented in table 9.4.

Overarm throwing should be analyzed relative to the goal of the throw. The conditions at release of the ball are most strongly associated with accomplishing the goal of the throw. The critical feature the analyst can easily observe in evaluating this aspect of performance is the *angle of release* created by the initial trajectory of the ball. Like the basketball jump shot, the outcome of the throw is largely determined by the ball speed, spin, and most importantly by the angle of release. Biomechanical research has shown that air resistance plays a major role in the flight of most balls. The optimal angles of projection for throwing balls for horizontal distance in most sporting

Table 9.4
Critical Features and Cues for the High-Speed Overarm Throw

Critical feature	Cues
Leg drive and opposition	Step with the opposite foot; turn your side to the target
Sequential coordination	Uncoil the body
Strong throwing position	Align arm with shoulders
Inward rotation of arm	Roll the arm and wrist at release
Relaxation	Relax your upper body
Angle of release	Throw up an incline; throw over the cutoff's head

From "An integrated qualitative analysis of the overarm throw" by D. Knudson and C. Morrison. Adapted with permission from the *Journal of Physical Education, Recreation & Dance*, July/August, 1996, 17-22. JOPERD is a publication of the American Alliance for Health, Physical Education, Recreation and Dance, 1900 Association Drive, Reston, VA 22091.

situations are between 35 and 42 degrees above the horizontal (Dowell, 1978). A common error in young baseball players is to throw the ball with a very high trajectory. This limits the throw's effectiveness for baseball in two ways. It limits the length of the throw and increases the time it takes to cover the horizontal distance thrown.

Leg drive and opposition is the critical feature that combines the thrower's stance and step, setting up the rotations of the body to provide most of the power of the throw. The athlete creates opposition by turning the nonthrowing side of the body to the target as well as pushing off the back leg to step toward the target. Mature high-speed throwing uses a forward step greater than half the person's height (Roberton and Halverson, 1984). Research has shown that body rotation from good opposition contributes 40% to 50% of the ball speed, while the step contributes about 10% to 20% in skilled throwers (Miller, 1980). A vigorous leg drive that is channeled into body rotation is an essential technique point in high-speed throwing. Common errors are to rely too much (overstride) on leg action and to not transfer the energy from the stride to hip and trunk rotation.

Sequential coordination is the precise timing of accelerations of a proximal segment that transfer

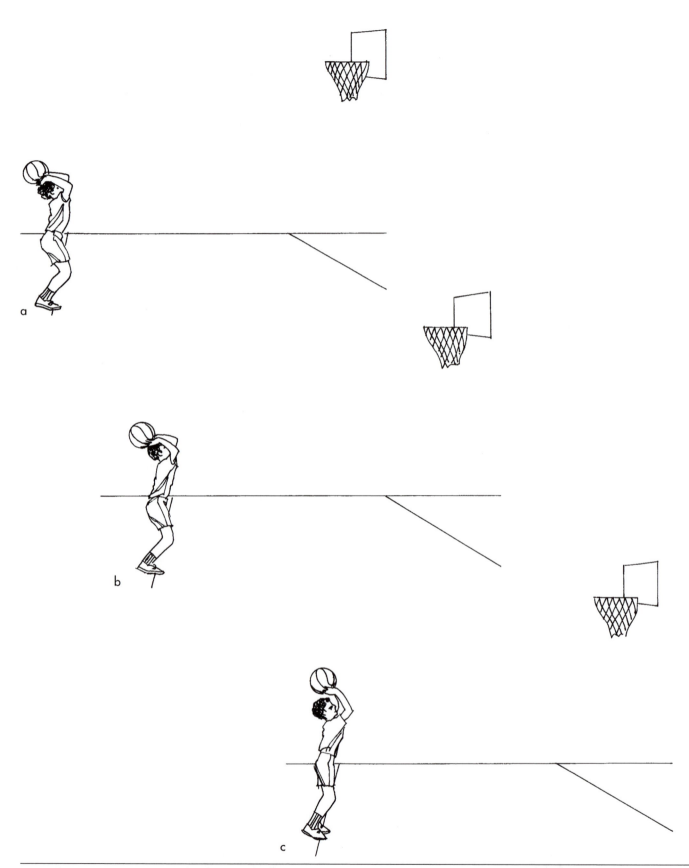

Figure 9.8   Sequence images of a child shooting a junior-size basketball at an 8-foot (2.44 meters) basket. A different intervention from the Knudson et al. (1993) critical features may be needed. What should the person work on and what information leads the analyst to this decision? Time between pictures is 0.1 seconds.

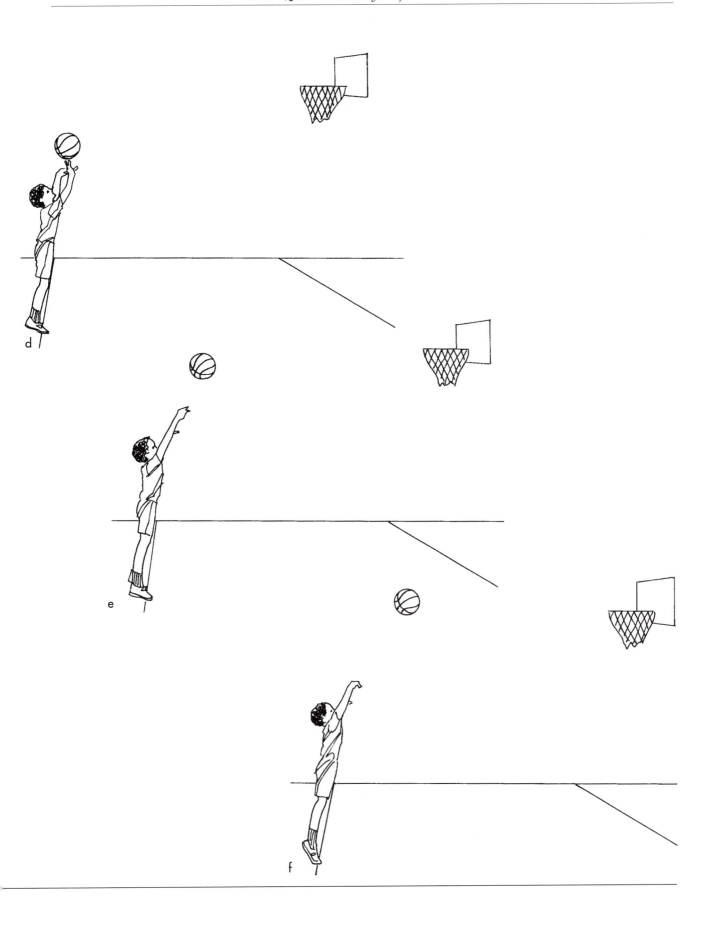

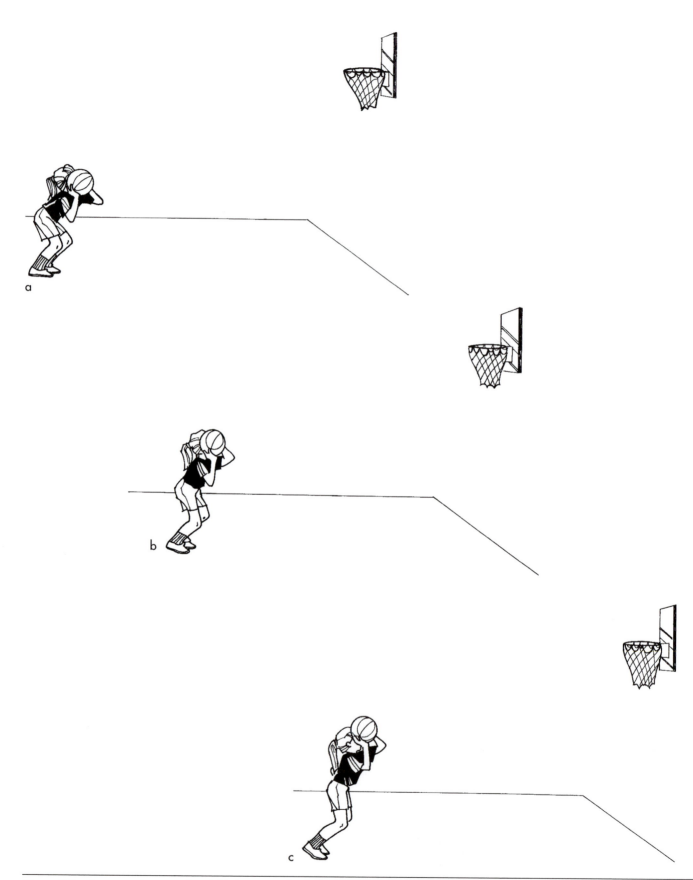

Figure 9.9 Sequence images of a child shooting a basketball at a 7-foot (2.13 meters) basket during a game. What intervention would be appropriate based on the qualitative analysis model presented? Time between pictures is 0.1 seconds.

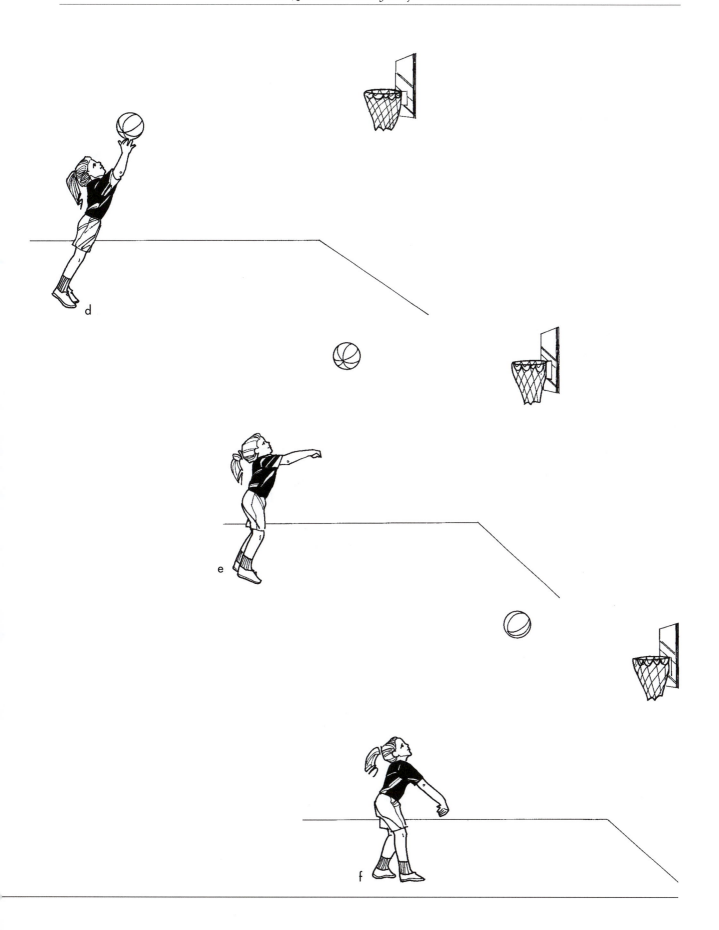

energy to distal segments to increase their speed. The forward acceleration of a proximal segment eccentrically loads agonists, and the later negative acceleration of the proximal segment uses joint forces or segmental interactions to speed up the distal segment. This concept of the interaction of a linked system of body segments has become known as the kinetic link or the kinetic chain (Kreighbaum and Barthels, 1985; Steindler, 1955). The sequential action of the leg drive, hip rotation, spinal rotation, arm, and forearm/hand action is required to generate high-speed throws. Roberton and Halverson (1984) have described the qualitative changes in various parts of the body in the development of sequential coordination in the overarm throw. Good form in the overarm throw is illustrated from two views in figures 9.10 and 9.11 (pages 144-145). This person is a highly skilled college baseball player.

A *strong throwing position* maintains alignment of the humerus at a right angle to the longitudinal axis of the spine (Plagenhoef, 1971). This position maximizes the speed transferred to the arm from the rotations of the hips and trunk. Atwater (1979) found this alignment (90 ± 15 degrees) to be a relatively invariant aspect of most throwing motions. In other words, there should be little difference in upper-arm position in sidearm or overarm throws, just differences in the lean of the trunk. The throwing position and trunk lean at release are observable from a rear view of the thrower (figure 9.11). The preparatory arm action in skilled overarm throwing typically involves a circular, downward backswing, with the upper arm aligned with the shoulders and the elbow maintaining a 90-degree angle after this backswing.

Inward rotation of the humerus and forearm is a major propulsive and injury protective action in the overarm throw (Atwater, 1979). The critical feature of *inward rotation of the arm* should be understood as the *combination* of humeral inward rotation, radio-ulnar pronation, and wrist flexion that provides the final propulsion of the ball. This and *relaxation* help create the final sequentially coordinated actions of the throw. A great deal of energy is transferred up the body, and good timing of the forearm pronation and wrist flexion can create that additional "pop," or great ball speed, of skilled throwers. Throwing with a "dead wrist" does not fully utilize the energy from the more proximal segments and fails to use the final joints in the kinetic chain of the throw. Recent biomechanical studies of the

kinetics of baseball pitching have increased our understanding of the stresses overarm throwing places on the upper extremity (Feltner and Dapena, 1986; Fleisig, Andrews, Dillman, and Escamilla, 1995).

Systematic Observational Strategy

We proposed a four-phase observational strategy for the qualitative analysis of the overarm throw (Knudson and Morrison, 1996). In the initial trials, look for timing, rhythm, signs of tension, and the trajectory of the throws. This is difficult to do from illustrations alone. Second, in the next few trials observe leg drive, opposition, and hip and trunk rotation. Third, observe the throwing position of the arm. Last, try to look for evidence of sequential coordination in the fast actions of the arm by looking for lag in the trunk, humerus, and forearm. This kind of observational strategy, focusing on body segments and actions, is similar to the Gangstead and Beveridge (1984) observational model. Figure 9.12 illustrates the movement of a woman throwing a softball for speed and accuracy, while figure 9.13 shows the overarm throwing pattern of a child. Analyze these sequences qualitatively and prescribe intervention to improve their performances.

Compare and contrast this observational strategy with the systematic observational strategies presented earlier using live or videotaped throwing performances. Compare differences in observational strategies with different critical features, especially the stages and components discussed in the motor development literature (Roberton and Halverson, 1984; Wickstrom, 1983). What aspects of other systematic observational strategies are incorporated into the Knudson and Morrison (1996) observational strategy?

Subject 1

The woman in figure 9.12 (pages 146-147) was a star college athlete, but not in a ball-throwing sport. Like many people, her throwing motor development stopped before a mature pattern had been achieved. Evaluation of performance could lead an analyst to praise the strengths of two critical features, strong throwing position and trajectory. The analyst must then diagnose the weaknesses in the remaining critical features. The major weaknesses are in her opposition and leg drive and the sequential coordination of the throw. Poor timing and coordination can be visually identified by the fact that the elbow and hand are well forward of the shoulder at release.

The best intervention for this performer may be to work on *opposition and leg drive* before sequential coordination. Much of the power for overarm throwing comes from a good opposition and leg drive, so the fine-tuning of sequential coordination will not be possible until the performer learns to move her legs, hips, and trunk forward powerfully as the arm moves backward. The weaknesses in a relaxed performance and inward rotation of the arm are less important and should be evaluated later, when coordination has improved.

Good feedback for this performer would be to praise some aspect of her throw (arm alignment and angle of release are good) and provide cues like "Turn your side to the target" or "Let's use that good leg to drive more by first turning sideways to the target, stepping forward, and powerfully rotating your trunk into the throw." The age of the performer allows the analyst to include more information with the feedback on this critical feature.

It is not likely that good *sequential coordination* would develop without strong leg drive and opposition to transfer energy to the arm from the legs and trunk. Motor learning and motor development literature suggest that after good leg drive and opposition, intervention could focus on relaxation and letting the sequential coordination (lag in the arm and forearm) develop with practice. It would be a good idea to provide feedback on the goal ahead and the practice required to improve throwing coordination.

Subject 2

Figure 9.13 (pages 146-147) illustrates the overarm throwing performance of a child throwing a softball for maximum distance in a competition. The goal of the performance is different from the goal in the previous example, so the analyst needs to know the desirable trajectory for throwing a ball for maximum horizontal distance. Qualitatively analyze the performance in figure 9.13 in order to help this performer throw farther.

The performer has several strong critical features of overarm throwing. He has good opposition and keeps his arm aligned with his shoulders. Improvements could be made in *leg drive*, *sequential coordination*, and the *angle of release* of the ball. The performer is trying so hard that he exaggerates the step, but he has limited weight transfer. It is hard to tell from the figure, but there is limited sequential coordination (simultaneous rotation of hip and trunk), and the angle of release is a little high.

If this boy were consistently throwing the ball with this technique, the best intervention would be to correct the leg action in the throw. Good initial verbal feedback would be to say, "That was a strong throw, John. I'd like you to concentrate on pushing your weight from your right foot to your left." Good leg drive will provide more energy that can be channeled into body rotation and eventually to the ball. The forward thrust of the weight shift may also pull the angle of release down. This feedback could be followed with a cue like "step" to help him remember in practice.

Let's see why focusing on the weight shift could be the best intervention. Remember that the prioritization of corrections depends on the performer's goals and the analyst's rationale for diagnosis. For many high-speed movements, sequential coordination is the last refinement for optimal performance. The development of sequential action will be limited until energy from the lower extremity can be channeled up the body. Correcting the angle of release will immediately improve performance because it is often an easy correction to make. But it may not be the best correction if the angle of release is related to the leg drive and subsequent loss of balance, rather than the typical child's perception that high throws go the farthest.

TENNIS SERVE

The qualitative analysis of the tennis serve provides an interesting contrast to the overarm throw. The overarm throw is the fundamental movement pattern associated with the tennis serve, and several authors have attempted to document the similarities between these two movements in order to examine the potential transfer of learning (Adrian and Enberg, 1971; Anderson, 1979; Miyashita et al., 1979; Rose and Heath, 1990; Zebas and Johnson, 1989). Much of the tennis service action is different due to the use of a racquet and rules restrictions on how the serve can be delivered. The ball must be tossed, must be hit in the air without the body changing position on court, and must travel over the net and land in the correct service court. Classic tennis instruction has a specific pattern for good

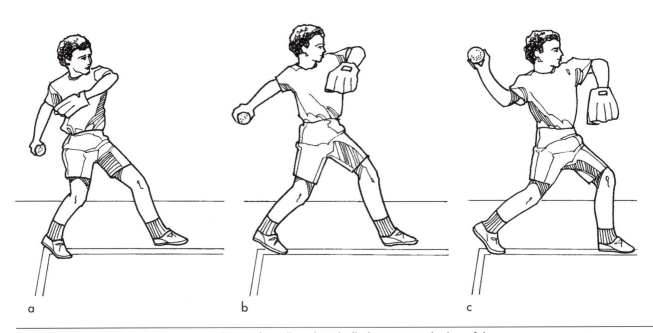

Figure 9.10 Side view of the overarm throw of a college baseball player. Note the lag of the upper arm one picture before release. Time between pictures is 0.1 seconds.

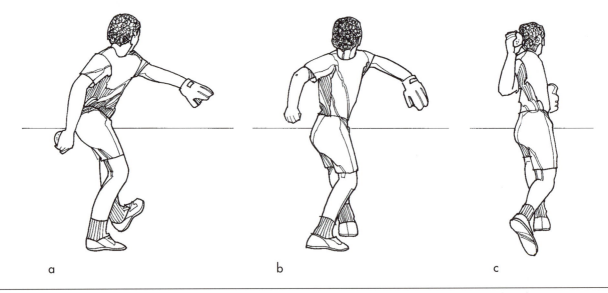

Figure 9.11 Rear view of the overarm throw of the same college baseball player. What aspects of performance are visible in this view that are not visible in figure 9.10? Time between pictures is 0.1 seconds.

form of the tennis serve, with small variations for different ball spins and match tactics. Note how the critical features of the tennis serve differ from overarm throwing.

Critical Features

A myriad of tennis books, magazines, and professional articles provide opinions on the important aspects of classic form for a good tennis serve.

Several models for the qualitative analysis of the tennis serve have been reported in the literature. Two physical education articles are noteworthy. Rose et al. (1990) proposed a model for the qualitative analysis of the tennis serve based on components similar to the motor development of the overarm throw. The integrated model for qualitative analysis of the tennis serve presented here is based on the paper by Knudson, Luedtke, and

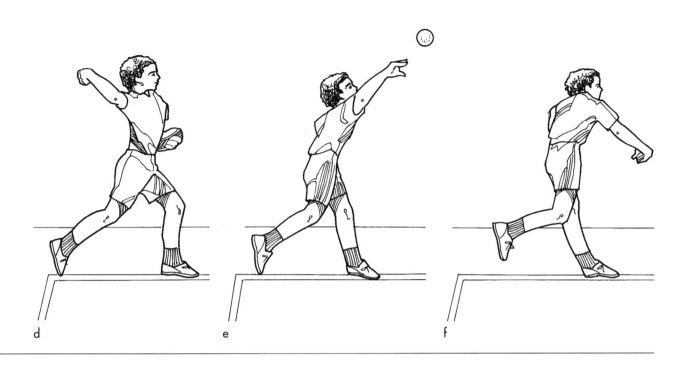

d   e   f

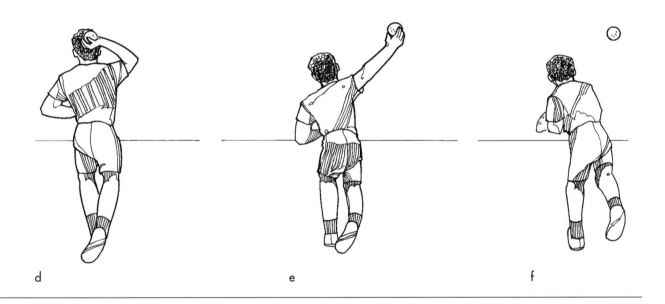

d   e   f

Faribault (1994). They proposed six critical features of the tennis serve and cues in order of importance. The critical features and a few of the cues suggested by the article are summarized in table 9.5.

Systematic Observational Strategy

If these critical features are in the correct order (ultimate importance in learning and serve performance), qualitative analysis is simplified. First, the systematic observation is based on the importance of the critical features; second, the diagnosis of performance is simplified because intervention can be provided in this order. Use the Knudson et al. (1994) qualitative analysis model for the tennis serve in the following two examples. Analyze the performance in figure 9.14 (pages 150-151), using the critical features listed

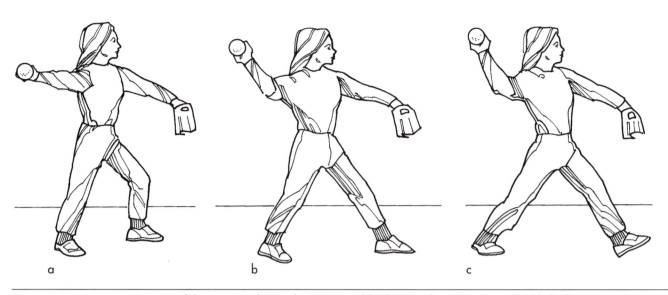

Figure 9.12   Sequence images of the overarm throw of a 20-year-old subject. What correction would help this person improve the most? Time between pictures is 0.1 seconds.

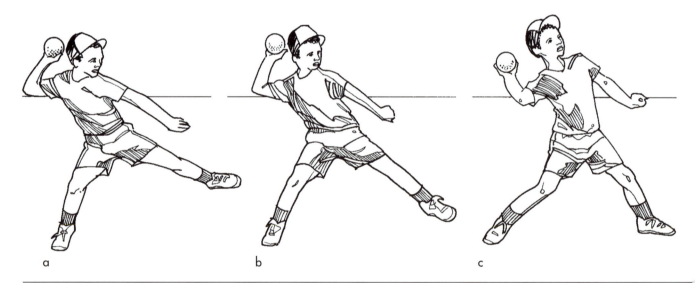

Figure 9.13   Photo sequence of the overarm throw of a boy throwing a softball for maximum distance. What correction would help this person improve the most? Time between pictures is 0.1 seconds.

in table 9.5 (page 148). This person was a beginning tennis player in a college tennis class when the video was made.

Subject 1

The woman in figure 9.14 does not fit into the desirable range of correctness for several critical features. Her major limitations are the use of a western (frying pan) *grip*, a *toss* that is not high enough, limited *upward* motion in the hitting action, and an abbreviated *follow-through*. This situation is common for many tennis instructors teaching novices. Many tennis novices will simplify the serve to make contact with the ball and increase the chance of hitting the ball in the

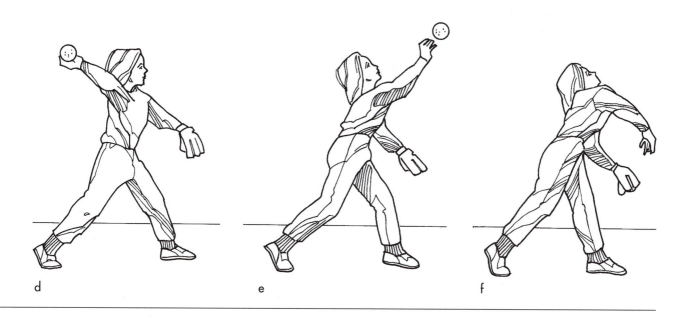

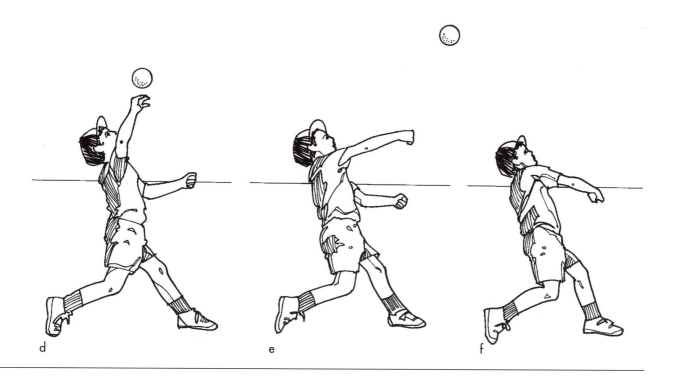

service court. What correction would help this performer improve the most? The Knudson et al. (1994) approach suggests that providing a cue like "Use a hammer grip" would be the most important feedback. The coach might say, "That serve had great timing! Check your grip, I think you need to slip your hand back to that hammer grip." Qualitative analysis of subsequent trials could help determine whether corrections were needed on the toss, upward hitting action, and follow-through.

Does the use of prioritized critical features make qualitative analysis easier? Does this qualitative analysis also have potential biases? The answer to both questions is probably yes. Diagnosis of performance is quite easy once weak

Table 9.5
Critical Features and Cues for the Tennis Serve

Critical feature	Cues
Grip	Hammer grip; loose and relaxed
Toss	Consistent placement; elevate the ball
Preparation	Trophy; coil the body; backscratch
Continuous upward motion	Uncoil; extend the wave
Follow-through	Release the wrist
Stance	Align your heels; slow and throw

Note. Critical features and cues are presented in order of importance to performance in the tennis serve. From "How to analyze the serve" by D. Knudson, D. Luedtke, and J. Faribault. Adapted with permission from *Strategies: A Journal for Sport and Physical Educators*, 7(8), 19-22. Copyright 1994 by the American Alliance for Health, Physical Education, Recreation and Dance, 1900 Association Drive, Reston, VA 22091.

critical features have been identified. The most important critical features are corrected first. This is also the potential bias of this approach. Some tennis instructors would not agree with the importance placed on the grip. For decades, there has been a controversy over which grip to teach beginning players—the best, advanced grip (continental grip) or the easier eastern forehand grip. There is a trade-off. Will the performer have the most difficulty as a beginner getting the ball into play with the best grip or later as an intermediate trying to improve to the next level by unlearning the eastern grip? The ideal situation would be to have research evidence that shows learning the continental grip is the most effective way to learn the serve. If this research has been done and the analyst has done his or her homework, the qualitative analysis will be unbiased. Potential bias is a concern when the analyst is not sure of the priority of the critical features of the movement.

Subject 2

Qualitatively analyze the tennis serve of the performer illustrated in figure 9.15 (pages 150-151). This person was also in a college tennis class, but she had more experience than the person in fig-

ure 9.14. Will the intervention suggested by your analysis be easier or harder for the performer because of that experience?

The weaknesses of this performer are more subtle and are related to two critical features. The performer's toss has an exaggerated style that creates a *toss* that is too high and consequently makes the serve hitch or pause. Note the large arm rotation in preparation to toss the ball compared to the performer in figure 9.14. Experienced tennis coaches might notice that the arm action in preparation is scissors-like, moving initially in opposite directions rather than the traditional "down and up together" motion of the arms.

The second critical feature with problems is a *continuous upward motion* of the body. The high toss creates a pause after the weight shift. The upward action of the serve then begins without the energy that the lower extremities created earlier. Another possible symptom of this pause, not visible in the figure, is a slight dragging of the right toe. The sound of a dragging toe or visual inspection of the court and the performer's shoes can be clues to this limitation in performance.

How to provide intervention in this situation is a classic example of a major difficulty of diagnosis, the interaction of many factors that affect performance. Slowing the toss and making it lower may not directly synchronize the service action. The performer's body will likely go through its normal action, pause, and attempt to hit a ball that is now much lower that it should be at the contact point. Unfortunately, the other alternatives for intervention may be worse. Slowing the body *preparation* may not create much energy to transfer up the kinetic chain of the body or provide much eccentric stretch of muscle to contribute to the hitting action. Attempting to modify *stance*, weight shift, or foot action affects balance, which in turn affects the other changes being made in the kinetic chain. The performance would clearly improve if a slow-and-throw rhythm replaced the player's rush, pause, hit coordination. The toss, preparation, hitting action, and stance all *interact* to create the rhythm and service action.

The high toss and hurried racquet preparation are clearly creating a hitch in the service action. Slowing down and simplifying the toss would improve performance in the long run. Good intervention would combine a demonstration and feedback. The analyst could demonstrate the serve, focusing the player's attention on a three-count rhythm. Good feedback would include cues like "Slow down your preparation. Remember to slow and throw." Or "Smoothly build up racket speed like an ocean wave." Improving service rhythm will be difficult and usually results in short-term decreases in service performance.

This is another situation where the performer is mature enough to handle more advanced feedback. During a break, she should be given a detailed breakdown of the strengths and weaknesses of her serve. The coach might explain that the hitting action of the serve is great, but adjusting the toss and racquet preparation can improve consistency and power. The how and why of these changes and a long-term plan for improvement should be discussed. This will help motivate the player to make difficult adjustments and tolerate the initial decrease in performance.

Subject 3

Qualitatively analyze the service of the player in figure 9.16 (pages 152-153). This person is a professional tennis player who was an ATP rookie of the year and has ranked in the top 20 in the world for several years. If you were this player's coach, what intervention would you try? You will have trouble persuading the player that your intervention is worthwhile, since his results have been good and you are working for him.

This player performs all the critical features of the tennis serve well. (Few players rate among the best of a world-class field in tennis without a strong serve.) There is only one aspect of his serve that could be improved, the timing of the racquet preparation and toss. This athlete's toss is very high because it is not synchronized with the racquet preparation. He also lifts the racquet straight up, rather than the usual circular drop and lift simultaneous with the toss. It is possible that the timing of the toss/preparation and the kind of arm backswing in his serve are style factors that do not limit performance. If the player were to change his service preparation, would that substantially improve his serve? If so, how difficult will it be? Will the improved performance be worth the difficulty and initial decrease in serving ability? With a highly skilled player like this, how much input should the athlete have in this decision? Professional athletes can fire their coach, while collegiate athletes cannot.

Let's assume that you decide that changing the player's serve will improve his performance. You decide that a lower toss will be less affected by wind, the faster delivery will be more difficult to return, and the traditional backswing will create a larger eccentric muscular stretch prior to the upward swing. Professional tennis players compete in a year-long season. There are few long breaks during which this player could work on changing his serve, but you convince him to extend a break in tournament play. This resting phase of his periodization training cycle is extended to a month and a half. What intervention would be appropriate in practice during this break from competition? How do you motivate the athlete? How do you gauge success in practice and during the tournament play to follow?

In a one-to-one coaching situation like this, the analyst has much more time to provide intervention to improve performance than most coaches. This athlete is typically more mature and knowledgeable about the sport. One approach would be to say, "Let's talk about some small serve changes to work on during your down cycle. You've been serving with a great first and second serve percentage, but I think with a few minor

PRACTICAL APPLICATION

Have a partner perform overarm throws and tennis serves. How are the overarm throw and tennis serve similar, and how are they different? Are similar critical features of the same importance in each of these skills? Do differences in the serve and throw remain consistent across different performers? Does the ability to qualitatively analyze transfer to other similar motor skills?

Perform your own mini-experiment by practicing qualitative analysis of live or videotaped tennis serves and overarm throws. Both activities are difficult to analyze because of their speed. What outcome variables (ball accuracy, speed, spin) may be useful in giving the analyst information about performance elements that are difficult to see? Do you think skill in qualitative analysis of the overarm throw will transfer to skill in qualitative analysis of the tennis serve? Do you think skill in observation of the overarm throw helps in the qualitative analysis of the tennis serve?

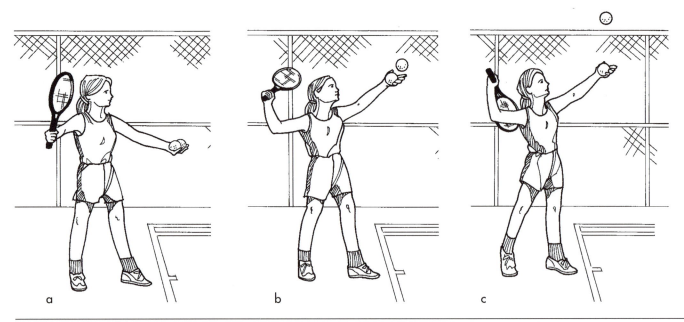

Figure 9.14 Sequence images of a beginning tennis player performing a high-speed tennis serve. What correction would the qualitative analysis system suggest is most appropriate? How similar is this tennis serve to the overarm throw? Time between pictures is 0.2 seconds.

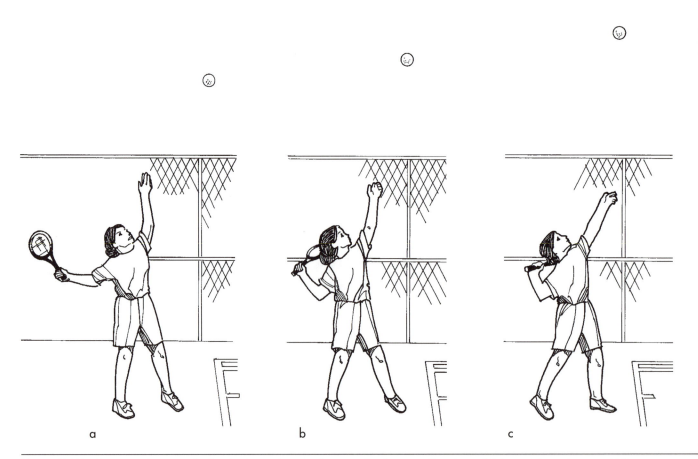

Figure 9.15 Sequence images of a beginning-to-intermediate tennis player performing a high-speed tennis serve. What correction would the qualitative analysis system suggest is most appropriate? Time between pictures is 0.2 seconds.

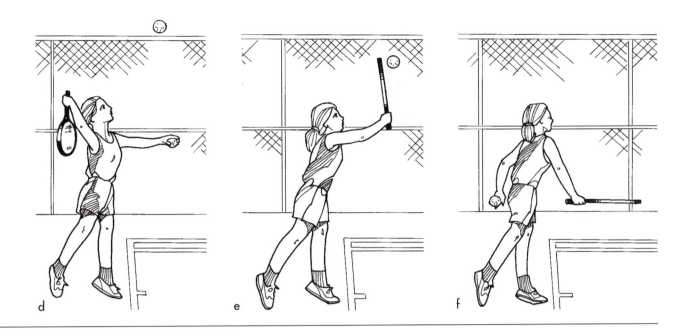

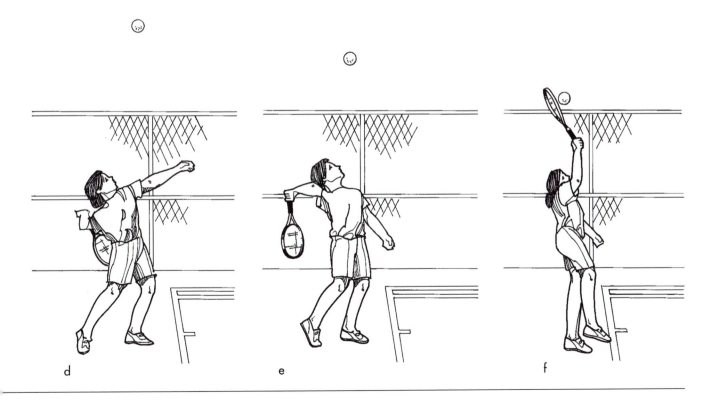

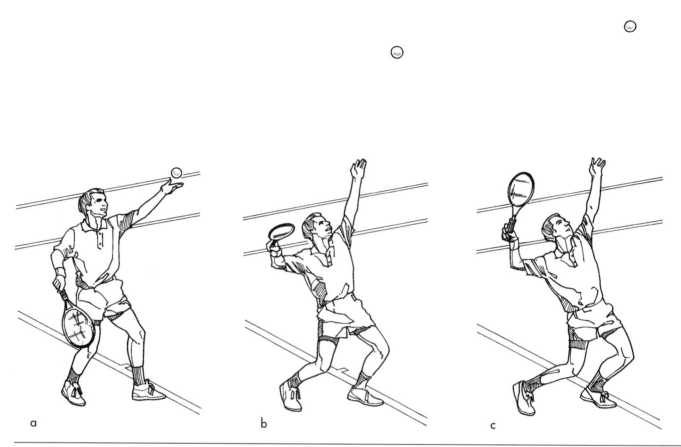

Figure 9.16   Sequence images of a professional tennis player performing a high-speed tennis serve. What correction would the qualitative analysis system suggest is most appropriate? Time between pictures is 0.2 seconds.

changes you could make your serve an even bigger weapon." After listening to his reply, you could propose, "The consistency and deception in your serve can be improved if we work on your toss. The power of your serve can be improved by changing your racket preparation to more of a drop and lift." Listen to the athlete's opinion on these suggestions, and together decide which corrections, if any, should be attempted.

As the coach, you should also lay out the long-term practice plan. Build the player's confidence so that he can improve his serve and so that it will pay off. Progress can be monitored by continual qualitative analysis of the serve, radar measurements of service speed, and results and serve statistics from practice matches. It is important to show the athlete that you have a plan to monitor his progress toward the goal.

HUMAN GAIT

Most people automatically perform some qualitative analysis of gait as they passively observe others walking. We have all experienced a situation where we recognized someone we knew by the walk long before we could see the person's face. Our visual attention is drawn to specific aspects of a person's gait. Qualitative analysis of gait in physical therapy is typically more complex than qualitative analyses for such activities as an overhand throw and a tennis serve. Walking, like other human movements, has important critical features. The integrated qualitative analysis system for human walking here is based on six critical features common in clinical analyses of gait. This model is simpler than the ones many therapists use. Qualitative analysis of gait in physical therapy involves greater depth of analysis into the musculoskeletal system because the therapist is knowledgeable about the patient's medical history, physical testing, and rehabilitation. In fact, the purpose of qualitative analysis of gait in physical therapy usually extends beyond observable function to what musculoskeletal limitations are affecting the patient.

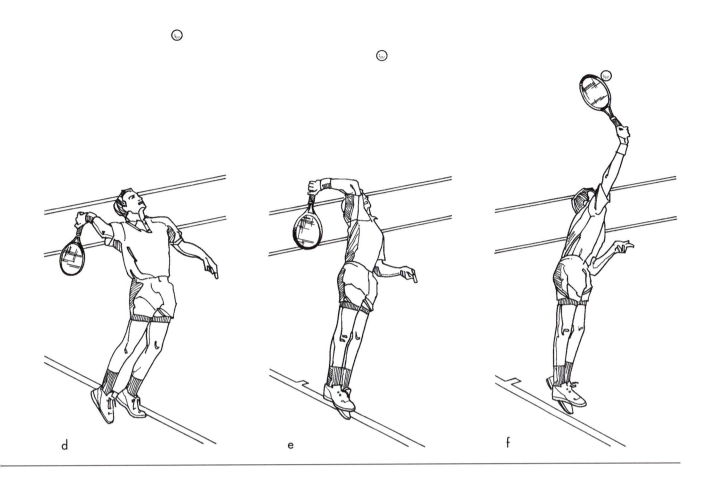

Characteristics of Human Gait

Human gait is an example of an overlearned fundamental movement pattern that, in normal situations, is performed with a great deal of efficiency and consistency. People start walking as infants struggling to control balance against gravity and later become children and then adults who can walk skillfully without conscious effort. The characteristics of normal gait have been extensively documented (Whittle, 1991; Winter, 1987, 1989; Woollacott and Shumway-Cook, 1989). Gait is a classic example of the flexibility of motor control provided by the brain. In normal gait, the kinematics (angles, distances, and speeds) of the lower extremity are highly consistent. The kinetics (muscle forces and torque), however, can be quite variable in creating the exact same kinematics or pattern of motion (Winter, 1984). This flexibility of neuromuscular control is an important ally of the therapist attempting to compensate for a patient's deficit, but it can be a difficult problem in the analysis and diagnosis of problems in gait.

The goals of qualitative analysis of human gait in typical clinical settings vary depending on the limitations and needs of each patient. Rehabilitation of minor injuries may require limited qualitative analysis and gait training, while more serious problems require extensive qualitative gait analysis, rehab, and gait training. In general, gait analysis has goals that vary from establishing safe gait to improving gait until it is more functional, and finally to more cosmetic gait. A cosmetically normal gait is very important to many patients. The issues that therapists usually try to evaluate are range of motion, strength, gait pattern, and the need for orthotic devices. Thus, gait qualitative analysis in physical therapy is essentially a biomechanical analysis to determine the cause of an observed gait abnormality.

A good review of typical gait analysis and common gait abnormalities can be found in Lehmann (1982). Eastlack et al. (1991) identified four major observational gait analysis systems that are used in physical therapy: the child prosthetic-orthotic studies observational gait analysis form (New

York University), the Rancho Los Amigos Hospital normal and pathological gait syllabus, the functional ambulation profile, and a guide to the visual examination of pathological gait (Temple University). Most of these analysis systems are organized around the biomechanical characteristics of normal gait.

Normal gait has a high-energy *stance phase* (60% of cycle) and a lower-energy *swing phase* (40% of cycle). There is a short period (25%) of double support, when both feet are in contact with the ground. The key events of the stance phase are typically called heel strike, foot flat, midstance, and toe-off. The important events of swing are acceleration, midswing, and deceleration.

The Biomechanics of Gait

The primary biomechanical trait of human gait may be efficiency. The motor development of walking begins with the instability, wide stance, and raised arms of an infant and gradually progresses to a precisely controlled and highly efficient movement pattern. Most of the upward or side-to-side movements in walking are typically less than two inches, which minimizes the energy expended to move the body. One of the most well-established descriptions of normal gait is the landmark "determinants of gait" proposed by Saunders et al. (1953). These six actions of the body in normal gait minimize the motion of the body's center of gravity to make walking efficient.

Normal gait involves *pelvic rotation* of about 4 degrees forward and backward in the transverse plane. This pelvic motion minimizes vertical motion of the body and the amount of hip flexion/extension in walking. The second determinant of gait is about a 5-degree downward *pelvic tilt* in the frontal plane to keep the body from rising as it is moved over the stance leg and the other leg swings through. Normal *knee flexion* in midstance is 10 to 20 degrees. A small amount of *ankle dorsiflexion* enhances the functional length of the leg and cushioning at heel strike. *Ankle plantar flexion at toe-off* helps smooth out the body's vertical motion. *Minimal lateral motion* of the body is the final determinant that helps maintain balance over the narrow base of support in normal walking.

Critical Features of Human Gait

Based on this review of human gait literature, we propose six critical features of human gait, which are related to the three dominant biomechanical features of human gait: maintenance of posture and balance, support actions, and control of foot recovery (Winter, 1989). Table 9.6 summarizes these critical features.

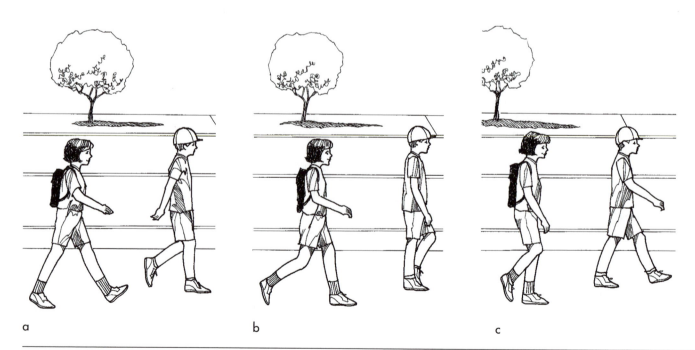

a   b   c

Figure 9.17 Sequence images of half a walking cycle in two young adults. Are all the features of normal gait apparent? What other views would be helpful? Time between pictures is 0.1 seconds.

Table 9.6 Critical Features and Cues for Human Gait	
Critical feature	**Cues**
Minimal sway	Body over base of support
Arm opposition	Opposite arm and leg
Minimal rise	Smooth recovery; smooth push-off
Cushioning	Give with the leg
Leg support	Push down and backward
Push off	Press with toes

Systematic Observational Strategy

These three areas also provide the basis for a good systematic observational strategy of human gait. Most of these critical features can be evaluated from a sagittal plane view. An analyst might look at a person's overall posture and balance by visually focusing on the trunk in the first few steps. To observe the next several steps, focus on one leg in the support phase and then in the swing phase of the gait cycle. Use this observational strategy to qualitatively analyze the gait illustrated in figure 9.17. You can easily practice qualitative analysis of gait in shopping malls or other public areas where you can observe people inconspicuously. It is important that they not notice you so they will use their natural gait (and not be alarmed that someone is watching them).

Examples of Normal Gait

The sequential images in figure 9.17 illustrate half a cycle of normal walking of two young adults. Are all the critical features of gait previously discussed exhibited? Which person do you think was walking faster? Why? What critical features are difficult to evaluate and what other vantage points would be helpful for observation?

The people illustrated in figure 9.17 are in different phases of the gait cycle. The female (wearing a backpack) begins in double support with left foot toe off and right foot strike, while the male begins in midstance on his left foot. Both persons walk smoothly with upright trunks, have their arms moving in opposition to the legs, flex the knee and hip in stance, and vigorously push off. The female is walking faster as evidenced by the extension in the legs (compare both subjects near double support). Note that their heads become closer in successive images. A rear view is essential to evaluating the width of the base of support, lateral motion, and pelvic tilt. This sagittal plane view is an effective vantage point for

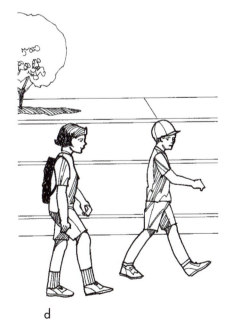

d

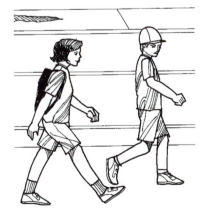

e

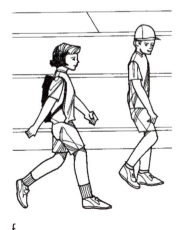

f

evaluating step lengths, joint actions, opposition, and vertical motion of the body. How might gait change if the backpack were very heavy, they were walking uphill, or the ground were very slippery?

A way to practice the evaluation and diagnosis of gait analysis is to create artificial gait situations. Videotape fellow students walking on the ice one winter morning. Create different foot pains by placing a small stone in a subject's sock. Taping or bracing joints can also create an artificial injury that analysts can study by qualitatively analyzing the resulting gait. Gait can be observed or videotaped on hills and after the performer has fatigued a muscle group with exercises. Care must be taken to insure performer safety when setting these situations up for qualitative analysis practice.

LIVE PERFORMANCES

The best practice is to analyze live performances. You may be able to observe unobtrusively at a neighborhood park, gym, or athletic field. Another good way to practice is to review videotaped performances. The videos need to be made following the recommendations in chapter 11. Most television coverage of sporting events is inadequate for practicing good qualitative analysis because you cannot change vantage points or distances, change the task, or have the performer repeat the task. You can practice qualitative analysis by watching network or cable sports coverage, but you will not have enough information to make a good integrated qualitative analysis.

SUMMARY

Training has been shown to improve qualitative analysis ability. We presented images of several human movements to illustrate the application of the integrated model of qualitative analysis. These examples illustrate many of the important factors in qualitative analysis of human movement. Your analytical skill will develop when you make a conscious effort to improve all four tasks of qualitative analysis (preparation, observation, evaluation/diagnosis, and intervention) and practice qualitative analysis of human movement. Readers should compare their analyses of the examples presented in the text and critically examine differences. Do various qualitative analysis models lead to the same intervention?

DISCUSSION QUESTIONS

1. What systematic observational strategies are difficult to employ with the sequence images presented in this chapter?

2. Discuss the advantages of diagnosing and providing intervention based on critical features that have been prioritized according to their importance to performance.

3. Identify possible problems of diagnosing and providing intervention based on critical features that have been prioritized according to their importance.

4. What information is missing in the drawings of the movements? How would your evaluation and diagnosis be different if additional information were available?

Theory
Into Practice Situations

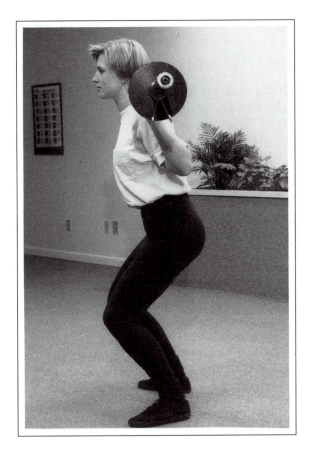

An adult at your health club is becoming very interested in weight training and has asked for your help in doing squats. She has never done squats before and wants you to evaluate her technique and give her a lesson on the finer points. Precise body positioning and technique are essential in weight training to make sure that the muscle groups targeted by the exercises are the muscle groups that are primarily involved. Use the science of biomechanics to qualitatively analyze the squat in the photograph. If she were to do several repetitions and begin to have more forward trunk lean, what differences in muscle group involvement would you expect (Hint: Look at the moment arm, or horizontal distance from the load to the joints)? What back position (amount of lumbar arch) is associated with even or safe spinal loading?

Chapter Objectives

1. Develop skill in applying integrated qualitative analysis to a variety of real-world problems.
2. Identify subdisciplines of kinesiology that provide relevant information for making decisions within qualitative analysis of human movement.

Many situations arise where a professional must integrate information from several subdisciplines of kinesiology. This chapter presents some scenarios from various kinesiology professions where an integrated qualitative analysis can be applied to help a performer.

Think through each of the tasks of an integrated qualitative analysis (preparation, observational strategies, evaluation and diagnosis, and intervention) for each situation presented in this chapter. These situations are useful for generating discussions. Only the first situation is developed as an example. Use a separate sheet of paper for notes summarizing relevant information for each task. Your notes can be in point form or in text, like the example that follows.

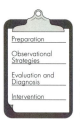

Preparation

Observational Strategies

Evaluation and Diagnosis

Intervention

"CLEARED TO PLAY"

A sophomore coming off an anterior cruciate ligament (ACL) knee injury has asked to return to your junior college volleyball team. As head coach, you have to decide if she is ready for practice and match play because there is no athletic trainer to monitor her rehab. What aspects of volleyball skills should qualitative analysis focus on? What physical tests can you give this athlete to help you make this decision? Do the athlete's personality traits have any bearing on this decision?

Preparation

In the preparation task of qualitative analysis, you should review any preinjury information you may have on this athlete. Your research into her injury, rehab, and previous history should suggest which critical features of volleyball movements you should observe to evaluate this athlete's ability to play. Since the ACL is an important knee ligament limiting forward motion of the tibia on the femur, you should plan to ob-

serve the control of knee flexion and extension. Important volleyball movements that may stress the ACL are jumping, landing, and making vigorous changes of direction. You should also plan to focus on the player's facial expressions and body language for signs of knee pain.

Beyond observing for signs of injury, you may want to analyze the amount of recovery of previous ability. If quantitative information (jump height, speed trials, agility measures) is not available, use your memory to compare the athlete's volleyball movements to those of other players. You may also plan to perform your typical qualitative analysis of selected volleyball skills to look for changes in technique.

Observational Strategies

Plan to observe carefully the athlete's control of knee flexion in landing, jumps, and changes of direction. Your observational strategy should also focus on the athlete's expression for any signs of discomfort. A good plan for observation might begin with the usual team warm-up routine so you'll know what movements are coming and can be sure of a gradual, safe increase in movement intensity. Some volleyball movements you should plan to observe are jumps and landings in spiking and blocking. Intensity should be gradually increased. Since the ACL checks forward motion of the tibia, you might ask the athlete to hop forward and backward as far as possible on each foot six times. Landing in backward hopping creates a forward force on the lower leg that tends to stress the ACL. A major difference in distance jumped or control of the knee between the injured and uninjured legs is an important point for your observation. Finally, plan to monitor the athlete's affected knee for swelling after any practice or physical tests.

Evaluation and Diagnosis

Your focus in evaluation is on the quality of the athlete's control of the knee during the high-energy phases of jumping, landing, and cutting movements. Evaluating the focal points of observation may be simpler than in many qualitative analyses, because you are primarily interested in detecting injury-related weaknesses that would prohibit participation. The buckling or giving of the knee or unusual knee motions may merely need to be detected. Evaluating the athlete's recovery of ability relative to other athletes or evaluating her technique in the various volleyball skills is more difficult. Judging the quality of a spike is more difficult than merely detecting differences in distances or heights of jumps.

The diagnosis of the weaknesses identified in evaluation depends on your philosophy regarding the return of injured players. Since tissues that have not fully healed are more easily reinjured, some coaches might keep diagnosis simple by not allowing a player to return if she shows any signs of weakness or loss of knee control. This diagnosis of performance could also be tricky because the athlete might experience some discomfort associated with higher-intensity activity rather than overuse of tissue that is not fully healed. Here you must apply your knowledge of sports medicine and biomechanics to make sure critical features you have identified in evaluation are not related to reinjury or to limiting volleyball performance. Clearly, the injury risk to the athlete is the first priority of diagnosis, with level of performance being the second priority.

Intervention

As the coach, you have many options in dealing with this athlete. If the diagnosis indicates that she is ready to return, you should provide positive feedback on her effort in rehabilitating the injury. It would also be wise to express confidence in the player's recovery and ability. Remind her that her timing and teamwork will take time to recover. Express confidence in the athlete, but ask her to be careful and caution her that most athletes tend to rush the recovery process.

If the diagnosis indicates that the athlete should not return to the team, there are also several approaches to intervention. It is very important to be sensitive when you tell the athlete she needs to continue rehab before she can join the team. You might say, "You've made a lot of progress, but I would like you to come back in two weeks for another tryout." Another option

would be to allow limited practice with the team. You could also recommend that the athlete consider a knee brace.

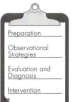

"BUT I CAN SCORE"

A high school basketball player is having great success driving to the left and scoring during a preseason practice. However, he uses his right hand to execute lay-ups and is successful only because of his speed and superior jumping ability. What feedback or intervention would be appropriate? What will happen if taller/faster opponents guard this player or weak-side defense rotates to defend the lay-up?

"THE SLUMP"

A college softball player is struggling with her hitting. At midseason she was leading the team, but now she has been hitless in several games. What would be a good approach to the qualitative analysis of her hitting? Should intervention focus on technique or the hitter's confidence? Assume there is a video of her hitting from earlier in the season.

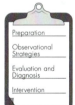

"BUT THE CHAMP DOES IT THIS WAY"

As a tennis coach, you notice that a promising junior tennis player is using more open-stance forehand drives during practice and matches. You think he is emulating many tennis professionals, who are using more open-stance strokes rather than the traditional square stance. What intervention do you provide to this 12-year-old player?

"BUT I CAN LIFT MORE"

An athlete is struggling with a plateau in chest strength and asks for your help with training. During his bench press you notice the body position illustrated in figure 10.1. What intervention is appropriate for an athlete of any age with the technique illustrated? The athlete senses he

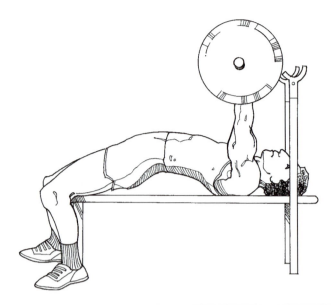

Figure 10.1   Incorrect bench press form. What intervention is appropriate?

can lift more with this technique, but what parts of the body does it put at risk of injury? Are there variations to the bench press that would be safer? Are there alternative exercises isolating specific muscle groups that can be used together to replace the bench press? What intervention strategy will you use to motivate the use of a safer lifting technique?

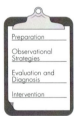

"THE PARENT DISTRACTION"

An overzealous parent keeps yelling at one of your players, "Box out!" Defensive rebounding has not been a problem in this game and you have coached the team to emphasize the fast break against this team. How can qualitative analysis be used to evaluate which player this parent is yelling at and whether the players are being affected? What intervention would be appropriate?

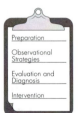

"FINAL JUDGMENT/ AUTHORITY"

You are asked to be a judge for a diving demonstration given by a local swim club. The divers will be children ages 10 to 16 who are first- and second-year students preparing for future competition. How

can you increase the accuracy and consistency of your qualitative analyses of the dives? How can you avoid bias related to dive difficulty, age of the performer, and the order within the demonstration?

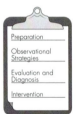

"MACHINES VERSUS FREE WEIGHTS"

You are asked to be part of a panel discussion on weight training at the state convention. The panel has chosen to discuss the differences between weight training with free weights and with a machine. How can you use qualitative analysis to compare free-weight arm curls with machine arm curls? You have a videotape of lifters using machines and free weights. What subdisciplines of kinesiology are most relevant in analyzing each exercise?

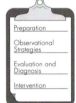

"FINISHING STRONG"

You are a basketball coach. Your best shooter has been shooting the lights out all game long, but suddenly near the end of the game her shots are falling short. You may have only one or two looks at her form before you can call a time out in the final minutes of the game. What physical factors are involved, and how can they be evaluated? How can you evaluate how game pressure is affecting the athlete? What factors in shooting and other basketball skills should be observed? What interventions are best for different causes of this problem? Does this athlete's psychological make-up affect your intervention?

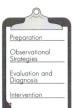

"CHOKE?"

Two of the best tennis players in your junior development program have signed up for group lessons through the summer. One player excels in practice, where there are few observers and little crowd noise. This player has had difficulty in tournaments because of the crowd noise and pressure. The other player is just the opposite. He seems unmotivated in practice but thrives on pressure and has pulled off some big wins in tournaments. What can be done in practice and competition to help both performers? How can qualitative analysis be used to address the needs of each player?

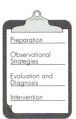

"PUSH AND GLIDE"

You are teaching in-line skating at a summer camp. One student is having difficulty with turns to the left. Your intial intervention focused on the push-off and recovery of her right leg. Like a good analyst, you immediately return to observation from intervention and find that the student is still having difficulty. Could your initial evaluation and diagnosis be incorrect? Should you plan to evaluate the right leg again, or focus on the left leg? What aspects of leg action and balance might provide clues to the skater's problem? Could changing the task provide other clues for your evaluation?

SUMMARY

This chapter presented several real-life situations where an integrated qualitative analysis would be appropriate for a kinesiology professional to use to help a performer. Simultaneous consideration of information from several subdisciplines of kinesiology is needed in analyzing each situation. The unique nature of each situation demands thoughtful consideration in integrating information from many subdisciplines. For example, the qualitative analysis of the squat relied heavily on biomechanics, but information from exercise physiology and psychology were also vital in shaping the appropriate intervention. These situations are useful in stimulating discussion among professionals about the qualitative analysis of human movement.

Videotape Replay
Within Qualitative Analysis

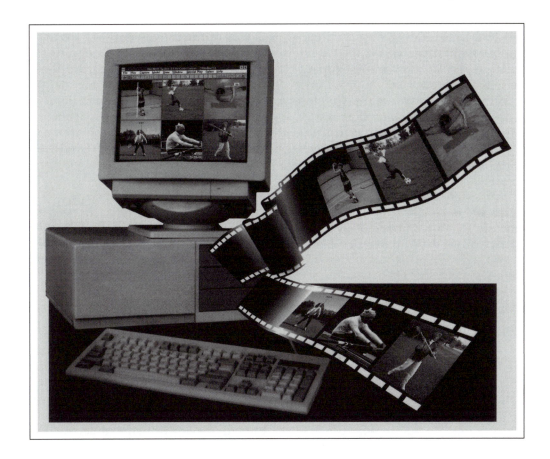

PREVIEW

You are a coach who has used video to record and qualitatively analyze your athlete's performance. You receive information on a newly-released video and computer system with new features. Can use of this system improve your qualitative analyses? Videotape replay has often been used to extend observational power, but what are the limitations of this system? For which of the four tasks of qualitative analysis will the video system be of most benefit?

Chapter Objectives

1. Describe the uses of videotape replay for extending observational power within qualitative analysis.
2. Explain how to use videotape to maximize qualitative analysis ability.
3. Describe spatial and temporal limitations of commercial and consumer video equipment in documenting human movement.

An important tool in extending observational power within qualitative analysis is the use of videotape replay, especially slow-motion replay. Video replay may be most useful in providing information to the analyst who is unavailable for real-time observation. Videotape can capture fast elements of the movement that are unobservable by the naked eye. This greater movement detail and unlimited capacity for replay makes video an important tool within qualitative analysis for extending the observational power of the teacher or coach. This chapter will review the factors that are important in using video to improve qualitative analysis of motor skills.

INTRODUCTION TO VIDEO IN KINESIOLOGY

Many of the early studies of videotape in teaching motor skills focused on its use as visual feedback. Reviews of these early studies found that video replay used as feedback to performers is not significantly different from regular practice and teacher-augmented feedback in improving motor skills (Rothstein, 1980; Rothstein and Arnold, 1976). Recent studies have begun to show that video replay may have some benefits due to the observational learning or modeling of the performer's behavior beyond the capacity of intrinsic feedback (Dowrick, 1991b; Gould and Roberts, 1982). Even when this visual feedback or KP is not very useful to the performer, video replay can provide important information to improve qualitative analysis.

Videotape replay may, however, have other potential benefits for improving motor skills if used correctly (Franks and Maile, 1991; Rothstein, 1980; Trower and Kiely, 1983). A major advantage of videotape replay is that it shows high-speed

details of the movement that are not easily discernible with real-time observation. Video recorded performances also have unlimited replay potential to increase observational power. This chapter discusses important issues in video technology, explains how to use it most effectively for the qualitative analysis of human movement, and gives advice on how to produce videos for qualitative analysis.

A Two-Dimensional Image

Before we discuss the use of videotape, teachers and coaches should know how video imaging works and be aware of the limitations of the medium. This section describes the basics of video imaging and how these technical facts shape the analyst's use of video within qualitative analysis.

A normal photographic or video image from one camera is a two-dimensional (2-D) representation of a three-dimensional (3-D) scene. This means that only objects oriented at right angles to the lens will be represented accurately in the two dimensions of the image. Anything aligned toward or away from the camera will be distorted in the image (2-D representation) taken from the real world (3-D reality).

For example, suppose three TV cameras were placed next to the runway of the gymnastics vault (figure 11.1). The coach believed that the angle between the gymnast's extended arms prior to the block on the horse should be a specific angle for this athlete. The coach could get an accurate estimate of the angle between the two arms of the gymnast only if the camera were at a right angle to the motion of the arms at the instant of interest (Camera B). The views from cameras A and C show an arm angle that is smaller than the actual angle between the gymnast's arms. You can visualize these 2-D distortions of a 3-D event by imagining the angles

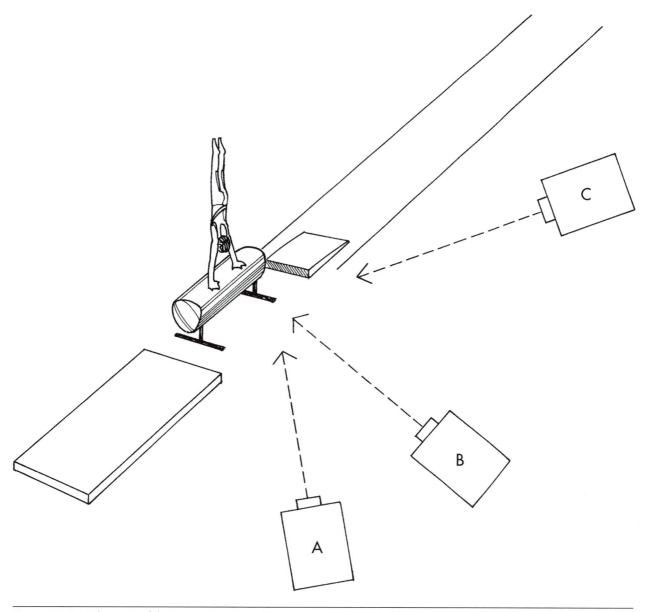

Figure 11.1 Schematic of three camera views of a gymnast vaulting. Only camera B provides an accurate image of the angle of the performer's arms as he blocks on the horse.

viewed by cameras A and C as the shadows cast by the gymnast's arms on the walls behind him that are parallel to the cameras (the imagined light source). This is why an athlete can look as if he or she is stepping on a boundary line in one camera view, while a camera view down the boundary line shows that the athlete is inside the line.

The point to remember is that video images are 2-D representations of a 3-D world. There are some predictable distortions of the image caused by the position and orientation of the objects in the field of view. People who use videotape for

qualitative analysis should set up taping sessions to minimize these distortions and should know when these distortions may affect judgments about the performances.

> *The two-dimensional images created by normal photography or video provide distorted representations of the three-dimensional world. For example, objects not parallel to the camera can appear smaller than they actually are.*
>
> **KEY POINT**

The Video Image

Video images are also limited representations of reality because they are made up of a 2-D array of dots. These dots that comprise each picture are called *pixels* (short for picture elements). Each picture element is given a shade on the gray scale (from black to white) for a black-and-white video picture. Color video is made up of pixels that have been given an intensity or mix of red, green, and blue light. A video picture is called a *frame* and is made up of two halves, or *fields*. One field is odd-numbered, horizontal lines of pixels and the other field is even-numbered, horizontal lines. This is why normal video is called *interlaced* video. The more pixels and lines of pixels in a video frame, the higher the resolution and the better the image.

Resolution

The number and size of these pixels determine the quality of the video picture. The television production video equipment can have 525 (NTSC) or 625 (PAL) horizontal lines of pixels (Feldman, 1988). The number of pixels for a given field of view determines the *resolution* of the video picture and thus the image quality. Resolution in all directions is a critical issue when video is used for actual measurements (quantitative analysis), but it is still important in qualitative analyses if the images are of poor quality or the subject of the analysis is small in a large videotaped field of view.

Video picture format is determined by broadcasting conventions that vary around the world. National Television Standards Committee (NTSC) standards are used in North America and Japan. The United Kingdom and European countries use Phase Alternation Line (PAL) video picture format, while the French and Russians use Sequential Couleur a Memorie (SECAM) video. NTSC video has 30 frames or pictures each second; PAL and SECAM video have 25 frames per second. There is video equipment available that can switch among these international formats.

When consumer electronics are used to tape and display human movement, the resolution of the video images suffers. There is often a difference between the resolution of one video component (camera) and the resolution of the whole system. For example, even a professional NTSC video signal may show up on a good TV as only 490 horizontal lines since it takes time to jump from the bottom of one frame to the top of the next. Camcorder video signals may have less

horizontal and vertical resolution than professional video. NTSC video produced by consumer camcorders, for example, generally creates images with 300 to 330 horizontal lines, with 235 to 245 pixels in each line. High-band consumer video formats (Super VHS [S-VHS] or Hi8mm) typically have 400 to 480 lines of horizontal resolution, with up to 640 pixels per line. A problem with higher resolution video is that many TVs and VCRs in the United States follow "broadcast standard" TV and cable formats of only 330 horizontal lines in a video frame. To take advantage of the improvements in resolution of high-band video systems, one must factor in the added cost of special tapes, camcorders, and monitors.

Note that the vertical resolution (the number of horizontal lines) is essentially fixed by the format of the video. The horizontal resolution (number of pixels in each horizontal line) varies according to how the analog video signal is sampled. When a video ad claims 400 lines of resolution, this typically means the equipment can create 400 pixels in each horizontal line.

Some large-screen televisions are based on improved-definition television (IDTV), which creates a better-quality picture. In the future, high-definition television (HDTV) video with thousands of horizontal lines and thousands of pixels in each line may be available, but it will probably be years before HDTV is phased into broadcasts and becomes widely available to consumers.

Paused Video Image

The resolution of video, and consequently the quality of the picture, becomes worse when the VCR is put in *freeze-frame* or pause mode. When most consumer VCRs are put in pause mode, only one field is shown in order to prevent a flickering picture. Flicker is caused when there is motion between the two halves of a video frame (1/60th or 1/50th of a second apart), making the image seem to vibrate between the two positions on the screen. Some VCRs effectively give a person 60 half-pictures (fields) to look at when the frame-advance or slow-motion features are activated. Unfortunately, most VCRs jump from the first field of a frame to the first field of the next frame when the frame advance is pushed. Video pictures are physically bigger horizontally than vertically, but this is nowhere near the horizons of normal vision. Normal video has an *aspect ratio* (field width divided by height) of 4 to 3. This difference in field of view, combined with pixel resolution and lost resolution in freeze-frame mode, affects the quality of objects represented in these directions on the image.

When consumer video is used for slow-motion or frame-by-frame qualitative analysis, you are most often looking at a video field with half the vertical resolution of a normal video frame. If the video images were created with poor lighting, a small image size for the performer, a noncontrasting background, an unfavorable camera location, or some other problem, the video would probably not provide a good medium for the observation of small details. For example, if a subject's image is small and her arm rotates out of parallel with the camera, it may be impossible to tell what position or angle the arm is in.

> **KEY POINT**
>
> *The quality of a video image is strongly related to the number of picture elements (pixels) used to create that image. Many aspects of video technology affect the quality of video images that are used to extend observation within qualitative analysis.*

Measurement From Video

Biomechanics research has been using video for precise kinematic measurements, or *quantitative analysis*, for many years. Careful setup and procedural techniques are needed to collect images and to digitize, scale, and make calculations from video data. Many of these video systems are based on digital and commercial video that break the video signal into each field (noninterlaced video) and may use sophisticated image processing to create subpixel resolution. Stereo-photogrammetric techniques and computers are needed to generate 3-D data from synchronized multiple camera images (Allard, Stokes, and Blanchi, 1995).

Readers should use video for primarily qualitative analysis and not attempt measurements from video unless they are trained in these techniques or technical assistance is available. Making videos for qualitative analysis is less complicated than for quantitative analysis. The following sections discuss important information in video technology and procedures for using video to enhance qualitative analysis.

VIDEO TECHNOLOGY

This section will summarize the basics of video technology. Two important characteristics of normal video that analysts need to be familiar with will be presented: frame rate and features of camcorders and VCRs.

Frame Rate

A modern camcorder generates a video picture by using a charge-coupled device (CCD), a photosensitive array that assigns the appropriate gray

---

PRACTICAL APPLICATION

You are a first-year football coach at Metro High School and the head coach assigns you to coach the punters. Since many of the important actions of kicking are too fast to observe reliably in real time, you bring your camcorder to practice and videotape the punters trying out. You record side views of the punters, maximizing the size of the punter in the field of view so the tapes can be reviewed in freeze-frame and slow-motion replay.

As you review the "film," you can identify differences in knowledge of performance (KP), like punting technique, impact position, and ball position on the foot. Several strengths and weaknesses can be identified, and one punter looks the closest to the desirable punting form you expect. The problem is that you realize you did not create a written or auditory account—have no knowledge of results (KR)—of the distance, hang time, and accuracy of each punt. Slow-motion video replay can extend observational power of only some of the critical features of punting. If videos are shot from a position above the press box, coaches can document distance, accuracy, and hang time of the punts. In short, video replay can extend observational power in qualitative analysis, but it is not a magic bullet.

scale or color to the pixels of a video frame. In the United States, the alternating current (AC) electrical power has a frequency of 60 hertz, so video standards are set up so the phases of the current are used to scan each field of video. This gives NTSC video an effective frame rate of 30 frames per second. Normal film frame rates are 24 frames per second. Compared to real-time visual observation, stop-action or slow-motion video dramatically increases the ability to see details of human movement. PAL and SECAM videos have an effective frame rate of 25 frames per second.

The *sampling rates* of human vision and normal video are important to understand because they help determine what aspects of human movement can be observed. For very high-speed movements like pitching, tennis serving, or golf, normal video may sample at a high enough rate to consistently capture some details of interest. A good example of distortions created by inadequate sampling would be the motion of the wheels of a stagecoach or wagon recorded by the typical frame rates in old Westerns. When you watch these old movies, it appears that the wagon wheels are rotating backwards because the frame rate is too slow to represent their actual rotation. The wheels rotate too fast, making the spoke position of sequential frames appear behind the initial position, when in reality the spoke has rotated all the way around to a position behind the previous image.

Special *high-speed video* cameras are commercially available for research and other specialized tasks. Video cameras and support equipment capable of hundreds to several thousand frames per second are unnecessary for most qualitative analyses of human movement—and out of the price range of most teachers, coaches, and therapists. These high-speed video cameras would be necessary for a video analysis of the stiffness of various golf-club shafts, ball rotation in baseball pitching, or the dynamics of a foot striking the ground in running.

Be aware that some consumer camcorders are described as "high-speed cameras" that are not high-speed video. They are really just 30 frames per second, but with very small exposure times for each picture (e.g., 1/10,000th of a second). There is a marked difference in the kinematic information created between video with 30 frames per second and video with 200 or 1,000 frames per second (fps) . Compare the temporal identification of impact in the illustrations in figure 11.2 that were taken from high-speed film (100 fps). Even 100 fps cannot guarantee that an image will contain impact (image b), but notice how far the racket can move (image a to c) when capturing images at 30 fps. The importance of the shutter speed will be discussed in the next section on camcorders.

Some companies market video equipment specifically for sports instructors and coaches. Special

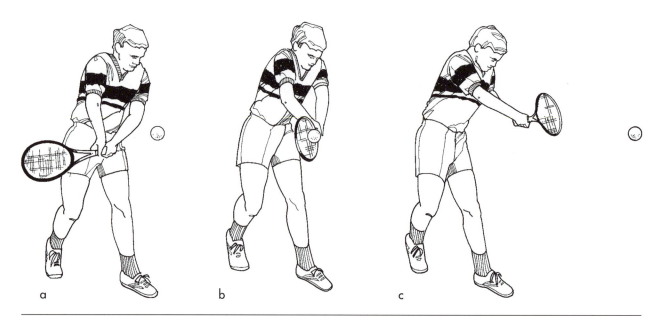

Figure 11.2   The difference between video sampling (30 frames per second) and high-speed imaging. High-speed imaging (100 fps) can usually identify impact (b), an event that lasts only 0.005 seconds. The sampling of normal video can miss events of short duration. Frames a and c are 1/30th of a second apart.

video cameras, VCRs, editing equipment, and computer interfaces have been the state of the art in the imaging of football games for coaches to evaluate game plans and opponents. These game tapes have replaced the old 16-millimeter films that were used to record games and scout opponents. Many camcorders are marketed as appropriate video equipment for the analysis of sports. In fact, most camcorders have focusing, white balance, and shutter features that make them suitable for making video images for qualitative analysis. Let's look at the desirable camcorder features for qualitative analysis.

The Camcorder

The camcorder is the combination of two machines that were separate in the early versions of video technology, the video camera and the recorder or machine to code the video signal on magnetic tape. Factors that help determine a camcorder's suitability include the shutter, image quality, and format.

Shutter

Perhaps the most important feature for imaging human movement for qualitative analysis is a *shutter*, which limits the exposure time that each field is scanned by the CCD. Capturing a field in 1/500 or 1/1,000 of a second ensures that moving objects do not move much as the image is being captured. This allows the imaging of high-speed movements without blurring. The term "high-speed shutter" is a misnomer, since the shutter prevents image blurring but does not allow the camera to capture more images per second. In other words, the same 30 frames per second with crisp images of fast movements does not make a camera high-speed.

The problem a shutter may create is a need for extra light when exposure times are very small. This is rarely a problem in using a camcorder outside in natural lighting, but indoors shuttered video may be underexposed unless extra light is used. Current camcorders have shutters that can generate exposure times as small as 1/10,000 of a second. These settings are rarely necessary in capturing human movement. In fact, videotaping slower movements may not require the use of a shutter at all. Table 11.1 lists several common human movements and sports and the corresponding exposure times that may be needed to freeze the action.

It is also important to check how the camcorder operates in the stop mode. Some camcorders have

Table 11.1
Recommended Exposure Times for Videotaping Typical Human Movements

Activity	Exposure time (shutter setting)
Walking	1/60 (off)
Sit to stand	1/60 (off)
Bowling	1/60 (off)
Basketball	1/100
Vertical jump	1/100
Jogging	1/100 to 1/200
Sprinting	1/200 to 1/500
Baseball pitching	1/500 to 1/1,000
Baseball hitting	1/500 to 1/1,000
Soccer kicking	1/500 to 1/1,000
Tennis	1/500 to 1/1,000
Golf	1/1,000 or smaller

a short rewind or roll-up of a couple of seconds after the tape is stopped. A good practice is to stop taping a couple of seconds after and start a couple of seconds before the action of interest.

Image Quality

Since an analyst may not have complete control over the situation being videotaped (weather, competition, logistics, etc.), the camcorder selected should have several automated features that help create good video images. These features should also be manually adjustable. Camcorders should have *low light sensitivity* and *autoexposure*. Many camcorders have low light sensitivity down to 1 lux. The camcorder should be able to create clear video pictures with the low levels of illumination that may be due to poor lighting, camera position, or the small exposure times created by a shutter. Some camcorders have a button adjustment for low-level lighting.

Other important image quality features include *autofocus, autowhite balance,* and a *backlighting* adjustment. Camcorders often automatically adjust the color sensitivity (white balance) to get uniform color in different lighting conditions. Especially important is a manual override on the autofocus feature. If the subject cannot be videotaped with the sun behind the camcorder, the backlighting adjustment is needed to prevent the light behind the subject from washing out the image with light.

Most camcorders use infrared beams directed at the center of the field of view to automatically focus the lens. Several conditions may not maintain a focused image, so the camcorder should have a manual override of the autofocus. An analyst may want the subject not to be in the center of the video picture to keep something else in the field of view, or other objects behind or in front of the subject may interfere with the autofocus. To focus manually, zoom in on the subject and focus, then adjust the zoom lens to the desired field of view. The camcorder should be as stable as possible to maximize image quality. A tripod is highly desirable, but some camcorders have stabilizing features to help limit motion of the field of view.

Formats for Camcorders

One of the most important factors in choosing a camcorder is the format of the magnetic cassette tape that will be used. Since the 1960s large cassettes with 3/4-inch tape have been used. Two smaller 1/2-inch versions began competing for the portable/home video market: Video Home System (VHS) and a scaled-down version of professional video (Beta). Several other formats have evolved from these two videocassette formats. These newer formats focus on two improvements, smaller size and greater resolution. High-band formats (ED-BETA, Hi-8, and S-VHS) all have better resolution, while some formats accommodate smaller cassettes for very small camcorders. The high-band versions are not necessary for qualitative analysis, but they are desirable if the tapes and other video equipment are within your budget. In the following paragraphs, the high-band formats are in parentheses.

Two formats provide the smallest videocassettes. One format uses 8-millimeter tapes (Hi-8) that can store about 2 hours of video. This format requires that you use the recorder part of your camcorder to run the video signal to display or copy the images. Another format is VHS-C (or S-VHS-C), a compact version of the VHS format that can also hold up to 2 hours of video. These tapes have adapters so they can be used in VCRs, which use the standard 1/2-inch magnetic tape. These two formats have made the miniature, handheld camcorders very popular.

The most popular format in the United States is VHS, whose high-band version is Super VHS (S-VHS). VHS has been more popular than Beta for years and is less expensive because of the competition with smaller camcorders. Beta's high-band version is ED-BETA (extended definition). Current VHS and Beta camcorders are larger than compact models but are not heavy or cumbersome.

Another important camcorder feature for qualitative analysis is a *zoom lens*. Often a camcorder cannot be placed in a desirable position because of facility or competition limitations. A zoom lens, which can accommodate a variety of distances from the subject, solves that problem. Lens focal lengths are specified in millimeters, but the range of a zoom lens is usually expressed as a ratio. Current camcorders have a zoom lens with a ratio above 12:1, meaning that an object will appear 12 times larger in full zoom than in full wide-angle. A zoom lens may allow the analyst to create video images from locations distant from the performer or from electrical power. Since electrical outlets are not always available, a long-life battery and a spare are essential.

> *Some of the most important camcorder features related to qualitative analysis are a shutter, low-light sensitivity, and a zoom lens.*
>
> **KEY POINT**

Some camcorders provide valuable editing features. Date, titles, or time codes can be added to the image. Analysts should look up repair histories and reviews of these features in consumer publications (*Consumer Reports*, 1995) or trade magazines like *Videomaker* and *Video Review*. More on editing features will be discussed in the next section on VCRs. Good reviews of video technology are available (Dowrick, 1991a; McGrain, 1984).

When selecting a camcorder format for qualitative analysis, think about how and where you will be making the videos. How much time do the events take? How will the tapes be viewed? How accessible is equipment that will be needed to view, copy, or store the video? All these questions and others affect the choice of video format and camcorder features.

The VCR

The VCR (videocassette recorder) is the machine that reads the videotape and generates the video signal that can be shown on various monitors,

TVs, screens, projectors, or computers. A VCR can also code a video signal on the magnetic tape of a videocassette. Most recent models have slow-motion replay. This section discusses the important features you should evaluate when selecting a VCR for use in qualitative analysis. It does not address commercial VCRs designed for professional use.

Formats for VCRs

Buying a VCR can be a confusing task. Modern VCRs have a bewildering array of features that may be desirable for consumers taping their favorite shows (stereo, programmability) but may not be critical for qualitative analysis. A VCR that can be used for real-time or slow-motion qualitative analysis of human movement should have several key features. The first choice to make is the tape format. All the tape formats are adequate for qualitative analysis. Check the most recent *Consumer Reports* review of video equipment to see what makes and models are the best and most reliable. VCRs range in price from less than $200 to thousands of dollars for commercial equipment.

Number of Heads

You need a *four-head* VCR to read enough video-tape to obtain a clear image in freeze-frame, pause, or still mode. Look for a model that has a field advance in both directions. Some VCRs advance a whole frame, showing only the first field of each frame. Make a tape of a digital clock to take along to stores so you can evaluate picture quality and frame advance differences. Often these features are not very important to consumers, so try things out rather than relying on sales personnel. With many VCRs, to advance the frame, you must repeatedly press the pause or still button or use the jog-shuttle dial.

Playback Speeds

The VCR should also have *variable-speed* slow-motion, which can show the action at different rates of slow motion. Variable slow motion used to be a button feature, but now it is more like professional VCRs, with a *jog-shuttle dial* that you can turn forward or backward to change tape speeds from still to frame-by-frame, slow-motion, normal, and search. This helps you find key events in the movement and select the speed of replay.

Time Codes

Other features in consumer VCRs relevant to qualitative analysis are title generators, time code

(address) generators, and index/search functions. An analyst may want to add titles or words of reminder to a video image. A particularly good or bad trial can be electronically marked by the index function so the VCR can search for it at a later viewing. VCRs that can display or generate SMPTE time codes (hour, minute, second, frame) on the field of view are valuable for temporal analysis and finding specific frames. Picture mixing, split-screen, or PIP (picture-in-picture) can be used to compare multiple video images on one screen. These high-end VCRs are modeled after expensive video editing equipment used by professionals.

> *The most important VCR features for qualitative analysis are four heads, freeze-frame, and a jog-shuttle dial.* **KEY POINT**

MAKING VIDEOS FOR QUALITATIVE ANALYSIS

Videotaping patients or athletes for qualitative analysis has been popular for several decades. There are many different objectives for capturing human movement on video. For example, many parents tape their children's practice routines or competitions and send the tape to coaches to evaluate for possible athletic scholarships. These "daddy videos" are often of little value because of their technical quality. The video may not be made from a vantage point of interest, or the conditions of the performances may not be adequate for qualitative analysis by the coaches.

Replay Options

Naturally, the procedures for making a video to analyze performance qualitatively depend on the objectives of the analysis. A tape made to analyze technique in the tennis service or volley may be very different from a tape made to evaluate court movement or service return ability. Video images for qualitative analysis can be made for *real-time replay* and feedback to the performer or for *slow-motion* analysis to improve the observational power of the teacher, coach, or therapist.

Real-Time Replay

One approach to using videotape for qualitative analysis is to view or replay the recorded images at normal speed. This is called real-time analysis of videotape. Creating video for real-time replay for performers or qualitative analysis by a teacher or coach requires a certain approach. The field of view needs to be several times larger than the moving subject. This gives a stable background for the subject to move against. A good rule of thumb is to have the subject take up between one-third and one-half of the field height.

It is important to give the observers of your real-time video a field of view that accurately represents the environment the performer is moving in. Some of these tapes are made to diagnose how the performer responds to dynamic game conditions (tennis, basketball, volleyball), and analyzing the form of the performer is not the primary interest. In this situation, the field size is maximized to allow observation of the whole court. Most real-time replay of video for qualitative analysis is used in this fashion by coaches or motor skill instructors to assist in the observation of performance, though sometimes it is used as feedback or intervention to improve performance.

KEY POINT

Video images created for real-time qualitative analysis should have a large field of view with background features for the subject to move against. This approach is designed to simulate live qualitative analysis of human movement.

Research on the use of real-time video replay as intervention or feedback to performers has a long history in kinesiology. Numerous studies over the past 30 years show that video replay is no more effective than traditional teacher-augmented feedback (Rothstein and Arnold, 1976).

More recent studies confirm these early results but also suggest that video replay may provide useful information as intervention to improve performance. Based on her meta-analysis of videotape feedback research, Rothstein (1980) proposed that seven factors are important for using video replay for augmented feedback. It should be used with *verbal cues* that focus the performer's attention. It should be used *frequently* (at least five replays). Video feedback is most effective for *advanced beginners and intermediates*, not complete novices or expert players. Some research has shown that unstructured video replay

can negatively affect learning in beginners (Ross, Bird, Doody, and Zoeller, 1985). Provide *practice immediately following* the video feedback. Possibly *zoom in on the aspect of performance* you want to provide feedback about. When taping, *vary the camera angle* and capture a field of view that is *consistent with the goals and nature of the activity.* For example, a close-up shot of the tennis serve would be helpful in this closed motor skill, while a view of the whole court would be helpful in analyzing how the groundstroke techniques selected relate to the environment (open motor skills).

Other recent papers review the use of videotape in the qualitative analysis or teaching of motor skills (Franks and Maile, 1991; Jambor and Weekes, 1995; Trinity and Annesi, 1996). One of the most important functions of video replay for performers has been its use for self-modeling (Dowrick, 1991b). A performer should be compared to a model of skilled performance who is similar to the performer in age, skill level, appearance, and the like. Some people exaggerate negative perceptions of themselves compared to models who are too different from them (Trower and Kiely, 1983). Most motor skills instructors who have used video have experienced the keen interest of people watching themselves on video.

Care must be taken to monitor subject motivation and the psychological impact of anyone else who may also be watching. Some rather interesting comments and behaviors from an audience arise during video replay. The most desirable situation is one-on-one with the performer, eliminating extraneous effects of an audience. If other performers are watching the replay, be sure to focus group attention on good points of performance and try to limit extraneous or negative comments.

Slow-Motion Replay

In general, video images generated for slow-motion analysis should focus on higher-speed movements that are difficult to see with the naked eye. Videos made for this kind of replay should maximize the size of the performer in the field of view. Zooming in on the subject is important for two reasons. First, the resolution of the video picture will be improved in the pause and slow-motion modes of the VCR. Second, perceptual problems with limited background information are reduced when the images are paused, slowed down, or repeated.

The ability to freeze the motion at key points in the movement and to slow down very fast movements greatly increases observational power. This is why slow-motion video analysis should not be limited to high-speed movements or sport skills. A coach struggling to make a key diagnostic decision might use slow-motion video replay to verify certain perceptions from live analyses of slow movements.

> **KEY POINT**
>
> *Video images created for slow-motion replay in qualitative analysis should zoom in on the subject to maximize the performer's size in the field of view.*

This greater observational power, however, comes at a cost. Slow-motion video analysis requires more time for the videotape to be positioned, played, and replayed. Time used in video analysis is often time lost in performer practice and the live qualitative analysis that could be performed.

Camera Position

Camera location should be carefully selected to make sure subject motion is as close to right angles to the camera as possible. Ideally, the camcorder should be mounted on a tripod. Panning should generally be avoided, but limited panning may be needed in certain conditions. To avoid perspective or lens distortions, the camcorder should be as far from the subject as possible, using the zoom lens to frame the subject. Extreme examples of such distortion are a peephole in a door and a camcorder's view of a tennis court from above the fence. Objects in the foreground appear very large; objects far away appear much smaller than normal. And objects moving to and from the camera are distorted. Motion of objects in the distance is underestimated, while motion of objects near the camera is exaggerated. The farther different-size objects are from the camera, the smaller the differences between their sizes appear.

Limit camera motion when capturing video images for any qualitative analysis. Observers of the video you generate are attempting to detect changes in the subject's position. Changes in camera angle or camera motion will distort the actual motion of the subject. It is important to understand how camera motion affects the images created. The most accurate video representation (2-D) of reality (3-D) would be a nonmoving camera positioned on a tripod, with the subject moving parallel to the camera lens. This situation will create images of the subject moving on a 2-D background that are representative of the actual motion.

It is not always possible to set up a stationary camera to record movements. A good real-world example of how camera motion can dramatically change the perception of motion is the Indianapolis 500. A stationary camera parallel to the straightaway would capture images (very few frames!) of the cars moving past. A camera mounted looking out the side of a car in the race would see a very different view of the speeds of the cars, like what you experience on the freeway.

Now imagine you are a race fan in the stands panning your camera as cars go by. Only at one instant, when the car is moving parallel to your seat, does your video picture accurately represent the movement of the car. The car moves toward you (and in the video) slowly, gets very fast near you, and slows again after the car passes you. The situation is analogous to the gymnastics example presented earlier. The motion of the car is underestimated as the car approaches. In effect, it becomes the proportional speed of the car as the car nears the camera angle of 90 degrees. The apparent length of the car is another example of this distortion. The car looks short in the distance, appears to get longer as it approaches you, and then shrinks as it moves away.

Taping Protocol

Precise control of the setting and technique of video capture are needed to generate images suitable for the qualitative analysis of interest. Although modern camcorders do well in various lighting conditions, the most desirable condition is even lighting from behind the camera. The camera location should strive for this lighting and for a contrasting background with a horizontal or vertical reference. The background should not hide the motion of the subject and should provide a directional frame of reference on which to place the subject's motion. The protocol should provide subject identification information and some way to identify trials. Verbal cueing to the tape audio, time codes, or clocks in the field of view will help you identify key events or trials in later playback.

It is very important to make a written record of the subject, date, and notes on performance and keep it with the video. Any information about the performance or results that is not visible in the field of view should be written down. With written records, the analyst does not have to play the tape to identify places to start. VCR counter numbers and indexing information can be added to the written record to help access video images quickly.

THE FUTURE OF VIDEO AND COMPUTERS IN QUALITATIVE ANALYSIS

The observational power of analysts can be improved by videotape replay, especially the slow-motion replay of human movement. Current video equipment with advanced features useful in qualitative analysis is often very expensive. A coach who wanted to use split-screen video to compare a performer's trial with a prototype performance would not be able to buy the right equipment inexpensively off the shelf. Even more expensive are computer-assisted video systems that can place drawings or graphics on the video to illustrate key points on the movement. Advances in computer and video technology will eventually make many of these new video features affordable for kinesiology professionals.

The future of video imaging will be strongly related to developments in cameras and computers. Increases in the speed and storage capabilities of computers may make the tape storage of video obsolete. There are already cameras that interface directly with computers so the CCD video data are digitized and stored directly in the computer. Technical advances in cameras to capture video and in computers to store and enhance the video images may make concerns about resolution and the speed of video less of a problem. Hardware and software are now available that sample the analog signal of video at a higher rate, allowing computers to grab or digitize higher-resolution video still images.

Video images and sound can also be stored on optical or videodisks (12-inch optical disks). Advances in writing and erasable optical disks, video and digital data compression, and more powerful computers may make video image storage on cassette tapes obsolete.

In the future, the line between video technology and computers will get thinner and thinner. In the past, research has focused on how separate computer technology could be used to assist in the coding and analysis of the movements of athletes on a team from video recordings of sport (Franks and Goodman, 1986; Franks and Nagelkerke, 1988; Patrick and Lowdon, 1987). Researchers and commercial vendors are looking at ways to integrate computer and video/imaging technologies. Overlays or split screens with current performance versus desirable form are possible with present technology. The main questions are these: When will good qualitative analysis video/computer support equipment be available at a reasonable cost? When will the advantages of each technology be combined and readily available?

> *Technological advances and the integration of video and computer technology may dramatically influence the impact and use of video for the qualitative analysis of human movement.*
>
> **KEY POINT**

Companies that specialize in high-speed and research videography have developed products for qualitative analysis of sport skills. The *Video Illustrator* (Peak Performance Technologies, Englewood, CO) has a 60-hertz video camera, commercial-grade VCR, computer, frame grabber, and software (figure 11.3). The user can split the screen into two, four, or eight images for easy comparison or sequence illustration. On-screen illustration and calculation capabilities allow the coach to highlight various aspects of performance. Since calculations from the video image require careful setup and have many technical limitations, special care must be taken to make sure that the angle or speed calculations are accurate (Allard, Stokes, and Blanchi, 1995). The *Video Illustrator* system can also handle high-speed video.

The *Video Expert* system (Motion Analysis Corp., Santa Rosa, CA) is another qualitative analysis video system similar to the *Video Illustrator* system. Unfortunately, this system is too expensive ($12,000-$30,000) for most teachers and coaches. A less expensive system, the *Neat* system (Neat Systems Inc., Annapolis, MD; figure 11.4), costs around $5,000. It can grab video from any camcorder, store it on a computer's hard drive, and use software to replay and manipulate the video.

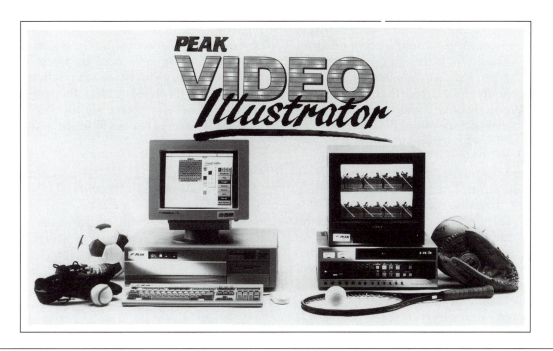

Figure 11.3 The *Video Illustrator* system allows the user to customize video for teaching and qualitative analysis. Courtesy of Peak Performance Technologies, Englewood, CO.

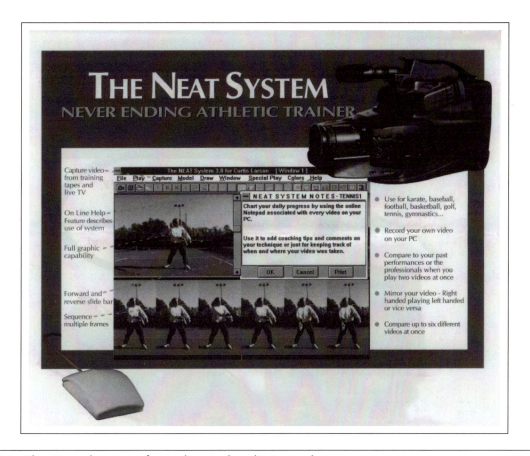

Figure 11.4 The *Neat* video system for teaching and qualitative analysis. Courtesy of Neat Systems Inc., Annapolis, MD.

Improvements in videotape technology, HDTV, and the increased integration of imaging and computers will make for an exciting future for the use of imaging for qualitative analysis. The video systems of the future that are designed for qualitative analysis will have many attractive features to help teach motor skills. The systems will be portable with extended battery power; screens will be large, flat, antiglare color monitors; and the computer-controlled camera can be run by remote control or programmed to follow the athlete. Currently, the only barriers to this technology are the cost of the equipment and the expertise of the teacher, coach, or therapist. We expect the cost of advanced computer and video technology to come down and that kinesiology research will give some insight into how best to use these tools together to improve the qualitative analysis of human movement.

SUMMARY

Videotape is an important tool in extending observational power for qualitative analysis. Although video replay has been used as feedback for performers, the research has not shown it to be superior to teacher feedback. Slow-motion video replay, however, dramatically extends the observational ability of analysts. The ability to replay movements again and again also improves observation. Video equipment and technical information were reviewed to assist teachers/ coaches in using videotape for qualitative analysis. Many advanced video features that are currently very expensive should become available because of advances in video and computer technology.

DISCUSSION QUESTIONS

1. What views would be desirable for a qualitative analysis of a pitcher's form versus the ball flight in baseball pitching?

2. What compromises must be made in setting up the field of view for videotaping the approach for a long jump?

3. Compare and contrast the sampling rates of the human eye, normal video, and high-speed video.

4. A TV station would like to shoot a special on the dramatic improvement of a local pole vaulter. What advice would you give the show's producer on how to videotape some of the athlete's practice vaults? How do views that exaggerate the motion for TV viewers differ from views that are good for observation of performance?

GLOSSARY

augmented feedback—Feedback that goes beyond the information normally available to a performer.

closed motor skills—A classification of motor skills that have few environmental restrictions because the performer has minimal temporal and environmental restrictions on the movement selected.

common errors—Errors that are typically observed in people learning a motor skill.

critical features—The key features of a movement that are necessary for optimal performance.

cues—Short, descriptive words or phrases used to communicate ideas about movement to learners.

deterministic model—A model linking mechanical variables with the goal of the movement, used in the Hay and Reid (1988) approach to qualitative analysis.

developmental sequence—The classification of typical phases or stages that people exhibit in the development of a movement.

diagnosis—Critical scrutiny of the strengths and weaknesses identified in evaluation being done to prioritize possible means of intervention in qualitative analysis.

dynamic visual acuity (DVA)—The accuracy of visual discrimination when there is relative movement between the observer and an object.

evaluation—The judgment of the quality of human movement to identify strengths and weaknesses of performance within qualitative analysis.

exaggeration—An intervention technique in which a performer is encouraged to overcorrect or overcompensate for a persistent movement error in the hope that this feedback might bring about the desired change in technique.

feedback—Information about human movement.

field—Half of a video picture, composed of the even- or odd-numbered horizontal lines of a video frame (but not both).

field dependence—A way of processing information in which the background information is necessary for accurate interpretation. An analyst might use this perceptual style since it relies heavily on the frame of reference.

field independence—A way of processing information without reference to any sources of information except the object or movement being observed. With this perceptual style, the observer does not need background information to make sense of the movement.

filters—Processes in the brain that deal with different information—intensity, color, lines, shapes, shades, sounds—to help make sense of sensory information.

fixation—The focusing of the eyes on an object in the visual field.

frame—A single video picture that is composed of two halves called fields. There are 25 or 30 frames for each second of normal video.

freeze-frame—A mode of video replay that stops and holds a video image so it can be shown on a monitor.

fundamental movement pattern—A general category of human movements (e.g., lift, run, jump, throw).

fusion—Putting together the two-dimensional visual information from two eyes to create the three-dimensional perception of vision.

gestalt—A way of processing visual spatial information to get an overall impression. In a gestalt way of looking at things, the whole is greater than the sum of its parts. This impression of the event uses features such as region, proximity, continuation, and closure. Gestalt is also a field of study in psychology.

high-speed video—Special video technology used to create more video pictures (frames) per second than the 25 or 30 frames in normal video.

information processing—The cognitive process of organizing and making sense of sensory information, and the decision making based on that sensory information.

intervention—The fourth task of the integrated model of qualitative analysis. It involves the administration of feedback, corrections, or other change in the environment provided by the analyst to improve performance.

intrinsic feedback—Information about movement that is readily available to the performer (e.g., sensory information about the result, kinesthetic information, and proprioceptive information).

jog-shuttle dial—A key VCR feature that uses a dial to allow multiple-speed playback, either forward or backward.

knowledge of performance (KP)—Information about the movement of the body.

knowledge of results (KR)—Information about the outcome or results of a movement.

manual guidance—A mode of intervention within qualitative analysis in which the analyst physically positions or assists the performer in making the desired movement.

mechanical guidance—A mode of intervention within qualitative analysis that uses an aid or mechanical device to help the performer make the desired movement.

moment of inertia—A mechanical term that describes an object's resistance to being rotated (angular acceleration).

motor program—The essential cognitive information needed to perform a movement.

observation—The second task of an integrated qualitative analysis. In this task, sensory information is gathered about performance with a systematic observational strategy.

observational learning—The use of visual models (pictures or demonstrations) to provide information about a movement.

open motor skills—A classification of motor skills that are strongly influenced by their environment because it is unpredictable.

perception—The organization and interpretation of stimuli from our environment, mediated by our senses.

performance—The quality of a movement in achieving a goal, or the short-term and long-term effectiveness of a person's movement in achieving a goal.

pixel—Short for a picture element. The small dots of light that form a video image.

qualitative analysis—The systematic observation and introspective judgment of the quality of human movement for the purpose of providing the most appropriate intervention to improve performance.

reinforcement—Feedback that supports a behavior so that it will be repeated and eventually learned.

reliability—The consistency of a measurement or a qualitative assessment.

resolution—The number of lines of pixels that make up a video image.

sampling rate—The temporal resolution of a measurement or qualitative analysis of a continuous event. The sampling rate of normal video is 30 frames (pictures) per second.

shutter—A photo or video technique to limit the exposure time of an image. This limits the chances of significant motion of the object during image capture, which would create a blurry image.

skill—An adapted fundamental movement pattern for a specific activity or goal. For example, a baseball pitch is a skill related to overarm throwing.

smooth pursuit—The simultaneous rotation of both eyes to track a slow-moving object.

spatial ability—The ability to deal with spatial relationships and to use this information in different contexts.

static visual acuity (SVA)—The accuracy of visual discrimination in static, high-contrast conditions.

style—Aspects of movement that are personal differences, idiosyncrasies, or actions related to a specific performer.

systematic observational strategy (SOS)—A plan to gather all the relevant information about a human movement within qualitative analysis.

task modification—An intervention strategy that improves performance by changing a performer's practice tasks to make them more appropriate for the performer.

technique—A kind of motor skill that has a more specific purpose. For example, a curveball is a technique related to the skill of baseball pitching.

validity—The extent to which a measurement or a qualitative analysis accurately assesses a variable.

vergence—Medial and lateral eye movements that adjust for movements of objects toward and away from the observer.

zoom lens—A key feature in video camcorders that allows the field of view to be adjusted for objects at different distances.

BIBLIOGRAPHY

Abendroth-Smith, J., Kras, J., & Strand, B. (1996). Get aboard the B-BOAT: Biomechanically based observation and analysis for teachers. *Journal of Physical Education, Recreation and Dance,* **67**(8), 20-23.

Abernethy, B. (1988). Visual search in sport and ergonomics: Its relationship to selective attention and performer expertise. *Human Performance,* **1**, 205-235.

Abernethy, B. (1989). Expert-novice differences in perception: How expert does the expert have to be? *Canadian Journal of Sport Sciences,* **14**, 27-30.

Abernethy, B. & Russell, D.G. (1987). The relationship between expertise and visual search strategy in a racquet sport. *Human Movement Science,* **6**, 283-319.

Adrian, M.J. & Cooper, J.M. (1989). *Biomechanics of human movement.* Indianapolis, IN: Benchmark Press.

Adrian, M.J. & Cooper, J.M. (1995). *Biomechanics of human movement* (2nd ed.). Madison, WI: Brown & Benchmark.

Adrian, M.J. & Enberg, M.L. (1971). Sequential timing of three overhead patterns. In C. Widule (Ed.). *Kinesiology Review.* Washington, DC: AAHPER, 1-9.

Adrian, M. & House, G. (1987a). Sporting miscues: Part one. *Strategies,* **1**(1), 11-14.

Adrian, M. & House, G. (1987b). Sporting miscues: Part two. *Strategies,* **1**(2), 13-15.

Alfano, P.L. & Michel, G.F. (1990). Restricting field of view: Perceptual and performance effects. *Perceptual and Motor Skills,* **70**, 35-45.

Allard, P., Stokes, I., & Blanchi, J. (Eds.) (1995). *Three-dimensional analysis of human movement.* Champaign, IL: Human Kinetics.

Allison, P.C. (1985a, August). The development of the skill of observing during field experiences of pre-service physical education teachers. Paper presented at the meeting of the Association Internationale des Ecoles Superieures d'Education Physique, Garden City, NY.

Allison, P.C. (1985b). Observing for competence. *Journal of Physical Education, Recreation and Dance,* **60**(6), 50-51, 54.

Allison, P.C. (1986, April). Laban's movement framework as a descriptor of change in students' movement response observations. Paper presented at the national convention of the American Alliance for Health, Physical Education and Dance, Cincinnati, OH.

Allison, P.C. (1987a, April). The impact of varying amounts of lesson responsibility on pre-service physi-

cal education teachers' ability to observe. Paper presented at the national convention of the American Alliance for Health, Physical Education, Recreation and Dance, Las Vegas, NV.

Allison, P.C. (1987b). What and how pre-service physical education teachers observe during an early field experience. *Research Quarterly Exercise and Sport,* **58**, 242-249.

Allison, P.C. (1988). Strategies for observing during field experiences. *Journal of Physical Education, Recreation and Dance,* **59**(2), 28-30.

Allison, P.C. (1990). Classroom teachers' observations of physical education lessons. *Journal of Teaching in Physical Education,* **4**, 272-283.

Ammons, R.B. (1956). Effects of knowledge of performance: A survey and tentative theoretical formulation. *Journal of General Psychology,* **54**, 279-299.

Anderson, J.R. (1990). *Cognitive psychology and its implications.* New York, NY: W.H. Freeman & Co.

Anderson, M.B. (1979). Comparison of muscle patterning in the overarm throw and tennis serve. *Research Quarterly,* **50**, 541-553.

Annett, J. (1993). The learning of motor skills: Sports science and ergonomics perspectives. *Ergonomics,* **37**, 5-16.

Arend, S. & Higgins, J.R. (1976). A strategy for the classification, subjective analysis and observation of human movement. *Journal of Human Movement Studies,* **2**, 36-52.

Armstrong, C.W. (1977a). Skill analysis and kinesthetic experience. In R.E. Stadulis (Ed.). *Research and practice in physical education.* Champaign, IL: Human Kinetics, 13-18.

Armstrong, C.W. (1977b). Effects of teaching experience, knowledge of performer competence and knowledge of performance outcome on performance error identification. *Research Quarterly,* **48**, 318-327.

Armstrong, C.W. (1986). Research on movement analysis: Implications for the development of pedagogical competence. In M. Pieron & G. Graham (Eds.). *Sports pedagogy.* Champaign, IL: Human Kinetics, 27-32.

Armstrong, C.W. & Hoffman, S.J. (1979). Effects of teaching experience, knowledge of performer competence, and knowledge of performance outcome on performance error identification. *Research Quarterly,* **50**, 318-327.

Arnell, P. & Bauker, P. (1991). The accuracy of visual gait assessment. In *Proceedings of the 11th International*

Congress of the World Confederation for Physical Therapy. London: WCPT, 431.

Arnold, P.J. (1993). Kinesiology and the professional preparation of the movement teacher. *Journal of Human Movement Studies, 25*, 203-231.

Arnold, R.K. (1978). Optimizing skill learning: Moving to match the environment. *Journal of Physical Education, Recreation, and Dance, 49*(9), 84-86.

Arrighi, M.A. (1974). The nature of game strategy observation in field hockey with respect to selected variables. Doctoral dissertation, University of North Carolina, Greensboro. Abstract in *Dissertation Abstracts International, 35*, 2030A.

Attinger, D., Luethi, S., & Stuessi, E. (1987). Comparison of subjective gait observation with measured gait asymmetry. In G. Bergmann et al. (Eds.). *Biomechanics: Basic and applied research.*Boston: M. Nijhoff, 563-568.

Atwater, A.E. (1979). Biomechanics of overarm throwing movements and of throwing injuries. *Exercise and Sport Sciences Reviews, 7*, 43-85.

Austin, S. & Miller, L. (1992). An empirical study of the cybervision golf videotape. *Perceptual and Motor Skills, 74*, 875-881.

Bahill, A.T. & LaRitz, T. (1984). Why can't batters keep their eyes on the ball? *American Scientist, 72*, 249-253.

Balan, C.M. & Davis, W.E. (1993). Ecological task analysis—An approach to teaching physical education. *Journal of Physical Education, Recreation, and Dance, 64*(9), 54-61.

Baluyut, R., Genaidy, A.M., Davis, L.S., Sehll, R.L., & Simmons, R.J. (1995). Use of visual perception in estimating static postural stresses: Magnitudes and sources of error. *Ergonomics, 38*, 1841-1850.

Bampton, S. (1979). *A guide to the visual examination of pathological gait.* Philadelphia, PA: Temple University Rehabilitation and Research Training Center No. 8., Moss Rehabilitation Hospital.

Bard, C. & Fleury, M. (1976). Analysis of visual search activity during sport problem situations. *Journal of Human Movement Studies, 3*, 214-222.

Bard, C., Fleury, M., Carriere, L., & Halle, M. (1980). Analysis of gymnastics judges' visual search. *Research Quarterly for Exercise and Sport, 51*, 267-273.

Barrett, K.R. (1977). We see so much but perceive so little: Why? In L.I. Gedvilas and M.E. Kneer (Eds.). *Proceedings of the NAPECW/NCPEAM National Conference.* Chicago: University of Illinois-Chicago Circle.

Barrett, K.R. (1979a). *Observation of movement—An assumed teaching/coaching behavior.* Unpublished manuscript, University of North Carolina, Greensboro.

Barrett, K.R. (1979b). Observation of movement for teachers—A synthesis and implications. *Motor Skills: Theory into Practice, 3*, 67-76.

Barrett, K.R. (1979c). Observation for teaching and coaching. *JOPER, 50*(1), 23-25.

Barrett, K.R. (1980, February). A system for describing and observing a spatial relationship movement task. Paper presented at the preconvention symposium on Physical Education for Children, Southern District of the American Alliance for Health, Physical Education and Recreation, Nashville, TN.

Barrett, K.R. (1981, October). Observation as a teaching behavior—Research to practice. Paper presented at the national meeting of the Canadian Association for Physical Education and Health Education.

Barrett, K.R. (1982, April). The content of observing—A model for curriculum development. Paper presented at the national convention of the American Alliance for Health, Physical Education, Recreation and Dance, Houston, TX.

Barrett, K.R. (1983). A hypothetical model of observing as a teaching skill. *Journal of Teaching in Physical Education, 3*, 22-31.

Barrett, K.R., Allison, P.C., & Bell, R. (1987). What preservice physical education teachers see in an unguided field experience: A follow-up study. *Journal of Teaching in Physical Education, 7*, 12-21.

Barthels, K. & Kreighbaum, E. (1988, April). A Western System of Analysis and Observation. Paper presented to the national convention of the American Alliance for Health, Physical Education, Recreation and Dance, Kansas City, MO.

Bayless, M.A. (1980). The effect of style of teaching on ability to detect errors in performance. *Wyoming Journal for Health, Physical Education, Recreation and Dance, 3*, 2-4, 15.

Bayless, M.A. (1981). Effect of exposure to prototypic skill and experience in identification of performance error. *Perceptual and Motor Skills, 52*, 667-670.

Behar, I. & Bevan, W. (1961). The perceived duration of auditory and visual intervals: Cross-model comparison and interaction. *American Journal of Psychology, 74*, 17-26.

Belka, D.E. (1988). What preservice physical educators observe about lessons in progressive field experiences. *Journal of Teaching in Physical Education, 7*, 311-326.

Bell, F.I. (1987). The effects of two training programs on the ability of preservice physical education majors to observe the developmental steps in the overarm throw for force. Doctoral dissertation, University of North Carolina, Greensboro. Abstract in *Dissertation Abstracts International, 48*, 1144A.

Bell, R., Barrett, K.R., & Allison, P.E. (1985). What preservice physical education teachers see in an unguided, early field experience. *Journal of Teaching in Physical Education, 4*, 81-90.

Berg, K. (1975). Functional approach to undergraduate kinesiology. *JOPER, 46*(7), 43-44.

Berger, J. (1987). *Ways of seeing.* London: British Broadcasting Corp. & Penguin Books.

Best, J.B. (1986). *Cognitive psychology.* St. Paul, MN: West Publishing Company.

Beveridge, S.K. & Gangstead, S.K. (1984). A comparative analysis of the effects of instruction on the analytical proficiency of physical education teachers and undergraduates. Paper presented at the Anaheim, California, Annual Convention for the American Alliance for Health, Physical Education, Recreation and Dance. (ERIC Document Reproduction Service No. ED 244, 939.)

Beveridge, S.K. & Gangstead, S.K. (1988). Teaching experience and training in the sports skill analysis process. *The Journal of Teaching in Physical Education, 7*, 103-114.

Bilodeau, I.M. (1969). Information feedback. In E.A. Bilodeau (Ed.). *Principles of skill acquisition.* London: Academic Press.

Bird, M. & Hudson, J. (1990). Biomechanical Observation: Visually Accessible Variables. In Nosek, M., Sojka, D., Morrison, P., & Susan, P. (Eds.). *Proceedings of the 8th International Symposium of the Society of Biomechanics in Sports.* Prague: Conex, 321-326.

Biscan, D.U. & Hoffman, S. J. (1976). Movement analysis as a generic ability of physical education teachers and students. *Research Quarterly, 47*, 161-163.

Blundell, N.L. (1985). The contribution of vision to the learning and performance of sports skills. Part 1: The role of selected visual parameters. *Australian Journal of Science and Medicine in Sport, 17*, 3-11.

Boehm, A.E. & Weinber, R.A. (1987). *The classroom observer: Developing observation skills in early childhood settings.* New York: Teachers College Press.

Bowers, L. & Klesius, S. (1991, April). Use of interactive videodisk in the analysis of skills for teaching. Paper presented to the American Alliance for Health, Physical Education, Recreation and Dance, San Francisco, CA.

Boyce, W.F., Gowland, C., Rosenbaum, P., Lane, M., Plews, N., Goldsmith, C., Russell, D., Wright, V., Poter, S., & Harding, D. (1995). The gross motor performance measure: Validity and responsiveness of a measure of quality of movement. *Physical Therapy, 75*, 603-613.

Boyer, E.L. (1990). *Scholarship reconsidered: Priorities of the professoriat.* Princeton, NJ: The Carnegie Foundation for the Advancement of Teaching.

Braden, V. (1983, May). Vic Braden's startling revelations about line calls. *Tennis*, 37-39.

Bressan, E.S., & Weiss, M.R. (1982). A theory of instruction for developing competence, self-confidence and persistence in physical education. *Journal of Teaching in Physical Education, 2*(1), 38-47.

Broadbent, D. (1958). *Perception and Communication.* Oxford: Pergamon.

Broer, M.R. (1960). *Efficiency of Human Movement.* Philadelphia: Saunders.

Broker, J.P., Gregor, R.J., & Schmidt, R.A. (1989). Extrinsic feedback and the learning of cycling kinetic patterns. *Journal of Biomechanics, 22*, 991. Abstract of XII Congress ISB.

Brophy, J. & Good, T. (1986). Teacher behavior and student achievement. In M. Wittrock (Ed.). *Handbook of research on teaching* (3rd ed.). New York: Macmillan, 328-375.

Brosvic, G.M. & Finizio, S. (1995). Inaccurate feedback and performance on the Muller-Lyer illusion. *Perceptual and Motor Skills, 80*, 896-898.

Brown, E.W. (1982). Visual evaluation techniques for skill analysis. *Journal of Physical Education, Recreation, and Dance, 53*(1), 21-26, 29.

Brown, E.W. (1984). Kinesiological analysis of motor skills via visual evaluation techniques. In R. Shapiro & J.R. Marett (Eds.). *Proceedings: Second National Symposium on Teaching Kinesiology and Biomechanics in Sports.* Colorado Springs, CO: NASPE, 95-96.

Brown, S. (1995). The effects of limited and repeated demonstrations of the development of fielding and throwing in children. Doctoral dissertation, University of South Carolina. Abstract in *Dissertation Abstracts International, 55*, 1868A.

Bunn, J.W. (1955). *Scientific principles of coaching.* Englewood Cliffs, NJ: Prentice-Hall.

Burg, A. (1966). Visual acuity as measured by static and dynamic tests: A comparative evaluation. *Journal of Applied Psychology, 50*, 460-466.

Campbell, F.W. & Wurtz, R.H. (1978). Saccadic omission: Why we do not see a gray-out during a saccadic movement. *Vision Research, 18*, 1297-1303.

Cappozzo, A., Marchetti, M., & Tosi, V. (Eds.) (1992). *Biolocomotion: A century of research using moving pictures.* Rome: Promograph.

Carpenter, R.H.S. (1988). *Movements of the eyes* (2nd ed.). London: Pion.

Catalano, J. (1995, June). The eyes have it. *Training & Conditioning*, 6-14.

Cavanagh, P.R. (1990). Biomechanics: A bridge builder among the sport sciences. *Medicine and Science in Sports and Exercise, 22*, 546-557.

Cavanagh, P.R. & Kram, R. (1985). The efficiency of human movement—A statement of the problem. *Medicine and Science in Sports and Exercise, 17*, 304-308.

Cayer, L. (1992). The skill of analysis and correction. In *Proceedings: 3rd National Tennis Seminar.* Melbourne: Tennis Australia, 1-15.

Chen, L. (1982). Topological structure in visual perception. *Science, 128*(12), 699-700.

Christina, R.W. & Corcos, D.M. (1988). *Coaches guide to teaching sport skills.* Champaign, IL: Human Kinetics.

Chung, T.W. (1993). The effectiveness of computer-based interactive video instruction on psychomotor skill analysis competency of preservice physical education teachers in tennis teaching. Doctoral dissertation, University of Northern Colorado. Abstract in *Dissertation Abstracts International, 53*, 2290A.

Clark, J.E., Stamm, C.L., & Urquia, M.F. (1979). Developmental variability: The issue of reliability. In G.C. Roberts & K.M. Newell (Eds.). *Psychology of motor behavior and sport—1978*. Champaign, IL: Human Kinetics, 253-257.

Cloes, M., Deneve, A., & Pieron, M. (1995). Interindividual variability of teacher's feedback. Study in simulated teaching conditions. *European Physical Education Review*, **1**, 83-93.

Cloes, M., Premuzak, J., & Pieron, M. (1995). Effectiveness of a video training programme used to improve error identification and feedback processes by physical education student teachers. *International Journal of Physical Education*, **32**(3), 4-10.

Cohn, T.E., & Chaplik, D.D. (1991). Visual training in soccer. *Perceptual and Motor Skills*, **72**, 1238.

Consumer Reports (1995, March). Your home-entertainment guide. *Consumer Reports*, 155-207.

Cook, D.A. (1990, Winter). Using the basic skills to organize your movement analysis. *Professional Skier*, 50-52.

Cooper, J.M. & Glassow, R.B. (1963). *Kinesiology*. St. Louis: Mosby.

Cooper, L.K. & Rothstein, A.L. (1981). Videotape replay and the learning of skills in open and closed environments. *Research Quarterly for Exercise and Sport*, **52**, 191-199.

Cox, R.H. (1987). An exploratory investigation of a signal discrimination problem in tennis. *Journal of Human Movement Studies*, **13**, 197-210.

Cozzallio, E.R. (1986). The development of assessment instruments for screening selected gross motor skills in kindergarten children. Doctoral dissertation, Florida State University. Abstract in *Dissertation Abstracts International*, **47**, 118A.

Craft, A.H. (1977). The teaching of skills for the observation of movement: Inquiry into a model. Doctoral dissertation, University of North Carolina, Greensboro. Abstract in *Dissertation Abstracts International*, **38**, 1975A.

Craik, R.L. & Oatis, C.A. (1995). *Gait analysis: Theory and application*. St. Louis: Mosby.

Dahle, L.K., Mueller, M., Delitto, A., & Diamond, J.E. (1991). Visual assessment of foot type and relationship of foot type to lower extremity injury. *Journal of Orthopaedic and Sports Physical Therapy*, **14**, 70-74.

Dale, E. (1984). *The Educator's Quotebook*. Bloomington, IN: A Publication of the Phi Delta Kappa Educational Foundation.

Damos, D. (1988) Determining the transfer of training using curve fitting. *Proceedings of the Human Factors Society*, 32nd Annual Meeting.

Daniels, D.B. (1984). Basic movements and modeling: An approach to teaching skill analysis in the undergraduate biomechanics course. In R. Shapiro & J.R. Marett (Eds.). *Proceedings: Second National Symposium on Teaching Kinesiology and Biomechanics in Sports*. Colorado Springs, CO: NASPE, 243-246.

Daniels, D.B. (1987). Qualitative analysis: The coach's most important tool. In Petiot, B. et al. (Eds.). *World identification systems for gymnastic talent*. Montreal: Sport Psyche Editions, 163-172.

Davis, J. (1980). Learning to see: Training in observation of movement. *JOPER*, **51**(1), 89-90.

Davis, W. E. (1984). Motor ability assessment of populations with handicapping conditions: Challenging basic assumptions. *Adapted Physical Activity Quarterly*, **1**, 125-140.

Davis, W. E. & Burton, A.W. (1991). Ecological task analysis: Translating movement behavior theory into practice. *Adaptive Physical Education Quarterly*, **8**, 154-177.

Day, M. C. (1975). Developmental trends in visual scanning. In H.W. Reese (Ed.). *Advances in child development and behavior*. New York: Academic Press, 154-193.

DeBruin, H., Russell, D.J., Latter, J.E., & Sadler, J.T.S. (1982). Angle-angle diagrams in monitoring and quantification of gait patterns for children with cerebral palsy. *American Journal of Physical Medicine*, **61**, 176-192.

Dedeyn, K. (1991). Error identification comparison between three modes of viewing a skill. In J. Wilkerson, E. Kreighbaum, & C. Tant (Eds.). *Teaching kinesiology and biomechanics in sports*. Ames, IA: NASPE Kinesiology Academy, 21-25.

DeLooze, M.P., Toussaint, H.M., Ensink, J., Mangnus, C., & Van der Beek, A.J. (1994). The validity of visual observation to assess posture in a laboratory-simulated, manual material handling task. *Ergonomics*, **37**, 1335-1343.

DePauw, K. & GocKarp, G. (1989, January). Systematic infusion of knowledge into the undergraduate curriculum. Paper presented at the National Association for Physical Education in Higher Education Conference, San Antonio, TX.

DeRenne, C., Ho, K., & Blitzblau, A. (1990). Effects of weighted implement training on throwing velocity. *Journal of Applied Sport Science Research*, **4**, 16-19.

DeRenne, C. & House, T. (1987, March). The 4 absolutes of pitching mechanics. *Scholastic Coach*, 79-83.

Deutsch, J. A. & Deutsch, D. (1963). Attention: Some theoretical considerations. *Psychological Review*, **70**, 80-90.

Donkelaar, P. & Lee, R.G. (1994). The role of vision and eye motion during reaching to intercept moving targets. *Human Movement Science*, **13**, 765-783.

Douwes, M. & Dul, J. (1991). Validity and reliability of estimating body angles by direct and indirect observations. In Y. Queinnec & F. Daniellou (Eds.). *Designing for Everyone: Proceedings of the International Ergonomics Association*. London: Taylor & Francis, 885-887.

Dowell, L.J. (1978). Throwing for distance: Air resistance, angle of projection, and ball size and weight. *Motor Skills: Theory into Practice*, **3**(1), 11-14.

Dowrick, P.W. (1991a). Equipment fundamentals. In P.W. Dowrick (Ed.). *Practical guide to using video in the behavioral sciences.*New York: John Wiley & Sons, 7-29.

Dowrick, P.W. (1991b). Feedback and Self-Confrontation. In P.W. Dowrick (Ed.). *Practical guide to using video in the behavioral sciences.* New York: John Wiley & Sons, 92-108.

Draper, J. (1986). Analyzing skill to improve performance. *Sports Coach, 9*(4), 33-35.

Duck, T. (1986, June). Applied sport biomechanics for advanced coaching. *Sports Science Periodical on Research and Technology in Sport,* 1-6.

Dunham, P. (1986). Evaluation for excellence. *Journal of Physical Education, Recreation and Dance, 57*(6), 34-36, 60.

Dunham, P. (1994). *Evaluation for Physical Education.* Englewood, CO: Morton.

Dunham, P., Reeve, E.J., & Morrison, C.S. (1989). *DISPE: A total instructional system for physical education.* Edina, MN: Alpha Editions.

Eastlack, M.E., Arvidson, J., Snyder-Mackler, L., Danoff, J.V., & McGarvey, C.L. (1991). Interrater reliability of videotaped observational gait analysis assessments. *Physical Therapy, 71,* 465-472.

Eastman Kodak Company (1979). *High speed photography standard book.* No. 0-87985-165-1.

Eckrich, J., Widule, C.J., Shrader, R.A., & Maver, J. (1994). The effects of video observational training on video and live observational proficiency. *Journal of Teaching in Physical Education, 13,* 216-227.

Eckrich, R. (1991). The effects of video observational training on video and live observational proficiency. Doctoral dissertation, Purdue University. Abstract in *Dissertation Abstracts International, 52,* 465A.

Emmen, H.H., Wesseling, L.G., Bootsma, R.J., Whiting, H.T.A., & Van Wieringen, P.C.W. (1985). The effect of video-modeling and video-feedback on the learning of the tennis service by novices. *Journal of Sports Sciences, 3,* 127-138.

Ericson, M., Kilbom, A., Wiktorin, C., & Winkel, J. (1991). Validity and reliability in the estimation of trunk, arm and neck inclination by observation. *Proceedings of the International Ergonomics Association Conference.* Paris, 245-247.

Eriksen, C. W. & Webb, J. M. (1989). Shifting of attentional focus within and about a visual display. *Perception and Psychophysics, 45,* 175-183.

Farah, M.J., Hammond, K.M., Levine, D.N., & Calvanio, R. (1988). Visual and spatial mental imagery: Dissociable systems of representation. *Cognitive Psychology, 20,* 439-462.

Feldman, L. (1988, April). Sony VCR ED-V9000. *Video Review,* 66-67.

Feltner, M.E. (1989). Three-dimensional interactions in a two-segment kinetic chain. Part II: Application to the throwing arms in baseball pitching. *International Journal of Sport Biomechanics, 5,* 420-450.

Feltner, M.E. & Dapena, J. (1986). Dynamics of the shoulder and elbow joints of the throwing arm during the baseball pitch. *International Journal of Sport Biomechanics, 2,* 235-259.

Fisher, G.H. (1981). Human information processing and a taxonomy of sporting skills. In I.M. Cockerill & W.W. MacGillivary (Eds.). *Vision and sport.* Cheltenham: Stanley Thornes.

Fisk, S.F. (1993, August). Seeing is believing. *Tennis,* 33.

Fitts, P.M. (1965). Factors in complex skill training. In R. Glaser (Ed.). *Training Research and Education.* New York: Wiley.

Fitts, P.M. & Posner, M.I. (1967). *Human Performance.* Belmont, CA: Brooks/Cole.

Fleisig, G.S., Andrews, J.R., Dillman, C.J., & Escamilla, R.F. (1995). Kinetics of baseball pitching with implications about injury mechanisms. *American Journal of Sports Medicine, 23,* 233-239.

Fleisig, G.S., Barrentine, S.W., Escamilla, R.F., & Andrews, J.R. (1996). Biomechanics of overarm throwing with implications for injuries. *American Journal of Sports Medicine, 23,* 233-239.

Fleming, L.K. (1980). Identifying performance errors and teaching cues in tennis: The effectiveness of an instruction program. Unpublished master's thesis, Brigham Young University, Provo, Utah.

Foster, S.L. & Cone, J.D. (1986). Design and use of direct observation procedures. In A.R. Ciminero, K.S. Calhounm, & H.E. Adams (Eds.). *Handbook of behavioral assessment.* New York: Wiley, 253-324.

Franck, F. (1979). *The awakened eye.* New York: Random House.

Franks, I.M. (1993). The effect of experience on the detection and location of performance differences in a gymnastic technique. *Research Quarterly for Exercise and Sport, 64,* 227-231.

Franks, I.M. & Goodman, D. (1986). A systematic approach to analyzing sports performance. *Journal of Sports Sciences, 4,* 49-59.

Franks, I.M. & Maile, L.J. (1991). The use of video in sport skill acquisition. In P.W. Dowrick (Ed.). *Practical guide to using video in the behavioral sciences.* New York: John Wiley & Sons, 231-243.

Franks, I.M. & Miller, G. (1991). Training coaches to observe and remember. *Journal of Sports Sciences, 9,* 285-297.

Franks, I.M. & Nagelkerke, P. (1988). The use of computer interactive video in sport analysis. *Ergonomics, 31,* 1593-1603.

Frederick, A.B. (1977). Using checklists and templates for analyzing gymnastic skills. In R.E. Stadulis (Ed.). *Research and practice in physical education.* Champaign, IL: Human Kinetics, 28-31.

French, C.A. & Plack, J.J. (1982). Effective communication: A rationale for skill instruction techniques. *Motor Skills: Theory into Practice*, **6**, 59-66.

Fronske, H. (1997). *Teaching Cues for Sports Skills*. Boston: Allyn & Bacon.

Fronske, H., Abendroth-Smith, J., & Blakmore, C. (1995). The effect of critical cues on throwing efficiency of elementary school children. *Research Quarterly for Exercise and Sport*, **66**(Suppl.), A-53.

Fronske, H. & Dunn, S.E. (1992). Cue your students in on good swimming. *Strategies*, **5**(5), 25-27.

Fronske, H., Wilson, R., & Dunn, S.E. (1992). Visual teaching cues for tennis instruction. *Journal of Physical Education, Recreation and Dance*, **63**(5), 13-14.

Gangstead, S.K. (1984). A comparison of three methodological approaches to skill specific analytical training. Jackson Wyoming, Northern Rocky Mountain Research Association. (ERIC Document Reproduction Service No. ED 255-471.)

Gangstead, S.K. (1987, June). Toward a pedagogical kinesiology: A training paradigm. Paper presented at the meeting of the International Congress of Health, Physical Education and Recreation, Vancouver, BC.

Gangstead, S.K. & Beveridge, S.K. (1984). The implementation and evaluation of a methodical approach to qualitative sports skill analysis instruction. *Journal of Teaching in Physical Education*, **3**(Winter), 60-70.

Gangstead, S.K., Cashel, C., & Beveridge, S.K. (1987). Perceptual style, visual retention and visual discrimination in qualitative sports skill analysis. Paper presented at the Annual Convention for the American Alliance for Health, Physical Education, Recreation and Dance. Research Consortium, Kansas City, MO.

Gavriyski, V. (1969). The colours and colour vision in sport. *Journal of Sports Medicine*, **4**, 49-53.

Genaidy, A.M., Simmons, R.J., Guo, L., & Hidalgo, J.A. (1993). Can visual perception be used to estimate body part angles? *Ergonomics*, **36**, 323-329.

Gentile, A.M. (1972). A working model of skill acquisition with application to teaching. *Quest*, **17**, 3-23.

Gibson, E.J. (1969). *Principles of perceptual development*. New York: Appleton-Century-Crofts.

Girardin, Y. & Hanson, D. (1967). Relationship between ability to perform tumbling skills and ability to diagnose performance errors. *Research Quarterly*, **38**, 556-561.

Gluck, M. & Kerr, L. (1982). *Mechanics for gymnastics coaching: Tools for skill analysis*. Springfield, IL: Charles C Thomas Publishers.

Godwin, S. (1975). Training powers of observation. In G. F. Curl (Ed.). *Human movement behavior: Conference report*. West Midlands, England: Association of Principals of Women's Colleges of Physical Education.

Goodkin, R. & Diller, L. (1973). Reliability among physical therapists in diagnosis and treatment of gait de-

viations in hemiplegics. *Perceptual and Motor Skills*, **37**, 727-734.

Gopher, D. & Donchin, E. (1986). Workload—An Examination of the Concept. In Boff, K.R., Kaufman, L., & Thomas, J.P. (Eds.). *Handbook of perception and human performance, Vol II*. New York, NY: John Wiley & Sons.

Gould, D. & Roberts, G. (1982). Modeling and motor skill acquisition. *Quest*, **33**, 214-230.

Gowland, C., Boyce, W.F., Wright, V., Russell, D., Goldsmith, C., & Rosenbaum, P. (1995). Reliability of the gross motor performance measure. *Physical Therapy*, **75**, 597-602.

Graham, K.C. (1988). A qualitative analysis of an effective teacher's movement task presentations during a unit of instruction. *The Physical Educator*, **11**, 187-195.

Graham, K.C., Hussey, K., Taylor, K., & Werner, P. (1993). A study of verbal presentations of three effective teachers. *Research Quarterly for Exercise and Sport*, **64**(Suppl.), 87A. (Abstract).

Gregg, J.R. (1987). *Vision and sports: An introduction*. Stoneham, MA: Butterworths Publishers.

Griffin, M.R. (1985). The utilization of product and process measures to compare the throwing, striking, and kicking proficiency of third and fifth grade students. Doctoral dissertation, Florida State University. Abstract in *Dissertation Abstracts International*, 45, 2797A.

Groot, C., Ortega, F., & Beltran, F.S. (1994). Thumb rule of visual angle: A new confirmation. *Perceptual and Motor Skills*, **78**, 232-234.

Groves, R. & Camaione, D.N. (1983). *Concepts in kinesiology* (2nd ed.). Philadelphia: Saunders.

Grunwald, H.A. (Ed.) (1986). *Artificial intelligence: Understanding computers*. Alexandria, VA: Time-Life Books.

Hall, J. (1993, Spring). Toward outcome-based movement analysis. *Professional Skier*, 10-12.

Halverson, L.E. (1983, April). Observing children's motor development in action. Paper presented at the national convention of the American Alliance for Health, Physical Education, Recreation and Dance, Minneapolis, MN.

Halverson, L.E., Roberton, M.A., & Harper, C.J. (1979, April). Learning to observe children's motor development. Paper presented to the national convention of the American Alliance for Health, Physical Education, and Recreation, New Orleans, LA.

Halverson, P.D. (1988). The effects of peer tutoring on sport skill analytic ability. Doctoral dissertation, Ohio State University. *Dissertation Abstracts International*, **48**, 2274A.

Hamburg, J. (1995). Coaching athletes using Laban movement analysis. *Journal of Physical Education, Recreation and Dance*, **66**(2), 34-37.

Harari, I. & Siedentop, D. (1990). Relationships among knowledge, experience and skill analysis ability. In D. Eldar & U. Simri (Eds.). *Integration or diversification of physical education and sport studies.* Wingate Institute: Emmanual Gill Publishing House, 197-204.

Harper, R.C. (1995). Effects of a videodisk instructional program on physical education majors' ability to observe the quality of performances of selected motor activities of pre-adolescents. Doctoral dissertation, The University of Alabama. Abstract in *Dissertation Abstracts International,* **55,** 3446A.

Harrison, J.M. (1973). A comparison of a videotape program and a teacher directed program of instruction in teaching the identification of archery errors. Unpublished doctoral dissertation, Brigham Young University, Provo, Utah.

Hartman, B.O. & Secrist, G.E. (1991). *Situational awareness is more than exceptional vision.* Alexandria, VA: Aerospace Medical Association.

Hatfield, F.C. (1972). Effects of prior experience, access to information, and level of performance on individual and group performance rating. *Perceptual and Motor Skills,* **35,** 19-26.

Hatze, H. (1976). Biomechanical aspects of a successful motion optimization. In P.V. Komi (Ed.). *Biomechanics VB.* Baltimore: University Park Press, 5-12.

Haubenstricker, J.L., Branta, C.F., & Seefeldt, V.D. (1983, May). *Standards of performance for throwing and catching.* East Lansing, MI: American Society for the Psychology of Sport and Physical Activity.

Hay, J. (1983). A system for the qualitative analysis of a motor skill. In G.A. Wood (Ed.). *Collected papers on sports biomechanics.* Perth: University of Western Australia Press, 97-116.

Hay, J.G. (1984). The development of deterministic models for qualitative analysis. In R. Shapiro & J.R. Marett (Eds.). *Proceedings: Second National Symposium on Teaching Kinesiology and Biomechanics in Sports.* Colorado Springs, CO: NASPE, 71-83.

Hay, J.G. (1993). *The biomechanics of sports techniques* (4th ed.). Englewood Cliffs, NJ: Prentice-Hall.

Hay, J.G. & Reid, J.G. (1982). *The anatomical and mechanical bases of human motion.* Englewood Cliffs, NJ: Prentice-Hall.

Hay, J.G. & Reid, J.G. (1988). *Anatomy, mechanics, and human motion* (2nd ed.). Englewood Cliffs, NJ: Prentice-Hall.

Haywood, K.M. (1984). Use of image-retina and eye-head movement visual systems during coincidence-anticipation performance. *Journal of Sport Sciences,* **2,** 139-144.

Haywood, K.M. (1993). *Life span motor development* (2nd ed.). Champaign, IL: Human Kinetics.

Haywood, K.M. & Williams, K. (1995). Age, gender, and flexibility differences in tennis serving among experienced older adults. *Journal of Aging and Physical Activity,* **3,** 54-66.

Haywood, K.M., Williams, K., & Van Sant, A. (1991). Qualitative assessment of the backswing in older adult throwing. *Research Quarterly for Exercise and Sport,* **62,** 340-343.

Henderson, D. (1971). The relationship among time, distance, and intensity as determinants of motion discrimination. *Perception and Psychophysics,* **10,** 313-320.

Hensley, L.D. (1983). Biomechanical analysis. *Journal of Physical Education, Recreation, and Dance,* **54**(8), 21-23.

Hensley, L.D., Morrow, J.R., & East, W.B. (1990). Practical measurement to solve practical problems. *Journal of Physical Education, Recreation, and Dance,* **61**(3), 42-44.

Higgins, J.R. (1977). *Human movement: An integrated approach.* St. Louis: Mosby.

Higgins, J. & Higgins, S. (1988, April). An Eastern System of Analysis and Observation. Paper presented at a national convention of the American Alliance of Health, Physical Education, Recreation and Dance, Kansas City, MO.

Hoare, D. (1992). Screening for gross motor coordination problems in primary school children. *Sports Coach,* **15**(2), 13-15.

Hoffman, S.J. (1974). Toward taking the fun out of skill analysis. *JOHPER,* **45**(9), 74-76.

Hoffman, S.J. (1977a). Toward a pedagogical kinesiology. *Quest,* **28,** 38-48.

Hoffman, S.J. (1977b). Competency based training in skill analysis. In R.E. Stadulis (Ed.). *Research and practice in physical education.* Champaign, IL: Human Kinetics, 3-12.

Hoffman, S.J. (1977c). Observing and reporting on learner responses: The teacher as a reliable feedback agent. In L.I.Gedvilas & M.E. Kneer (Eds.). *Proceedings of the NAPECW/NCPEAM National Conference.* Chicago: University of Illinois-Chicago Circle, 153-160.

Hoffman, S.J. (1983). Clinical diagnosis as a pedagogical skill. In T.J. Templin & J.K. Olson (Eds.). *Teaching in Physical Education.* Champaign, IL: Human Kinetics, 35-45.

Hoffman, S.J. (1984). The contributions of biomechanics to clinical competence: A view from the gymnasium. In Shapiro, R. & Marett, J.R. (Eds.). *Proceedings: Second National Symposium on Teaching Kinesiology and Biomechanics in Sports.* Colorado Springs, CO: NASPE, 67-70.

Hoffman, S.J. & Armstrong, C.W. (1975). Effects of pretraining on performance error identification. *Movement,* Actes due et symposium apprentissage psychomoteur et psychologie du sport, 207-214.

Hoffman, S.J., Imwold, C.H., & Koller, J.A. (1983). Accuracy and prediction in throwing: A taxonomic analysis of children's performance. *Research Quarterly for Exercise and Sport,* **54,** 33-40.

Hoffman, S.J. & Sembiante, J.L. (1975). Experience and imagery in movement analysis. In G.J.K. Alderson & D.A. Tyldesley (Eds.). *British Proceedings of Sports Psychology.* Salford, England: British Society of Sports Psychology, 288-293.

Holekamp, M.J. (1987). The effect of training on physical therapy student raters evaluating videotaped motor skill performances. Doctoral dissertation, University of Missouri-Columbia. Abstract in *Dissertation Abstracts International*, **48**, 1145A.

Hoshizaki, T.B. (1984). The application of models to understanding the biomechanical aspects of performance. In R. Shapiro & J.R. Marett (Eds.). *Proceedings: Second National Symposium on Teaching Kinesiology and Biomechanics in Sports.* Colorado Springs, CO: NASPE, 85-93.

Housner, L.D. & Griffey, D.C. (1985). Teacher cognition: Differences in planning and interactive decision-making between experienced and inexperienced teachers. *Research Quarterly for Exercise and Sport*, **56**, 45-53.

Housner, L.D. & Griffey, D.C. (1994). Wax on, wax off: Pedagogical content knowledge in motor skill acquisition, *Journal of Physical Education, Recreation, and Dance*, **65**(2), 63-68.

Howell, M.L. (1956). Use of force-time graphs for performance analysis in facilitating motor learning. *Research Quarterly*, **27**, 12-22.

Hubbard, A. & Seng, C.N. (1954). Visual movements of batters. *Research Quarterly*, **25**, 42-57.

Hudson, J. (1985, April). Possum: Purpose/observation system for studying and understanding movement. Paper presented at the AAHPERD National Convention, Atlanta, GA.

Hudson, J.L. (1987, April). "What goes up . . ." Paper presented at the AAPERD National Convention, Las Vegas, NV.

Hudson, J.L. (1990a). The value of visual variables in biomechanical analysis. In Kreighbaum, E. & McNeill, A. (Eds.). *Proceedings of the 6th International Symposium on Biomechanics in Sports.* Bozeman, MT: Color World Printers, 499-509.

Hudson, J.L. (1990b). Drop, stop, pop: Keys to vertical jumping. *Strategies*, **3**(6), 11-14.

Hudson, J.L. (1990c). Biomechanical observation: Visually accessible variables. In Nosek, M., Sojka, D., Morrison, W.E., & Susanka, P. (Eds.). *Proceedings of the VIIIth International Symposium of the Society of Biomechanics in Sports.* Prague: Conex, 321-326.

Hudson, J.L. (1995). Core concepts in kinesiology. *Journal of Physical Education, Recreation, and Dance*, **66**(5), 54-55, 59-60.

Huelster, L.J. (1939). Learning to analyze performance. *Journal of Health and Physical Education*, **10**(2), 84, 120-121.

Imwold, C.H. & Hoffman, S.J. (1983). Visual recognition of a gymnastic skill by experienced and inexperienced instructors. *Research Quarterly for Exercise and Sport*, **54**, 149-155.

Ishigaki, H. & Miyao, M. (1993). Differences in dynamic visual acuity between athletes and nonathletes. *Perceptual and Motor Skills*, **77**, 835-839.

Ishigaki, H. & Miyao, M. (1994). Implications for dynamic visual acuity with changes in age and sex. *Perceptual and Motor Skills*, **78**, 363-369.

Ishikura, T. & Inomata, K. (1995). Effects of angle of model demonstration on learning of motor skill. *Perceptual and Motor Skills*, **80**, 651-658.

Jambor, E.A. & Weekes, E.M. (1995) Videotape feedback: Make it more effective. *Journal of Physical Education, Recreation, and Dance*, **66**(2), 48-50.

James, R. & Dufek, J.S. (1993). Movement observation: What to watch . . . and why. *Strategies*, **6**(2), 17-19.

Janda, D.H. & Loubert, P. (1991). A preventative program focusing on the glenohumeral joint. *Clinics in Sports Medicine*, **10**, 955-971.

Janelle, C.M., Kim, J., & Singer, R.N. (1995). Subject-controlled performance feedback and learning of a closed motor skill. *Perceptual and Motor Skills*, **81**, 627-634.

Johnsson, G. (1975). Visual motion perception. *Scientific American*, **232**(6), 76-88.

Jones, P. (1987). The overarm baseball pitch: A kinesiological analysis and related strength-conditioning programming. *NSCA Journal*, **9**(1), 5-13, 78.

Jones-Morton, P. (1990a). Skill analysis series: Part I, analysis of the place kick. *Strategies*, **3**(5), 10-11.

Jones-Morton, P. (1990b). Skill analysis series: Part 2, analysis of the overarm throw. *Strategies*, **3**(6), 22-23.

Jones-Morton, P. (1990c). Skill analysis series: Part 3, analysis of running. *Strategies*, **4**(1), 22-24.

Jones-Morton, P. (1990d). Skill analysis series: Part 4, the standing long jump. *Strategies*, **4**(2), 26-27.

Jones-Morton, P. (1991a). Skills analysis series: Part 5, striking. *Strategies*, **4**(3), 28-29.

Jones-Morton, P. (1991b). Skills analysis series: Part 6, catching. *Strategies*, **4**(4), 23-24.

Kahneman, D. (1973). *Attention and effort.* Englewood Cliffs, NJ: Prentice-Hall.

Kamieneski, C.D. (1980). The effectiveness of an instructional unit in the analysis and correction of basketball skills. Doctoral dissertation, Brigham Young University. Abstract in *Dissertation Abstracts International*, **40**, 6191A.

Kay, H. (1970). Analyzing motor skill performance. In Connaly, K.J. *Mechanisms of motor skill development.* London: Academic Press, 139-159.

Keenan, A.M. & Bach, T.M. (1996). Video assessment of rearfoot movements during walking: A reliability study. *Archives of Physical Medicine and Rehabilitation*, **77**, 651-655.

Kelly, L.E. (1990, March). The effectiveness of computer managed interactive videodisk training on the development of sport skill competencies in teachers. Paper presented to the AAHPERD National Convention, New Orleans, LA.

Kelly, L.E., Dagger, J., & Walkley, J. (1989a). The effects of an assessment-based physical education program on motion skill development in preschool children. *Education and Treatment of Children*, **12**(2), 152-164.

Kelly, L.E., Reuschein, P., & Haubenstricker, J. (1989b). Qualitative analysis of overhand throwing and catching motor skills: Implications for assessing and teaching. *Journal of the International Council for Health, Physical Education and Recreation*, **25**, 14-18.

Kelly, L.E., Reuschlein, P., & Haubenstricker, J.L. (1990). Qualitative analysis of bouncing, kicking, and striking motor skills: Implications for assessing and teaching. *Journal of the International Council for Health, Physical Education, and Recreation*, **26**(2), 28-32.

Kelly, L.E., Walkley, J., & Tarrant, M.R. (1988). Developing an interactive videodisk application. *Journal of Physical Education, Recreation and Dance*, **59**(4), 22-26.

Kerner, J.F. & Alexander, J. (1981). Activities of daily living: Reliability and validity of gross vs. specific ratings. *Archives of Physical Medicine and Rehabilitation*, **62**, 161-166.

Kindig, L.E. & Windell, E.J. (1984). Analysis of sport skills. In R. Shapiro & J.R. Marett (Eds.). *Proceedings: Second National Symposium on Teaching Kinesiology and Biomechanics in Sports*. Colorado Springs, CO: NASPE, 231-232.

Kinesiology Academy (1980). Guidelines and standards for undergraduate kinesiology. *Journal of Physical Education, Recreation, and Dance*, **51**(2), 19-21.

Kinesiology Academy (1992, Spring). Guidelines and standards for undergraduate kinesiology. *Kinesiology Academy Newsletter*, 3-6.

Klatt, L.A. (1992). Biomechanics: Analyzing skills and performance. In J. Kindall (Ed.). *Science of Coaching Baseball*. Champaign, IL: Leisure Press, 49-83.

Klavora, P., Gaskovski, P., & Forsyth, R.D. (1994). Test-retest reliability of the dynavision apparatus. *Perceptual and Motor Skills*, **79**, 448-450.

Klavora, P., Gaskovski, P., & Forsyth, R.D. (1995). Test-retest reliability of three dynavision tasks. *Perceptual and Motor Skills*, **80**, 607-610.

Klesius, S. & Bowers, L. (1990). The I'm special interactive videodisk for training teachers of handicapped children. *Florida Educational Computing Quarterly*, **2**(4), 73-76.

Kluka, D.A. (1987). Visual skill enhancement. *Strategies*, **1**(1), 20-24.

Kluka, D.A. (1991). Visual skills: Considerations in learning motor skills for sport. *ASAHPERD Journal*, **14**(1), 41-43.

Kluka, D.A. (1994, Winter). Visual skills related to sport performance. *Research Consortium Newsletter*, 3.

Kniffin, K.M. (1985). The effects of individualized videotape instruction on the ability of undergraduate physical education majors to analyze select sport skills. Doctoral dissertation, Ohio State University. Abstract in *Dissertation Abstracts International*, **47**, 119A

Knudson, D. (1991). The tennis topspin forehand drive: Technique changes and critical elements. *Strategies*, **5**(1), 19-22.

Knudson, D. (1993). Biomechanics of the basketball jump shot: Six key teaching points. *Journal of Physical Education, Recreation, and Dance*, **64**(2), 67-73.

Knudson, D. (1995, April). An integrated model for the qualitative analysis of the tennis serve. Paper presented to the American Alliance for Health, Physical Education, Recreation, and Dance. Portland, OR.

Knudson, D., Luedtke, D., & Faribault, J. (1994). How to analyze the serve. *Strategies*, **7**(8), 19-22.

Knudson, D. & Morrison, C. (1996). An integrated qualitative analysis of overarm throwing. *Journal of Physical Education, Recreation, and Dance*, **67**(6), 31-36.

Knudson, D., Morrison, C., & Reeve, J. (1991). Effect of undergraduate kinesiology courses on qualitative analysis ability. In J. Wilkerson, E. Kreighbaum, and C. Tant (Eds.). *Teaching kinesiology and biomechanics in sports*. Ames, IA: NASPE Kinesiology Academy, 17-20.

Kovar, S.K., Mathews, H.M., Ermler, K.L., & Mehrhof, J.H. (1992). Feedback: How to teach how. *Strategies*, **5**(1), 21-25.

Kozak, W. (1989). Skill analysis. In Almstedt, J. et al. (Eds.). *Proceedings: National Coaching Certification Program Advanced II Seminar*. Gloucester, Ontario: Canadian Amateur Hockey Association, 51-77.

Kraft, R.E., & Smith, J.A. (1993). Throwing and catching: How to do it right. *Strategies*, **6**(5), 24-27, 29.

Krebs, D.E., Edelstein, J.E., & Fishman, S. (1985). Reliability of observational kinematic gait analysis. *Physical Therapy*, **65**, 1027-1033.

Kreighbaum, E. & Barthels, K.M. (1985). *Biomechanics: A qualitative approach for studying human movement* (2nd ed.). Minneapolis, MN: Burgess.

Kretchmar, R.T., Sherman, H., & Mooney, R. (1949). A survey of research in the teaching of sports. *Research Quarterly*, **20**, 238-249.

Kwak, E.C. (1993). The initial effects of various task presentation conditions on students' performance of the lacrosse throw. Doctoral dissertation, University of South Carolina. Abstract in *Dissertation Abstracts International*, **54**, 2507A.

Lafortune, M.A. & Cavanagh, P.R. (1983). Effectiveness and efficiency in bicycle riding. In H. Matsui & K. Kobayshi (Eds.). *Biomechanics VIII-B*. Champaign, IL: Human Kinetics, 928-936.

Landers, D. (1969). Effect of the numbers of categories systematically observed on individual and group performance ratings. *Perceptual and Motor Skills*, **29**, 731-735.

Landers, D.M. (1970). A review of research on gymnastic judging. *JOHPER*, **41**(7), 85-88.

Landin, D. (1994). The role of verbal cues in skill learning. *Quest*, **46**, 299-313.

Landin, D.K., Hebert, E., & Cutton, D.L. (1989). Analyzing the augmented feedback patterns of professional tennis instructors. *Journal of Applied Research in Coaching and Athletics*, **4**, 255-271.

Langley, D. (1993). Teaching new motor patterns—Overcoming student resistance toward change. *Journal of Physical Education, Recreation, and Dance*, **63**(1), 27-31.

Lappin, J.S. & Fuqua, M.A. (1983). Accurate visual measurement of three-dimensional moving patterns. *Science*, **221**, 480-482.

Larsson, L.E., Miller, M., Norlin, R., & Thaczuk, H. (1986). Changes in gait patterns after operations in children with spastic cerebral palsy. *International Orthopaedics*, **10**, 155-162.

Lee, A.M., Keh, N.C., & Magill, R.A. (1993). Instructional effects of teacher feedback in physical education. *Journal of Teaching in Physical Education*, **12**, 228-243.

Lehmann, J.F. (1982) Gait analysis: Diagnosis and management. In Kottke, F.J., Stillwell, G.K., & Lehmann, J.F. (Eds.). *Krusen's handbook of physical medicine and rehabilitation*. Philadelphia: Saunders, 86-101.

Leis, H.H. (1994). The effects of two instructional conditions on sport skill specific analytic proficiency of physical education majors. Doctoral dissertation, University of Southern Mississippi. Abstract in *Dissertation Abstracts International*, **54**(8), 2946A.

Locke, L. (1972). Implications for physical education. *Research Quarterly*, **43**, 374-386.

Locke, L.F. (1984). Research on teaching teachers: Where are we now? *Journal of Teaching Physical Education*, **2**(Summer), 63-85.

Lockhart, A. (1966, May). Communicating with the learner. *Quest*, **VI**, 57-67.

Logan, G.A. & McKinney, W.C. (1970). *Kinesiology*. Dubuque, IA: William C. Brown Co.

Long, G.M. (1994). Exercises for training vision and dynamic visual acuity among college students. *Perceptual and Motor Skills*, **78**, 1049-1050.

Long, G.M. & Rourke, D.A. (1989). Training effects on the resolution of moving targets—Dynamic visual acuity. *Human Factors*, **31**, 443-451.

Luttgens, K. & Wells, K.F. (1982). *Kinesiology: Scientific basis of human movement* (7th ed.). Philadelphia, PA: Saunders.

MacLeod, B. (1991). Effects of Eyerobics visual skills training on selected performance measures of female varsity soccer players. *Perceptual and Motor Skills*, **72**, 863-866.

Magill, R.A. (1993). Augmented feedback in skill acquisition. In R.N. Singer, M. Murphey, & L.K. Tennant (Eds.). *Handbook of research on sport psychology*. New York: Macmillan, 193-212.

Magill, R.A. (1994). The influence of augmented feedback on skill learning depends on characteristics of the skill and learner. *Quest*, **46**, 314-327.

Magill, R.A. & Parks, P.F. (1983). The psychophysics of kinesthesis for positioning response: the physical stimulus-psychological response relationship. *Research Quarterly for Exercise and Sport*, **54**, 346-351.

Malina, R.M. & Bouchard, C. (1991). *Growth, maturation, and physical activity*. Champaign, IL: Human Kinetics.

Malkia, E., Huhtinen, J., & Luthanen, P. (1991). A qualitative analysis of walking in children with CP. In *The 11th International Congress of the World Confederation for Physical Therapy: Proceedings*. London: World Confederation for Physical Therapy, 1160.

Marett, J.R., Pavlacka, J.A., Siler, W.L., & Shapiro, R. (1984). Kinesiology status update: A national survey. In R.Shapiro & J.R. Marett (Eds.). *Proceedings: Second National Symposium on Teaching Kinesiology and Biomechanics in Sports*. Colorado Springs, CO: NASPE, 7-15.

Marino, G.W. (1982). Qualitative biomechanical analysis of sports skills. *Coaching Science Update*, Coaching Association of Canada, **9**, 20-22.

Martens, R., Burwitz, L., & Zuckerman, J. (1976). Modeling effects on motor performance. *Research Quarterly*, **47**, 277-291.

Maschette, W. (1985). Correcting technique problems of a successful junior athlete. *Sports Coach*, **9**(1), 14-17.

Masser, L. (1985). The effect of refinement on student achievement in a fundamental motor skill K-6. *Journal of Teaching in Physical Education*, **6**, 174-182.

Masser, L.S. (1993). Critical cues help first-grade students' achievement in handstands and forward rolls. *Journal of Teaching in Physical Education*, **12**, 301-312.

Matanin, M.J. (1993). Effects of performance principle training on correct analysis and diagnosis of motor skills. Doctoral dissertation, Ohio State University. Abstract in *Dissertation Abstracts International*, **54**, 1724A.

Mathers, S. (1990, Winter). Training your eyes: A method of learning ski movement analysis. *Professional Skier*, 30-31.

Matlin, M. (1983). *Cognition*. New York, NY: Holt, Rinehart and Winston, Inc.

McCormick, E.J. & Sanders, M.S. (1982). *Human factors in engineering and design* (5th ed.). New York: McGraw-Hill.

McCraw, P. (1995). The qualitative analysis of motor skills using multi-media software engineering techniques. Unpublished master's thesis, Deakin University, Melbourne, Australia.

McCullagh, P. (1986). Model status as a determinant of observational learning and performance. *Journal of Sport Psychology*, **8**, 319-331.

McCullagh, P. (1987). Model similarity effects on motor performance. *Journal of Sport Psychology*, **9**, 249-260.

McCullagh, P.M. & Caird, J.K. (1990). Correct and learning models and the use of model knowledge of results in the acquisition and retention of a motor skill. *Journal of Human Movement Studies*, **18**, 107-116.

McCullagh, P. & Little, W.S. (1990). Demonstrations and knowledge of results in motor skill acquisition. *Perceptual and Motor Skills,* **71**, 735-742.

McCullagh, P., Stiehl, J., & Weiss, M.R. (1990). Developmental modeling effects on the quantitative and qualitative aspects of motor performance. *Research Quarterly for Exercise and Sport,* **61**, 344-350.

McCullagh, P., Weiss, M.R., & Ross, D. (1989). Modeling considerations in motor skill acquisition and performance: An integrated approach. *Exercise and Sport Sciences Reviews,* **17**, 475-513.

McGrain, P. (1984). Videography: An inexpensive alternative to film analysis in kinesiology and biomechanics. In R.Shapiro & J.R. Marett (Eds.). *Proceedings: Second National Symposium on Teaching Kinesiology and Biomechanics in Sports.* Colorado Springs, CO: NASPE, 59-63.

McNaughton, L. (1986). Some drills to improve visual perception abilities in team sport players. *Sports Coach,* **9**(2), 47-49.

McPherson, M.N. (1988a, April). Who: The physical education teacher as diagnostician. Paper presented to the national convention of the American Alliance for Health, Physical Education, Recreation and Dance. Kansas City, Missouri.

McPherson, M.N. (1988b). The development, implementation, and evaluation of a program designed to promote competency in skill analysis. Doctoral dissertation, University of Alberta. *Dissertation Abstracts International,* **48**, 3071A.

McPherson, M.N. (1990). A systematic approach to skill analysis. *Sports Science Periodical on Research and Technology in Sport,* **11**(1), 1-10.

McPherson, M.N. (1996). Qualitative and quantitative analysis in sports. *American Journal of Sports Medicine,* **24**, S85-S88.

McPherson, M.N. & Bedingfield, E.W. (1985). Development of instructional videotape for qualitative analysis. In J. Terauds & J.N. Barham (Eds.). *Biomechanics in Sports II: Proceedings of ISBS 1985.* Del Mar, CA: Research Center for Sports, 385-389.

McPherson, M. & Walsh, J. (1990). Application of the skill analysis approach to the nordic two skate. *Sports Coach,* **13**(3), 3-7.

Meehan, J.W. & Day, R.H. (1995). Visual accommodation as a cue for size. *Ergonomics,* **38**, 1239-1249.

Melville, D.S. (1993). Videotaping: An assist for large classes. *Strategies,* **6**(4), 26-28.

Messick, J.A. (1991). Prelongitudinal screening of hypothesized developmental sequences for the overhead tennis serve in experienced tennis players. *Research Quarterly for Exercise and Sport,* **62**, 249-256.

Messier, S.P. & Cirillo, K.J. (1989). Effects of a verbal and visual feedback system on running technique, perceived exertion and running economy in female novice runners. *Journal of Sports Sciences,* **7**, 113-126.

Metzler, M. (1989). A review of research on time in sport pedagogy. *Journal of Teaching in Physical Education,* **6**, 271-285.

Michigan Education Assessment Program. (1984). *Physical education assessment administration manual, 1984-1985.* Lansing, MI: Michigan Department of Education.

Mielke, D. & Morrison, C. (1985). Motor development and skill analysis: Connections to elementary physical education. *Journal of Physical Education, Recreation, and Dance,* **56**(9), 48-51.

Mielke, D. & Chapman, D. (1987). Effectiveness of education majors in assessing children on the test of gross motor development. *Perceptual and Motor Skills,* **64**, 1249-1250.

Miller, D.I. (1980). Body segment contributions to sport skill performance: Two contrasting approaches. *Research Quarterly for Exercise and Sport,* **51**, 219-233.

Miller, G. & Gabbard, C. (1988). Effects of visual aids on acquisition of selected tennis skills. *Perceptual and Motor Skills,* **67**, 603-606.

Minas, S. (1977). Memory coding for movement. *Perceptual and Motor Skills,* **45**, 787-790.

Miyashita, M., Tsunoda, T., Sakurai, S., Nishizono, H., & Mizuno, T. (1979). The tennis serve as compared with overarm throwing. In J. Groppel (Ed.). *Proceedings of a National Symposium on the Racket Sports.* Champaign, IL: University of Illinois, 125-140.

Miyazaki, S. & Kubota, T. (1984). Quantification of gait abnormalities on the basis of continuous foot-force measurement: Correlation between quantitative indices and visual rating. *Medical and Biological Engineering and Computing,* **22**, 70-76.

Montagne, G., Laurent, M., & Ripoll, H. (1993). Visual information pick-up in ball-catching. *Human Movement Science,* **12**, 273-297.

Moody, D.L. (1967). Imagery differences among women of varying levels of experience, interests, and abilities in motor skills. *Research Quarterly,* **43**, 55-61.

Morris, G. (1977). Dynamic visual acuity: Implications for the physical educator and coach. *Motor Skills: Theory Into Practice,* **2**, 15-20.

Morrison, C.S. (1976). The effect of vision, motion and laterality in wrist shooting accuracy in ice hockey. Unpublished master's thesis, Springfield College, Springfield, MA.

Morrison, C.S. (1994, August). Comparison of nationality, gender and type of instruction on the acquisition and retention of the qualitative analysis of movement ability. In F. Bell & G Van Gyn (Eds.). *Proceedings of the 10th Commonwealth and International Scientific Congress.* Victoria, BC, 169-173.

Morrison, C.S., Gangstead, S.K., & Reeve, J. (1990, March). Two approaches to qualitative analysis: Implications for future directions. Paper presented at the AAHPERD National Convention, New Orleans, LA.

Morrison, C.S. & Harrison, J.M. (1985). Movement analysis and the classroom teacher. *CAHPER Journal,* **51**(5), 16-19.

Morrison, C.S. & Harrison, J.M. (in press). Integrating qualitative analysis of movement into the university physical education curriculum. *The Physical Educator.*

Morrison, C.S. & Reeve, E.J. (1986). Effect of instruction units on the analysis of related and unrelated skills. *Perceptual and Motor Skills,* **62**, 563-566.

Morrison, C.S. & Reeve, E.J. (1988). Effect of undergraduate major and instruction on qualitative skill analysis. *Journal of Human Movement Studies,* **15**, 291-297.

Morrison, C. & Reeve, J. (1988, November). Effect of different instructional videotape units on undergraduate physical education majors' skill analysis ability. Paper presented to the Texas Association for Health, Physical Education, Recreation and Dance, San Antonio, TX.

Morrison, C. & Reeve, J. (1989). Effect of different videotape instructional units on undergraduate physical education majors' qualitative analysis of skill. *Perceptual and Motor Skills,* **69**, 111-114.

Morrison, C. & Reeve, J. (1992). Perceptual style and instruction in the acquisition of qualitative analysis of movement by majors in elementary education. *Perceptual and Motor Skills,* **74**, 579-583.

Morrison, C. & Reeve, J. (1993). A framework for writing and evaluating critical performance cues in instructional materials for physical education. *The Physical Educator,* **50**(3), 132-135.

Morrison, C.S., Reeve, E.J., & Harrison, J.M. (1984, February). The effect of two methods of teaching skill analysis and skill performance. Paper presented to the Southern District, American Alliance of Health, Physical Education, Recreation and Dance, Biloxi, MS.

Morrison, C., Reeve, E., & Harrison, J.M. (1992). The effect of instruction on the ability to qualitatively analyze and perform movement skills. *CAHPER Journal,* **58**(2), 18-20.

Morton, P. (1990). Effects of training in skill analysis on generalization across age levels. Doctoral dissertation, Ohio State University. Abstract in *Dissertation Abstracts International,* **50**, 2424A.

Mosher, R.E. & Schutz, R.W. (1983). The development of a test of overarm throwing: An application of generalizability theory. *Canadian Journal of Applied Sport Science,* **8**(1), 1-8.

Mosston, M. & Ashworth, S. (1986). *Teaching physical education.* (3rd ed.). Columbus, OH: Merrill.

Naatanen, R. (1990). The role of attention in auditory information processing as revealed by event-related potentials and other brain measures of cognitive function. *Behavioral and Brain Sciences,* **13**, 201-288.

National Association for Sport and Physical Education. (1992). *NASPE/NCATE Physical Education Guidelines: An instructional manual* (3rd ed.). Reston, VA: American Alliance for Health, Physical Education, Recreation and Dance.

Nelson, M.A. (1991). Developmental skills and children's sports. *Physician and Sportsmedicine,* **19**(2), 67-79.

Neumaier, A. (1982). Unterschung zur funktion des blickverhaltens bei visuellen wahrnehmungsprozessen im sport. *Sportweissenschaft,* **12**(1), 78-91.

Newell, K.M. (1976). Knowledge of results and motor learning. *Exercise and Sport Sciences Reviews,* **4**, 195-228.

Newell, K.M. (1990). Kinesiology: The label for the study of physical activity in higher education. *Quest,* **42**, 269-278.

Newell, K.M., Morris, L.R., & Scully, D.M. (1985). Augmented information and the acquisition of skill in physical activity. *Exercise and Sport Sciences Reviews,* **13**, 235-261.

Newell, K.M., Quinn, J.T., Sparrow, W.A., & Walter, C.B. (1983). Kinematic information feedback for learning a rapid arm movement. *Human Movement Science,* **2**, 235-269.

Newell, K.M., Sparrow, W.A., & Quinn, J.T. (1985). Kinetic information feedback for learning isometric tasks. *Journal of Human Movement Studies,* **11**, 113-123.

Newtson, D. (1976). The process of behavior observation. *Journal of Human Movement Studies,* **2**, 114-122.

Nielson, A.B. & Beauchamp, L. (1992). The effect of training in conceptual kinesiology on feedback provision patterns. *Journal of Teaching in Physical Education,* **11**, 126-138.

Norman, R.W. (1975). Biomechanics for the community coach. *Journal of Physical Education, Recreation, and Dance,* **46**(3), 49-52.

Norman, R.W. (1977). An approach to teaching the mechanics of human motion at the undergraduate level. In C.J. Dillman & R.G. Sears (Eds.). *Proceedings: Kinesiology, A National Conference on Teaching.* Champaign, IL: University of Illinois, 113-123.

O'Donnell, R.D., Moise, S.L., Warner, D.A., & Secrist, G.E. (1994). *Enhancing soldier performance: A nonlinear model of performance to improve selection, testing and training.* (Tech. report ARL-CR-1993). U. S. Army Research Institute, VA.

Ormond, (1992). The prompt/feedback package in physical education. *Journal of Physical Education, Recreation, and Dance,* **63**(1), 64-67.

Osborne, M.M. & Gordon, M.E. (1972). An investigation into the accuracy of rating of a gross motor skill. *Research Quarterly,* **43**, 55-61.

O'Sullivan, M. (1988, April). How: The Ohio State University model. Paper presented to the national convention of the American Alliance of Health, Physical Education, Recreation and Dance, Kansas City, MO.

Overdorf, V.G. (1990). Timing—in life and in sports—is everything. *Journal of Physical Education, Recreation, and Dance,* **61**(7), 66-69.

Painter, M.A. (1990). A generalizability analysis of observational abilities in the assessment of hopping using two developmental approaches to motor skill sequencing. Doctoral dissertation, Michigan State University. Abstract in *Dissertation Abstracts International*, **50**, 3888A.

Palmer, S.E. (1992). Common region: A new principle of perceptual grouping. *Cognitive Psychology*, **24**, 436-447.

Palmer, S. & Rock, I. (1994). Rethinking perceptual organization: The role of uniform connectedness. *Psychomomic Bulletin and Review*, **1**(1), 29-55.

Partridge, D. & Franks, I.M. (1986, Winter). Analyzing and modifying coaching behaviors by means of computer aided observation. *The Physical Educator*, 8-23.

Patrick, J. & Lowdon, B.J. (1987). Computer controlled video replay of player activity in sport. *Sports Coach*, **10**(3), 20-22.

Pellett, T.L., Henschel-Pellett, H.A., & Harrison, J.M. (1994). Feedback effects: Field-based findings. *Journal of Physical Education, Recreation, and Dance*, **65**(9), 75-78.

Petrakis, E. (1986). Visual observation patterns of tennis teachers. *Research Quarterly for Exercise and Sport*, **57**, 254-259.

Petrakis, E. (1987). Analysis of visual search patterns of dance teachers. *Journal of Teaching in Physical Education*, **6**, 149-156.

Petrakis, E. & Romjue, M.K. (1990). Cognitive processing of tennis teachers/coaches during skill observation. Paper presented to the Central District Association for Health, Physical Education, Recreation and Dance, Denver, Colorado.

Philipp, J.A. & Wilkerson, J.W. (1990). *Teaching team sports: A coeducational approach*. Champaign, IL: Human Kinetics.

Phillips, S.J. & Clark, J.E. (1984). An integrative approach to teaching kinesiology: A lifespan approach. In R. Shapiro & J.R. Marett (Eds.). *Proceedings: Second National Symposium on Teaching Kinesiology and Biomechanics in Sports*. Colorado Springs, CO: NASPE, 19-23.

Phillips, S.J., Roberts, E.M., & Huang, T.C. (1983). Quantification of intersegmental reactions during rapid swing motion. *Journal of Biomechanics*, **16**, 411-417.

Pinheiro, V.E.D. (1990). Motor skill diagnosis: Diagnostic processes of expert and novice coaches. Doctoral dissertation, University of Pittsburgh. Abstract in *Dissertation Abstracts International*, **50**(11), 3516A.

Pinheiro, V. (1994). Diagnosing motor skills—A practical approach. *Journal of Physical Education, Recreation, and Dance*, **65**(2), 49-54.

Pinheiro, V. & Simon, H.A. (1992). An operational model of motor skill diagnosis. *Journal of Teaching in Physical Education*, **11**, 288-302.

Piscopo, J. & Bailey, J.A. (1981). *Kinesiology, the science of movement*. New York: Wiley.

Plagenhoef, S. (1971). *Patterns of human motion: A cinematographic analysis*. Englewood Cliffs, NJ: Prentice-Hall.

Platt, B.B. & Warren, D.H. (1972). Auditory localization: The importance of eye movements and a textured visual environment. *Perception and Psychophysics*, **12**, 245-248.

Pomeroy, V. (1990). Development of an ADL oriented assessment-of-mobility scale suitable for use with elderly people with dementia. *Physiotherapy*, **76**, 446-448.

Portman, P.A. (1989). Parent intervention program. *Strategies*, **3**(2), 13-19.

Pribram, K.H. & McGuinness, D. (1975). Arousal, activation and effort in the control of attention. *Psychological Review*, **82**, 116-149.

Prinzmetal, W. & Gettleman, L. (1993). Vertical-horizontal illusion: One eye is better than two. *Perception and Psychophysics*, **53**, 81-88.

Proctor, R.W. & Dutta, A. (1995). *Skill acquisition and human performance*. Thousand Oaks, CA: Sage Publications.

Putnam, C.A. (1991). A segment interaction analysis of proximal-to-distal sequential segment motion patterns. *Medicine and Science in Sports and Exercise*, **23**, 130-144.

Radford, K.W. (1988). Observation—A neglected teaching skill. *CAHPER Journal*, **54**(6), 45-47.

Radford, K.W. (1989). Movement observation in physical education: A definitional effort. *Journal of Teaching in Physical Education*, **9**, 1-24.

Radford, K.W. (1991). For increased teacher effectiveness: Link observation, feedback and assessment. *CAHPER Journal*, **57**(2), 4-9.

Reeve, J. & Morrison, C. (1986). Teaching for learning: The application of systematic evaluation. *Journal of Physical Education, Recreation, and Dance*, **57**(6), 37-39.

Reiken, G.B. (1982). Description of women's gymnastic coaches' observations of movement. Doctoral dissertation, Teachers College, Columbia University. Abstract in *Dissertation Abstracts International*, **43**, 397A.

Revlen, L. & Gabor, M. (1981). *Sports vision*. New York: Workman Publishing.

Reynolds, A. (1992). What is competent beginning teaching? A review of the literature. *Review of Educational Research*, **G2**(1) 1-35.

Riggs, L.A. (1971). Vision. In J.W. Kling & L.A. Riggs (Eds.). *Woodworth and Schlosberg's Experimental Psychology* (3rd ed). New York: Holt, Rinehart and Winston.

Ripoll, H. & Fleurance, P. (1988). What does keeping one's eye on the ball mean? *Ergonomics*, **31**, 1647-1654.

Roberton, M.A. (1978). Longitudinal evidence of developmental stages in the forceful overarm throw. *Journal of Human Movement Studies*, **4**, 153-167.

Roberton, M.A. (1983). Changing motor patterns during childhood. In J.R. Thomas (Ed.). *Motor development during childhood and adolescence*. Minneapolis, MN: Burgess Publishing, 48-90.

Roberton, M.A. & Halverson, L.E. (1984). *Developing children—Their changing movement*. Philadelphia: Lea & Febiger.

Roberts, E.M. (1971). Cinematography in biomechanical investigation. In J.M. Cooper (Ed.). *Selected Topics on Biomechanics. Proceedings of CIC Symposium on Biomechanics.* Chicago, IL: The Athletic Institute, 41-50.

Robinson, D.A. (1981). Control of eye movements. In V.B. Brooks (Ed.). *Handbook of physiology. Section 1: The nervous system.* Vol. II, Part 2, Bethesda, MD: American Physiological Society, 1275-1320.

Robinson, S.M. (1974). Visual assessment of children's gross motor patterns by adults with backgrounds in teacher education. Unpublished doctoral dissertation, University of Wisconsin, Madison.

Roemmich, J.N. & Rogol, A.D. (1995). Physiology of growth and development: Its relationship to performance in the young athlete. *Clinics in Sports Medicine,* **14,** 483-502.

Romance, T.J. (1985). Observing for confidence. *Journal of Physical Education, Recreation, and Dance,* **56**(6), 47-49.

Rose, D.J. & Heath, E.M. (1990). The contribution of a fundamental motor skill to the performance and learning of a complex sport skill. *Journal of Human Movement Studies,* **19,** 75-84.

Rose, D. J., Heath, E., & Megale, D. (1990). Development of a diagnostic instrument for evaluating tennis serving performance. *Perceptual and Motor Skills,* **71,** 355-363.

Rose, G.K. (1983). Clinical gait assessment: A personal view. *Journal of Medical Engineering and Technology,* **7,** 273-279.

Ross, D., Bird, A.M., Doody, S.G., & Zoeller, M. (1985). Effects of modeling and videotape feedback with knowledge of results on motor performance. *Human Movement Science,* **4,** 149-157.

Rothstein, A.L. (1980). Effective use of videotape replay in learning motor skills. *Journal of Physical Education, Recreation, and Dance,* **51**(2), 59-60.

Rothstein, A.L. & Arnold, R.K. (1976). Bridging the gap: Application of research on videotape feedback and bowling. *Motor Skills: Theory into Practice,* **1,** 35-62.

Runeson, S. & Frykholm, G. (1981). Visual perception of lifted weight. *Journal of Experimental Psychology: Human Perception and Performance,* **7,** 733-740.

Rush, D.A. (1991). Improving skill analysis for diving. Doctoral dissertation, Ohio State University. Abstract in *Dissertation Abstracts International,* **51,** 2313A.

Sage, G.H. (1984). *Motor learning and control: a neurophysiological approach.* Dubuque, IA: W.C. Brown.

Saleh, M. & Murdoch, G. (1985). In defense of gait analysis. *Journal of Bone and Joint Surgery* (British), **67,** 237-241.

Sanders, R.H. (1995). Can skilled performers readily change technique? An example, conventional to wave action breaststroke. *Human Movement Science,* **14,** 665-679.

Sanders, R. & Wilson, B. (1989). Some biomechanical tips for better teaching and coaching: Part 1. *New Zealand Journal of Health, Physical Education and Recreation,* **23**(4), 14-15.

Sanders, R. & Wilson, B. (1990a). Some biomechanical tips for better teaching and coaching: Part 2. *New Zealand Journal of Health, Physical Education and Recreation,* **24**(1), 16-17.

Sanders, R. & Wilson, B. (1990b). Some biomechanical tips for better teaching and coaching: Part 3. *New Zealand Journal of Health, Physical Education and Recreation,* **24**(2), 19-21.

Sanderson, D.J. & Cavanagh, P.R. (1990). Use of augmented feedback for the modification of the pedaling mechanics of cyclists. *Canadian Journal of Sport Sciences,* **15,** 38-42.

Sanderson, F.H. & Whiting, H.T.A. (1974). Dynamic visual acuity and performance in a catching task. *Journal of Motor Behavior,* **6,** 87-94.

Satern, M.N. (1986, April). Apparent and actual use of observational frameworks by experienced teachers. Paper presented at the national convention of the American Alliance for Health, Physical Education, Recreation and Dance, Cincinnati, OH. (ERIC Document Reproduction Service No. ED 273-588.)

Satern, M.N., Coleman, M.M., & Matsakis, M.H. (1991). The effect of observational training on the frequency of skill-related feedback given by pre-service teachers during two peer teaching experiences. *KAHPERD Journal,* **60**(2), 12-16.

Saunders, J., Inman, V., & Eberhart, H. (1953). The major determinants in normal and pathological gait. *Journal of Bone and Joint Surgery,* **35A,** 543-558.

Schleihauf, R.E. (1983). An analysis of skill acquisition in swimming. In G.A. Wood (Ed.). *Collected papers on sports biomechanics.* Perth: University of Western Australia Press, 117-141.

Schmidt, R.A. (1991). *Motor learning & performance: From principles to practice.* Champaign, IL: Human Kinetics.

Schneider, W. & Shiffrin, R, W. (1977). Controlled and automatic human information processing: Decision research and attention. *Psychological Review,* **84,** 1-66.

Scott, M.G. (1942). *Analysis of human motion.* New York: F.S. Crofts & Co.

Scully, D.M. (1986). Visual perception of technical execution and aesthetic quality in biological motion. *Human Movement Science,* **5,** 185-206.

Seat, J.E. & Wrisberg, C.A. (1996). The visual instruction system. *Research Quarterly for Exercise and Sport,* **67,** 106-108.

Secrist, G.E. & Hartman, B.O. (1993). Situated awareness: the trainability of the near-threshold information acquisition dimension. *Aviation, Space and Environmental Medicine,* **64,** 885-897.

Seefeldt, V.D. & Haubenstricker, J.L. (1982). Patterns, phases, or stages: An analytical model for study of developmental movement. In J.A.S. Kelso & J.E. Clark (Eds.). *The Development of Movement Control and Coordination*. New York: Wiley & Sons, 309-318.

Sharpe, T. (1993). What are some guidelines on giving feedback to students in physical education? *Journal of Physical Education, Recreation, and Dance*, **64**(9), 13.

Shea, C.H. & Northan, C. (1982). Discrimination of visual linear velocities. *Research Quarterly for Exercise and Sport*, **53**, 222-225.

Shea, C.H., Shebilske, W.L., & Worchel, S. (1993). *Motor learning and control*. Englewood Cliffs, NJ: Prentice-Hall.

Sherman, A. (1980). Overview of research information regarding vision and sports. *Journal of the American Optometric Association*, **51**, 661-666.

Shields, B.C. (1995, Sept.) Successful "Q"munication. *IDEA Today*, 62-63.

Shigehia, P.M.J., Shigehia, T, & Symons, J.R. (1973). Effects of intensity of auditory stimulation on photopic visual sensitivity in relation to personality. *Japanese Psychological Research*, **15**, 164-172.

Shigehia, T. & Symons, J.R. (1973). Effect of intensity of visual stimulation on auditory sensitivity in relation to personality. *British Journal of Psychology*, **64**, 205-213.

Siedentop, D. (1991). *Developing teaching skills in physical education* (3rd ed.). Mountain View, CA: Mayfield.

Silverman, S. (1994). Communication and motor skill learning: What we learn from research in the gymnasium. *Quest*, **46**, 345-355.

Simon, H.A. (1979). *Models of Thought*. New Haven, CT: Yale University Press.

Sinclair, G.D. (1988). Pedagogical considerations. *CAHPER Journal*, **54**(3), 32-36.

Skrinar, G.S. & Hoffman, S.J. (1979). Effect of outcome information on analytic ability of golf teachers. *Perceptual and Motor Skills*, **48**, 703-708.

Smolensky, P. (1986). Formal modeling of sub-symbolic processes: An introduction to harmony theory. In Ellis Horwood (Ed.). *Advances in cognitive science*. New York: Ellis Horwood Ltd., 204-235.

Solso, R.L. (1979). *Cognitive psychology*. New York, NY: Harcourt Brace Jovanovich, Inc.

Spaeth, R.K. (1972). Maximizing goal attainment. *Research Quarterly*, **43**, 337-361.

Steinberg, G.M., Frehlich, S.G., & Tennant, L.K. (1995). Dextrality and eye position in putting performance. *Perceptual and Motor Skills*, **80**, 635-640.

Steindler, A. (1955). *Kinesiology of the human body under normal and pathological conditions*. Springfield, IL: Charles C Thomas.

Ste-Marie, D.M. & Lee, T. (1991). Prior processing effects on gymnastic judging. *Journal of Experimental Psychology: Learning Memory and Cognition*, **17**, 126-136.

Stephenson, D.A. & Jackson, A.S. (1977). The effects of training on judges' ratings of a gymnastic event. *Research Quarterly*, **48**, 177-180.

Stoner, L.J. (1984). Is this performer skilled or unskilled? In R. Shapiro & J.R. Marett (Eds.). *Proceedings: Second National Symposium on Teaching Kinesiology and Biomechanics in Sports*. Colorado Springs, CO: NASPE, 233-234.

Strand, B. (1988). The development of checkpoints for skill observation. *New Jersey Journal of Physical Education, Recreation, and Dance*, **62**(1), 19-21.

Strohmeyer, H.S., Williams, K., & Schaub-George, D. (1991). Developmental sequences for catching a small ball: A prelongitudinal screening. *Research Quarterly for Exercise and Sport*, **62**, 257-266.

Stuberg, W., Straw, L., & Deuine, L. (1990). Validity of visually recorded temporal-distance measures at selected walking velocities for gait analysis. *Perceptual and Motor Skills*, **70**, 323-333.

Swinnen, S. (1984a). Role of field dependence in perception of movements. *Perceptual and Motor Skills*, **57**, 319-325.

Swinnen, S. (1984b). Some evidence to the hemispheric asymmetry model of lateral eye movements. *Perceptual and Motor Skills*, **58**, 79-88.

Swinnen, S. (1984c). Field dependence/independence as a factor in learning complex motor skills and underlying sex differences. *International Journal of Sports Psychology*, **15**, 236-249.

Tant, C. (1990). A kick is a kick—Or is it? *Strategies*, **4**(2), 19-22.

Taylor, J.K. (1995). Developing observational abilities in preservice physical education teachers. Doctoral dissertation, University of South Carolina. Abstract in *Dissertation Abstracts International*, **55**, 1872A.

Taylor, J.K., Hussey, K.G., Werner, P.H., Rink, J.E., & French, K.E. (1993). The effects of strategy, skill and strategy and skill instruction on skill and knowledge in ninth grade badminton. *Research Quarterly for Exercise and Sport*, **64**(Suppl.), 96A (Abstract).

Theios, J. & Amarhein, P.C. (1989). Theoretical analysis of the cognitive processing of lexical and pictorial stimuli: Reading, naming and visual conceptual comparisons. *Psychological Review*, **96**(1), 5-24.

Thorndike, E.L. (1927). The law of effect. *American Journal of Psychology*, **39**, 212-222.

Tieg, D. (1983, July). Eyes on the PGA tour. *Golf Digest*, 85-89.

Tobey, C. (1992). The best kind of feedback. *Strategies*, **6**(2), 19-20.

Torrey, L. (1985). *Stretching the limits: Breakthroughs in sports science that create superathletes*. New York: Dodd, Mead, & Company.

Treisman, A. (1986). Features and objects in visual processing. *Scientific American*, **255**(5), 114B-125.

Treisman, A.M. & Gelade, G.L. (1980). A feature integration theory of attention. *Cognitive Psychology, 12*, 97-136.

Trinity, J. & Annesi, J.J. (1996). Coaching with video. *Strategies, 9*(8), 23-25.

Trower, P. & Kiely, B. (1983). Video feedback: Help or hindrance? A review and analysis. In P. Dowrick & S. Briggs (Eds.). *Using video: Psychological and social applications.* Chichester, UK: Wiley, 181-197.

Ulrich, B. (1977). A module of instruction for golf swing error detection. In R.E. Stadulis (Ed.). *Research and Practice in Physical Education.* Champaign IL: Human Kinetics.

Ulrich, D.A. (1984). The reliability of classification decisions made with the objectives-based motor skill assessment instrument. *Adapted Physical Activity Quarterly, 1*, 52-60.

Ulrich, D.A. (1985). *Test of Gross Motor Development.* Austin, TX: PRO-ED, Inc.

Ulrich, D.A., Ulrich B.D., & Branta, C.R. (1988). Developmental gross motor skill ratings: A generalizability analysis. *Research Quarterly for Exercise and Sport, 59*, 203-209.

Vanderbeck, E. (1979). "It isn't right but I don't know what's wrong with it": An approach to error identification. *JOPER, 50*(5), 54-56.

Van Wieringen, P.C.W., Emmen, H.H., Bootsma, R.J., Hoogesteger, M., & Whiting, H.T.A. (1989). The effect of video-feedback on the learning of the tennis service by intermediate players. *Journal of Sports Sciences, 7*, 153-162.

Vickers, J.N. (1989). *Instructional design for teaching physical activities: A knowledge structures approach.* Champaign, IL: Human Kinetics.

Vincent, R.H. (1984, March). In or out? See if you can make this line call. *Tennis*, 35-37.

Walkley, J.W. & Kelley, C.E. (1989). The effectiveness of an interactive videodisk qualitative assessment training program. *Research Quarterly for Exercise and Sport, 60*, 280-285.

Warren, D.H. (1970). Inter-modality interactions in spatial localization. *Cognitive Psychology, 1*, 114-133.

Watkins, M.A., Riddle, D.L., Lamb, R.L., & Personius, W.J. (1991). Reliability of goniometric measurements and visual estimates of knee range of motion obtained in a clinical setting. *Physical Therapy, 71*, 90-96.

Watts, R.G. & Bahill, A.T. (1990). *Keep your eye on the ball—The science and folklore of baseball.* New York: W.H. Freeman and Company.

Weiss, M.R. (1982). Developmental modeling enhancing children's motor skill acquisition. *Journal of Physical Education, Recreation, and Dance, 53*(9), 49-50, 67.

Welch, R.B., & Warren, D.H. (1980). Immediate perceptual response to intersensory discrepancy. *Psychological Bulletin, 88*, 638-667.

Werder, J.K. & Kalakian, L.H. (1985). *Assessment in adapted physical education.* Minneapolis, MN: Burgess Publishing.

Werner, P. & Rink, J.E. (1987). Case studies of teacher effectiveness in second grade physical education. *Journal of Teaching in Physical Education, 8*, 280-297.

Whittle, M.W. (1991). *Gait analysis: An introduction.* Oxford: Butterworth-Heinemann.

Wickens, C.D. (1981). *Processing resources in attention, dual task performance, and workload assessment.* Engineering-Psychology Research Laboratory, University of Illinois, Technical Report EPL-81—3/ONR-81-3.

Wickens, C.D. (1984a). *Engineering psychology.* Columbus, OH: Merrill.

Wickens, C.D. (1984b). Processing resources in attention. In R. Parasuraman & R. Davies (Eds.). *Varieties of attention.* New York: Academic Press, 63-102.

Wickstrom, R.L. (1983). *Fundamental motor patterns* (3rd ed.). Philadelphia, PA: Lea & Febiger.

Wiese-Bjornstal, D.M. (1993). Giving and evaluating demonstrations. *Strategies, 6*(7), 13-15.

Wild, M. (1938). The behavior pattern of throwing and some observations concerning its course of development in children. *Research Quarterly, 9*, 20-24.

Wilkerson, J.D. (1985, April). Application of concepts—A second look. Paper presented to the AAHPERD National Convention, Atlanta, GA.

Wilkerson, J.D., Kreighbaum, E., & Tant, C.L. (Eds.) (1991). *Teaching kinesiology and biomechanics.* Ames, IA: Iowa State University.

Wilkinson, S. (1986). The effects of a visual discrimination training program on the acquisition and maintenance of physical education students' volleyball skill analytic ability. Doctoral dissertation, Ohio State University. Abstract in *Dissertation Abstracts International, 47*, 1650A.

Wilkinson, S. (1990, March). Skill analysis: Past, present and future perspectives. Paper presented to the AAHPERD National Convention, New Orleans, LA.

Wilkinson, S. (1991). The effect of an instructional videotape on the ability of physical education majors to diagnose errors in the overarm throwing pattern. In W. Liemohn (Ed.). *Abstracts of Research Papers 1991.* Reston, VA: AAHPERD, 74.

Wilkinson, S. (1992a). Effects of training in visual discrimination after one year: Visual analysis of volleyball skills. *Perceptual and Motor Skills, 75*, 19-24.

Wilkinson, S. (1992b). A training program for improving undergraduates' analytic skill in volleyball. *Journal of Teaching in Physical Education, 11*, 177-194.

Wilkinson, S. (1996). Visual analysis of the overarm throw and related sport skills: Training and transfer effects. *Journal of Teaching in Physical Education, 16*, 66-78.

Williams, E.W. (1996). Effects of a multimedia performance principle training program on correct analysis and diagnosis of throwlike movements. *Dissertation Abstracts International, 56*, 3504A.

Williams, J.G. (1987). Visual demonstration and movement sequencing: Effects of instructional control of the eyes. *Perceptual and Motor Skills, 65*, 366.

Williams, J.G. (1989a). Throwing action from full-cue and motion-only video-models of an arm movement sequence. *Perceptual and Motor Skills, 68*, 259-266.

Williams, J.G. (1989b). Visual demonstration and movement production: Effects of timing variations in a models action. *Perceptual and Motor Skills. 68*, 891-896.

Williams, J.G. (1992). Catching action: Visuomotor adaptations in children. *Perceptual and Motor Skills, 75*, 211-219.

Williams, K. (1980). Developmental characteristics of a forward fall. *Research Quarterly for Exercise and Sport, 51*, 703-713.

Williams, K., Haywood, K., & VanSant, A. (1996). Force and accuracy throws by older adults: II. *Journal of Aging and Physical Activity, 4*, 194-202.

Wilmore, J.H. & Costill, D.L. (1994). *Physiology of sport and exercise.* Champaign, IL: Human Kinetics.

Wilson, S.J., Glue, P., Ball, D., & Nutt, D. (1993). Saccadic eye movement parameters in normal subjects. *Electroencephalography and Clinical Neurophysiology, 86*, 69-74.

Wilson, V.E. (1976). Objectivity, validity, and reliability of gymnastic judging. *Research Quarterly, 47*, 169-173.

Winter, D.A. (1984). Kinematic and kinetic patterns in human gait: Variability and compensating effects. *Human Movement Science, 3*, 51-76.

Winter, D.A. (1987). *Biomechanics and motor control of human gait.* Waterloo, Ontario: University of Waterloo Press.

Winter, D.A. (1989). Biomechanics of normal and pathological gait: Implications for understanding human locomotor control. *Journal of Motor Behavior, 21*, 337-355.

Witkin, H.A. (1954). *Personality through perception: An experimental and clinical study.* Westport, CT: Greenwood Press.

Witkin, H.A., Oltman, P.K., Raskin, E., & Karp, S.A. (1971). *A manual for the group embedded figures test.* Palo Alto: Consulting Psychologists Press.

Wood, C.A., Gallagher, J.D., Martino, P.V., & Ross, M. (1992). Alternate forms of knowledge of results: Interaction of augmented feedback modality on learning. *Journal of Human Movement Studies, 22*, 213-230.

Woollacott, M.H. & Shumway-Cook, A. (Eds.) (1989). *Development of posture and gait across the life span.* Columbia, SC: University of South Carolina Press.

Yantis, S. (1992). Multielement visual tracking: Attention and perceptual organization. *Cognitive Psychology, 24*, 295-340.

Youndas, J.W., Bogard, C.L., Suman, V.J. (1993). Reliability of goniometric measurements and visual estimates of ankle joint active range of motion obtained in a clinical setting. *Archives of Physical Medicine and Rehabilitation, 74*, 1113-1118.

Youndas, J.W., Carey, J.R., & Garrett, T.R. (1991). Reliability of measurements of cervical spine range of motion—Comparison of three methods. *Physical Therapy, 71*, 90-96.

Zajac, F.E. & Gordon, M.E. (1989). Determining muscle's force and action in multi-articular movement. *Exercise and Sport Sciences Reviews, 17*, 187-230.

Zebas, C. & Johnson, H.M. (1989). Transfer of learning from the overhand throw to the tennis serve. *Strategies, 2*(6), 17-18, 27.

Ziegler, S.G. (1987). Effects of stimulus cueing on the acquisition of groundstrokes of beginning tennis players. *Journal of Applied Behavior Analysis, 20*, 405-411.

Zollman, D. & Fuller, R.G. (1984). Interactive videodisks: New technology for the analysis of human motion. In R. Shapiro & J.R. Marett (Eds.). *Proceedings: Second National Symposium on Teaching Kinesiology and Biomechanics in Sports.* Colorado Springs, CO: NASPE, 53-56.

INDEX

ABOUT THE AUTHORS

Duane V. Knudson is an assistant professor of human performance at Baylor University in Waco, Texas, where he has taught since 1984. He received a PhD in biomechanics from the University of Wisconsin in 1988.

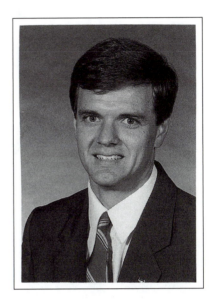

The author of numerous articles in research and professional journals, Dr. Knudson has expressed his interest in qualitative analysis by writing several papers on the topic. This work has appeared in *Strategies* and the *Journal of Physical Education, Recreation and Dance*. He has spoken on qualitative analysis at the 1995 and 1997 conventions of the American Association of Physical Education, Recreation and Dance (AAPHERD).

Dr. Knudson has published numerous papers on the applied biomechanics of sports and exercise. He is a member of both the International Society of Biomechanics in Sports and the Biomechanics Academy of AAPHERD. He reviews articles for journals such as the *Journal of Biomechanics, Physical Therapy,* and *Medicine and Science in Sports and Exercise*.

Dr. Knudson and his wife Lois live in Hewett, Texas. In his leisure time Dr. Knudson enjoys tennis, basketball, and volleyball.

Craig S. Morrison is associate professor of physical education at Southern Utah University in Cedar City, Utah. He received an EdD in physical education from Brigham Young University in 1982.

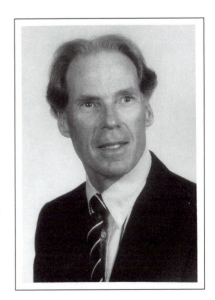

Dr. Morrison has researched qualitative analysis since 1979. He has published eight experimental studies and four review papers on qualitative analysis and has made numerous presentations on qualitative analysis at national and international conferences.

A recipient of a Distinguished Faculty of the Year Award from Southern Utah University for the 1995-1996 academic year, Dr. Morrison also won first place in the biomechanics division from the American Alliance of Health, Physical Education, Recreation and Dance (AAHPERD) in 1988 for the development of instructional, qualitative analysis videotapes. Dr. Morrison is a member of AAHPERD and the National Association for Physical Education in Higher Education.

For recreation, Dr. Morrison has competed in triathlons since 1983 and has finished five Hawaiian Ironman triathlons. He also enjoys cross country skiing, yoga, and building and playing guitars.

Sport mechanics made easy

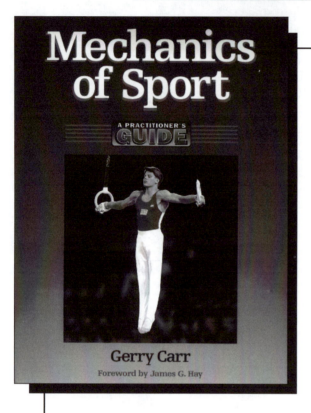

Mechanics of Sport

A PRACTITIONER'S GUIDE

Gerry Carr

Foreword by James G. Hay

1997 • Paper • 224 pp
Item PCAR0974 • ISBN 0-87322-974-6
$24.00 ($35.95 Canadian)

All great sport performances are based on the best use of the laws of physics and mechanics. Gerry Carr explains the mechanical concepts underlying performance techniques in a way that's easy to understand, showing readers how to observe, analyze, and correct sport technique for better performance. A wide variety of information on sports extends beyond the classroom for practitioners to actually *use* in their professional roles.

You'll find no confusing formulas or equations here. But you *will* find 19 real-life examples throughout the text that illustrate key principles. Plus, more than 200 superb illustrations highlight the author's explanations. Each chapter includes a summary of important points as well as study questions. A full glossary and answers to the study questions complete the text.

To request more information or to place your order, U.S. customers call **TOLL-FREE 1-800-747-4457.**
Customers outside the U.S. use appropriate telephone number/address shown in the front of this book.

Human Kinetics
The Information Leader in Physical Activity
http://www.humankinetics.com/

2335

Prices are subject to change.